THE EMT-BASIC EXAM REVIEW

KIRSTEN M. ELLING, BS, REMT-P

THOMSON

DELMAR LEARNING

Australia   Canada   Mexico   Singapore   Spain   United Kingdom   United States

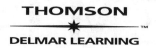

THOMSON
™
DELMAR LEARNING

The EMT-Basic Exam Review
by Kirsten M. Elling

Vice President,
Health Care Business Unit:
William Brottmiller

Editorial Director:
Cathy L. Esperti

Acquisitions Editor:
Maureen Rosener

Developmental Editor:
Darcy Scelsi

Editorial Assistant:
Elizabeth Howe

Marketing Director:
Jennifer McAvey

Marketing Channel Manager:
Heather Sisley

Marketing Coordinator:
Christopher Manion

Technology Director:
Laurie Davis

Technology Project Manager:
Mary Colleen Liburdi

Technology Project Coordinator:
Carolyn Fox

Production Director:
Carolyn Miller

Production Manager:
Barbara A. Bullock

Production Editors:
Bridget Lulay
Kenneth McGrath

Library of Congress Cataloging-in-
Publication Data

Elling, Kirsten M.
 The EMT-basic exam review /
Kirsten M. Elling.
    p. cm.
 Includes bibliographical references and
index.
  ISBN 1-4018-9152-7 (alk. paper)
 1. Emergency medicine--Examinations,
questions, etc. 2. Emergency medical
technicians--Examinations, questions, etc.
I. Title.
 RC86.9.E432 2005
 616.02'5--dc22
                                    2005014470

NOTICE TO THE READER

Dedication

This work is dedicated to my husband Bob. Thank you for always being there to support and encourage me in my educational and writing efforts.

—

Special Thanks

My deepest thanks to my close friend and colleague Mikel A. Rothenberg, M.D., for all his hard work, insight, and guidance during the development of the companion text, Why-Driven EMS Enrichment.

Contents

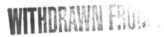

About the Author

Kirsten M. Elling, BS, REMT-P

Kirsten (Kirt) Elling is a career paramedic who works for the Town of Colonie in upstate New York. She began EMS work in 1988 as an EMT/firefighter and has been a National Registered Paramedic since 1991. She has been an EMS educator since 1990, teaching basic and advanced EMS programs at the Institute of Prehospital Emergency Medicine in Troy, New York. Kirt serves as Regional Faculty for the New York State Department of Health, Bureau of EMS, and the American Heart Association. She has written numerous scripts for the EMS training video series *PULSE: Emergency Medical Update;* is a co-author of *Why-Driven EMS Enrichment, The Paramedic Review, Principles of Assessment, Paramedic: Anatomy & Physiology,* and *Paramedic: Pathophysiology;* a contributing author of the IPEM *Paramedic Lab Manual;* and an adjunct writer for the 1998 revision of the National Highway Traffic Safety Administration, EMT-Paramedic, and EMT-Intermediate: National Standard Curricula.

Preface

Today there are many choices of books, magazines, videos, workbooks, and Web sites for instructors to use to prepare their students for EMS work on the streets. I sincerely hope you will agree that this book, *The EMT-Basic Exam Review,* is a valuable tool to help review and prepare for state and national examinations.

Previously, together with my husband Bob and our colleague Mikel Rothenberg, M.D., I completed the book *Why-Driven EMS Enrichment* and its companion text *The Paramedic Review. The EMT-Basic Exam Review* is the second in a series of review books designed to follow the organizational chapter format of the DOT curricula. The *Enrichment* book was designed for all levels of EMS providers, whereas the information in this book is specifically for EMT-Bs.

The EMT-Basic Exam Review consists of multiple-choice questions covering all topics and objectives (cognitive and affective) in the current EMT-B DOT National Standard Curriculum. For ease of reference and use, the chapter order follows that of the curriculum. *The EMT-Basic Exam Review* is the perfect resource for preparing for the National Registry written exam. The CD that accompanies the text has two full-length simulated practice examinations that mimic typical state and national exam formats. Included in this book is an appendix with the National Registry EMT-Basic level skills examination check-off sheets, as well as advice on how to prepare for each important skill. Blank answer forms are included at the end of each chapter.

Early in this project we decided that the questions would only be the multiple-choice style, with the standard format of three "distracters" (incorrect or less than optimal answers) and one correct answer to each question. Because this book will be used to prepare for both state and national EMT-B examinations, it makes the most sense to use the format and style of questions used on these types of exams.

You will find the answer key at the end of the book, in Appendix A, listing the letter of the correct answer and a corresponding rationale for the answer. If you would like a more detailed explanation of the questions in this book, as well as enrichment of advanced objectives, we suggest that you purchase the companion text, *Why-Driven EMS Enrichment* (ISBN 0-7668-2507-8).

For each question there is only one correct answer. When you have difficulty narrowing the choice down, always read through all four choices and select the best answer. There are nearly 1,500 questions in this book and another 300 on the CD. That's nearly 500 questions more than any other EMT-B review text currently on the market. I suggest that you tackle a chapter at a time; then, after taking each exam, check the answer key and mark the areas where you need to review the material.

I sincerely hope you will enjoy *The EMT-Basic Exam Review* and benefit from the test-taking review to expand your knowledge base. After all, the real test occurs in the field, where our patients rely on us to be prepared.

See you in the streets!

—*Kirt*

Acknowledgments

Thank you to all the editorial and production personnel who have contributed to this project, especially Maureen Rosener, Elizabeth Howe, Darcy Scelsi, Bridget Lulay, Brooke Graves, and special thanks to Mike Kennamer (technical reviewer).

Thank you to our reviewers for their invaluable feedback:

J. Alan Baker, AS, NREMT-P, LP
Assistant Director of EMSP
Victoria College
Victoria, TX

Tom Chartier, BAE, EMT-I
Western Iowa Tech Community College
Sioux City, IA
Woodbury Central High School
Moville, IA

Kevin Costa, Captain II
EMS Coordinator
Pasadena Fire Department
Pasadena, CA

Loren Deichman, NREMT-P, CCEMT-P, I/C
Clinical Coordinator
ENMU-R EMS Program
Roswell, NM

Michael Dant
EMT Program Supervisor
Health Careers & Public Services
Illinois Central College
Peoria, IL

Ken Davis NR/CCEMT-P, FP-C, I/C
Paramedic Coordinator
Eastern New Mexico University—Roswell
Roswell, NM

Bruce Evans, MPA, NREMT-P
Fire Captain, Fire Program Coordinator
Community College of Southern Nevada
Henderson, NV

Lynda Goerisch, MA, NREMT-P
EMT Coordinator/Instructor
Century College
White Bear Lake, MN

Michael Hastings MS, NREMT-P
EMS Program Director
Central Piedmont Community College
Charlotte, NC

Robbie Murray, NREMT-P. A.A.S.
Training Coordinator
Sussex County Emergency Medical Services
Georgetown, DE

M. Jane Pollock, EMT-P, CEN, Level II, EMD
Adjunct Clinical Instructor
Education and Training Specialist
Brody School of Medicine, East Carolina University
Department of Emergency Medicine, Division of EMS
Greenville, NC

J. Penny Shutts AEMT, NREMT-B, CIC
Educator
Sandy Creek, NY

Jean B. Will, Ed.D., RN, MSN, CED, EMT-P
Director of EMS Programs
Drexel University
Philadelphia, PA

Sandy Waggoner, EMT-P, FF, EMSI
Public Safety Coordinator
EHOVE Ghrist Adult Career Center
Milan, OH

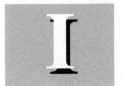
Preparatory

CHAPTER

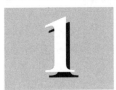

Introduction to Emergency Medical Care

1. Emergency medical service (EMS) system is defined as:
   a. a continuum of patient care that extends until discharge.
   b. everything that happens to an injured person before he reaches the hospital.
   c. a public service capable of transporting the disabled.
   d. patient care that begins at the scene of an injury or illness.

2. The emergency access telephone number 9-1-1 does not permit which of the following functions?
   a. reduced time for the caller to access EMS
   b. access to police, fire, and EMS with one number
   c. accelerated access to EMS with the use of cell phones
   d. instructions for life-saving emergency care over the phone

3. Which of the following levels of prehospital emergency medical training is absent from the list of nationally recognized levels of care?
   a. EMT-Assistant
   b. first responder
   c. EMT-Paramedic
   d. EMT-Intermediate

4. The emergency medical dispatcher (EMD) is trained to receive emergency calls, dispatch emergency services, and:
   a. determine when the caller is a minor.
   b. transcribe medical terminology.
   c. provide instructions for immediate emergency care.
   d. provide instruction for stabilizing non-life-threatening situations.

5. A respiratory therapist, a dental technician, and an oncology specialist are all examples of:
   a. EMDs.
   b. allied health personnel.
   c. bystanders.
   d. emergency department staff.

6. The health care provider who is typically the first person on the scene of an acute illness or injury in a non-health care related workplace is a:
   a. licensed practical nurse (LPN).
   b. first responder.
   c. paramedic.
   d. physician's assistant (PA).

7. During the transport of a patient, the EMT-B learns that the patient has some very specific concerns about possible treatment options for his present condition. Upon arrival at the hospital, the EMT-B conveys the patient's concerns to the nurse. This is an example of:
   a. patient advocacy.
   b. patient assessment.
   c. a Good Samaritan act.
   d. quality improvement.

8. An EMT-B should have good color vision because it can be critical to patient assessment, as well as to:
   a. taking the EMT-B certification exam.
   b. maintaining emergency equipment.
   c. keeping good documentation.
   d. operating an emergency vehicle.

9. The responsibilities of an EMT-B include:
   a. transfer of patient care.
   b. activation of the EMS system.
   c. issuing standing orders.
   d. registering with the National Association of EMTs.

10. In the field of emergency medicine, having _____ means identifying with and understanding the feelings, situations, and motives of your patients.
    a. integrity
    b. sympathy
    c. empathy
    d. honesty

11. Your ambulance is dispatched to stand by at the scene of a house fire. Upon arrival at the scene, your first priority is to:
    a. notify dispatch that your unit is the first on the scene.
    b. notify incoming emergency units of smoke or fire conditions.
    c. protect your own safety.
    d. establish EMS command and request additional resources.

12. The EMT-B who keeps his or her immunizations up to date is demonstrating:
    a. compliance with standing orders.
    b. personal safety.
    c. the use of PPE.
    d. continuous quality improvement.

13. Which of the following is an impractical role or responsibility of the EMT-B?
    a. safety of the crew, patient, and bystanders
    b. lifting and moving patients
    c. possessing good personal traits
    d. identifying every potential hazard on a scene

14. When an EMT-B relocates to another region, state, or territory, the process of obtaining the same certification is known as:
    a. reentrance.
    b. reciprocity.
    c. occupation barter.
    d. reactivation.

15. Which of the following is an example of an EMT-B advocating for a patient?
    a. ensuring a rapid response time and establishing a safe scene
    b. thoroughly documenting a refusal of medical attention (RMA)
    c. allowing a family member to ride in the ambulance with the patient when the patient does not want that
    d. collecting and safeguarding a patient's personal valuables while the patient is in the EMT-B's care

16. The practice of reviewing and auditing within an EMS system to ensure a high quality of care is referred to as:
    a. quality improvement.
    b. medical review.
    c. the National Highway Safety Act.
    d. medical direction.

17. The guidelines under which EMS personnel function are referred to as:
    a. protocols.
    b. quality control.
    c. online medical direction.
    d. state and local ordinances.

18. The EMT-B can help improve the quality of care by:
    a. participating in continuing education.
    b. washing his hands after each patient contact.
    c. carrying a portable radio whenever possible.
    d. avoiding direct contact with infectious patients.

19. Every EMS system has a/an _____ who assumes definitive responsibility for oversight of the patient care aspects of the EMS system.
    a. EMS supervisor
    b. medical director
    c. senior paramedic
    d. paramedic supervisor

20. An EMT-B who gives oral glucose to a patient who has signs and symptoms of hypoglycemia, per standing-orders protocol, is using:
    a. Red Cross guidelines.
    b. online medical direction.
    c. offline medical direction.
    d. national care standards.

21. An example of online (direct) medical control is:
    a. assisting a patient to take nitroglycerin per standing orders.
    b. contacting a physician by radio prior to performing a skill.
    c. obtaining feedback from the hospital staff after caring for a patient.
    d. administering a medication to a patient, then notifying the hospital to advise of the incoming patient and his status.

22. An on-duty EMT-B is operating _____ of the medical director for the EMS system.
    a. on Good Samaritan extension
    b. on advance directives
    c. as a designated agent
    d. for the scope of practice

23. The EMT-B is responsible for completing the prehospital care report (PCR), which contains two types of information: _____ and _____ information.
    a. regional, national
    b. behavioral, characteristic
    c. technical, supportive
    d. patient, administrative

24. The policies and procedures used by an EMS system may be authorized by a _____ agency.

    a. state

    b. regional

    c. local

    d. all of the above

25. Which of the following is not used by any state as an EMT-B state certifying examination?

    a. the National Registry

    b. written testing only

    c. some form of oral testing

    d. Prehospital Trauma Life Support (PHTLS)

Chapter 1 Answer Form

	A	B	C	D
1.	❏	❏	❏	❏
2.	❏	❏	❏	❏
3.	❏	❏	❏	❏
4.	❏	❏	❏	❏
5.	❏	❏	❏	❏
6.	❏	❏	❏	❏
7.	❏	❏	❏	❏
8.	❏	❏	❏	❏
9.	❏	❏	❏	❏
10.	❏	❏	❏	❏
11.	❏	❏	❏	❏
12.	❏	❏	❏	❏
13.	❏	❏	❏	❏

	A	B	C	D
14.	❏	❏	❏	❏
15.	❏	❏	❏	❏
16.	❏	❏	❏	❏
17.	❏	❏	❏	❏
18.	❏	❏	❏	❏
19.	❏	❏	❏	❏
20.	❏	❏	❏	❏
21.	❏	❏	❏	❏
22.	❏	❏	❏	❏
23.	❏	❏	❏	❏
24.	❏	❏	❏	❏
25.	❏	❏	❏	❏

CHAPTER 2

Well-Being of the EMT-B

1. Work in EMS comes with the peaks of high-stress situations and the valleys of total boredom. The EMT-B can reduce or prevent the development of chronic stress due to the job by:
   a. getting plenty of rest.
   b. alternating assignments.
   c. limiting exposure to high-stress incidents.
   d. all of the above.

2. After returning from a cardiac arrest call, which involved the unexpected death of a young patient, it would be normal and mentally healthy for the EMT-B to:
   a. talk about the call with crew members.
   b. become depressed.
   c. indulge in the use of alcohol.
   d. request more work hours or overtime.

3. Cumulative stress brought on by repeated exposure to emergency care situations can cause the EMT-B to:
   a. burn out.
   b. become bored.
   c. work longer hours.
   d. take a paramedic course.

4. The family of a woman in cardiac arrest is waiting at the emergency department (ED) when you arrive. After you turn the patient over to the staff, you realize that the family is looking at you and it is obvious that they want to talk to you. At this point you:
   a. avoid them until the ED physician has talked to them first.
   b. assume that they will be angry and prepare for the worst.
   c. listen to what they have to say, but do not give them any false hopes.
   d. tell them that you have no good news at this time and to wait to speak to the ED physician.

5. During a career in EMS, the EMT-B may have to help patients, or patients' family members, or even coworkers with the various stages of:
   a. confidentiality.
   b. working out a living will.
   c. developing a do not resuscitate order (DNR).
   d. the grieving process.

6. After being on the scene for 10 minutes with another crew that is working on a patient in cardiac arrest, you are getting ready to move the patient into the ambulance. Just then the patient's daughter arrives. She is very upset and appears to be in shock about her father. She keeps repeating that there is nothing wrong with him. What emotional stage of the death and dying process is she exhibiting?
   a. anger
   b. bargaining
   c. denial
   d. depression

7. The fire department was the first to respond to the scene of a cardiac arrest. When you arrive, they are performing CPR, although the patient appears to have obvious signs of lividity. The family is very upset and requests that you do everything possible to save the patient. What steps do you take in the approach to this family that is confronted with death and dying?
   a. Stop CPR and tell them that nothing else can be done.
   b. Keep doing CPR and begin transport of the patient.
   c. Stop CPR and show them the signs of irreversible death found on the patient.
   d. Keep doing CPR until the coroner arrives to convince the family that the patient is dead.

8. After being dispatched to a home on a cardiac arrest call, you arrive to find that the resident appears to have been dead for several hours. You notify dispatch that this is an unattended death and turn your attention to the family member who discovered the body. The relative tells you that the patient has been sick for a long time but has refused any help. The relative does not appear to be too upset. What stage of grieving does this represent?

   a. acceptance
   b. bargaining
   c. denial
   d. depression

9. Dispatch has sent you to a call for a sick person. When you arrive, the family tells you that the patient is terminally ill with lung cancer and that they need her transported to the hospital for a test. The approach to take with this patient is to:

   a. expect that the patient will be angry with you and verbally abuse you.
   b. let the family and patient know that the patient will not die on this transport.
   c. make the patient comfortable, maintain her dignity, and be respectful.
   d. call an ALS unit to do the transport, because the patient is medicated.

10. Your family is always complaining that your work takes all your time and that your job seems more important to you than they are. This reaction from your family is:

   a. a nuisance.
   b. uncommon and can be disregarded.
   c. a form of distrust.
   d. something you need to give priority attention to.

11. You are stuck on a late call again and have called your friends to tell them that you will not be able to go to the movies with them as planned. In the past they have been disappointed when this has happened, and this time they sound angry. How can you reasonably prevent this from occurring in the future?

   a. Avoid making any plans with your friends.
   b. Do not make plans for times near the end of your shift.
   c. Explain to your friends that this is the way it has to be.
   d. Consider quitting EMS and going into another type of work.

12. An EMT-B's spouse wants to understand the job of EMS; the spouse has never known anyone else in this profession. Despite the spouse's efforts to understand, there is constant frustration about the possible dangers of the job. This frustration is:

   a. very unusual and rarely occurs.
   b. more typical for female spouses.
   c. more typical for male spouses.
   d. most likely an added stressor for the EMT-B.

13. The EMT-B's possible reactions to critical-incident stress:

   a. are initially the same for everyone.
   b. always affect the EMT-B's family.
   c. are usually healthy and not a problem.
   d. are individual and are affected by previous exposures.

14. You are back at work after a two-week vacation. It does not take you long to see that your partner is acting different. She complains of a headache and nausea, and tells you that she has not been sleeping well and has distressing dreams. You recognize that these may be signs of:

   a. the flu.
   b. substance abuse or withdrawal.
   c. a stress reaction.
   d. feelings of incompetence.

15. Signs and symptoms of a crisis-induced stress reaction can occur during an incident or after. A stress reaction may typically produce all of the following *except:*

   a. plenty of rest.
   b. excessive dark humor.
   c. identifying with a victim.
   d. vision problems or sleep disturbance.

16. Each of the following is a recommended technique that the EMT-B can use for reducing or minimizing stress, *except:*

   a. coping.
   b. self-medication.
   c. problem solving.
   d. adaptation.

17. You are trying to reduce some of the environmental stress related to your job, so you decide to:

   a. let your partner drive on the calls requiring lights and sirens.
   b. only work with people you like.
   c. get a prescribed medication to help you adjust.
   d. avoid taking calls for children and the elderly.

18. This week you have decided to join a gym and begin an exercise program to help alleviate some of the stress in your life. Exercise is a great stress reliever because:
    a. finding time for yourself relieves stress.
    b. it provides a physical release of pent-up energy.
    c. it helps you focus on the positives.
    d. all of the above.

19. It is 2:00 a.m. and the house you have been dispatched to is completely dark. Why is this potentially a threat to the EMT-B?
    a. The patient may be blind.
    b. It may not be an actual EMS emergency.
    c. The patient may have fallen and been unable to turn on the lights.
    d. The patient may be unresponsive and alone.

20. A routine call for a sick person has suddenly become dangerous. The patient is refusing care and is threatening to take a swing at you. The safest way to handle this situation is to:
    a. quickly turn your back and run away.
    b. without raising your voice, state with authority that you will not allow any violence to occur here.
    c. call for the police and retreat if necessary.
    d. get the patient to sign a refusal-of-care form and leave.

21. Many scenes involve some type of possible hazard to the EMT-B, which can easily be controlled if recognized. Which of the following scenes should the EMT-B be able to control?
    a. an overturned motor vehicle that is leaking fuel
    b. a walkway to the house that is covered with ice
    c. a crime scene where the perpetrator is still present
    d. an ongoing domestic dispute between a mother and daughter

22. The efforts you take to protect yourself against disease transmission by bloodborne or airborne pathogens are:
    a. referred to as the scope of well-being.
    b. a form of sterilization.
    c. a low priority of the job.
    d. referred to as *body substance isolation*.

23. The use of body substance isolation (BSI) is of such paramount importance that EMS employers are required to have specific procedures in place and ensure that the necessary equipment is available. What component of BSI is the EMT-B responsible for?
    a. ensuring that proper BSI equipment is available for use on every call
    b. developing a written exposure control plan
    c. ensuring that handwashing is done after each call
    d. developing and enforcing a written plan of action in case of an exposure

24. When you arrive at work, your designated officer tells you that 2 days ago you transported a patient with a potentially life-threatening airborne disease. What action must be taken at this point?
    a. Your employer must arrange for you to be evaluated by a health care professional.
    b. You must go home until you are evaluated and cleared by a health care professional.
    c. Nothing has to be done until 48 hours have passed.
    d. Nothing has to be done until 90 days have passed.

25. An example of an airborne pathogen that EMT-Bs are at risk for exposure to during EMS calls is:
    a. hepatitis B.
    b. hepatitis C.
    c. German measles.
    d. staphylococcal skin infection.

26. Which of the following immunizations is not currently recommended for the EMT-B?
    a. polio
    b. tetanus
    c. hepatitis
    d. smallpox

27. In areas where tuberculosis is highly prevalent, TB screening for the EMT-B is recommended every _____ months.
    a. 6
    b. 12
    c. 18
    d. 24

28. Dispatch has sent you to a call for an assault. You are instructed to stand by one block from the address until the police call for you. While preparing for the call, you consider what PPE will be needed, and you:
    a. get out the bulletproof vests.
    b. decide that you will need gloves, at the very minimum.
    c. decide that you need nothing at this time without further information.
    d. put on your turnout jacket and helmet.

29. You have been assigned to perform a routine transport of a patient known to have bacterial meningitis. In preparation for the transport, which PPE and precautions will you need to take?
    a. gloves, eyewear, and surgical mask
    b. gloves, surgical mask, and handwashing after the call
    c. gloves, eye protection, and handwashing after the call
    d. gloves, HEPA respirator, and handwashing after the call

30. The county jail has requested transportation for an ill inmate, who is to be taken to the local hospital for evaluation of whooping cough. In preparation for this transport, which PPE and precautions will you need?
    a. gloves, eyewear, and surgical mask
    b. gloves, surgical mask, and handwashing after the call
    c. gloves, eye protection, and handwashing after the call
    d. gloves, HEPA respirator, and handwashing after the call

31. When responding to and working in a crime scene, the primary safety of the EMT-B is the responsibility of the:
    a. EMT-B.
    b. detective at the scene.
    c. safety officer.
    d. EMS supervisor.

32. During a severe thunderstorm, a loud burst of thunder and a lightning strike get your attention. When you look outside your station, you see that a power pole has been struck and wires are down in the road. You notify dispatch and request additional resources and then take which of the following safety precautions?
    a. Stay inside the building until the power company arrives.
    b. Put on rubber boots and investigate the area further.
    c. Stay inside the building until the fire department arrives.
    d. Establish a perimeter to keep people outside of the danger zone.

33. During the last call, blood from the patient dripped down onto a stretcher rail. Before putting the stretcher back into service, you make sure that the blood has been wiped off and the stretcher has been properly decontaminated. The reason for doing this right away is:
    a. you will maintain the cleanest ambulance and equipment in the department.
    b. that your next patient might come into contact with the dried blood if you wait until later.
    c. because the longer you wait to clean the blood off, the harder it is to disinfect the stretcher.
    d. because the longer you wait to clean the blood off, the higher the risk of it drying and turning into airborne particles.

34. The supervisor has asked you to help train two new employees. She has most likely chosen you to be a field-training officer because of your experience and how you routinely demonstrate:
    a. that there is never a need to call in sick.
    b. the importance of not showing any signs of stress.
    c. how an EMS professional should dress.
    d. the importance of taking protective measures against infectious diseases.

35. Each fall semester you help teach labs in the EMT-B original course. The instructor likes your style and has told you that she likes the way you advocate for the use of protective measures against infectious diseases and other hazards in each lab. One of the ways you do this is to:
    a. tell the students about all the times they will need to wear PPE in the field.
    b. spend a great deal of time talking about the use of PPE in various situations, as well as in rescue operations.
    c. have the students practice wearing gloves, eyewear, and masks in lab sessions.
    d. have the students wash their hands before and after each lab session.

Chapter 2 Answer Form

	A	B	C	D			A	B	C	D
1.	❑	❑	❑	❑		19.	❑	❑	❑	❑
2.	❑	❑	❑	❑		20.	❑	❑	❑	❑
3.	❑	❑	❑	❑		21.	❑	❑	❑	❑
4.	❑	❑	❑	❑		22.	❑	❑	❑	❑
5.	❑	❑	❑	❑		23.	❑	❑	❑	❑
6.	❑	❑	❑	❑		24.	❑	❑	❑	❑
7.	❑	❑	❑	❑		25.	❑	❑	❑	❑
8.	❑	❑	❑	❑		26.	❑	❑	❑	❑
9.	❑	❑	❑	❑		27.	❑	❑	❑	❑
10.	❑	❑	❑	❑		28.	❑	❑	❑	❑
11.	❑	❑	❑	❑		29.	❑	❑	❑	❑
12.	❑	❑	❑	❑		30.	❑	❑	❑	❑
13.	❑	❑	❑	❑		31.	❑	❑	❑	❑
14.	❑	❑	❑	❑		32.	❑	❑	❑	❑
15.	❑	❑	❑	❑		33.	❑	❑	❑	❑
16.	❑	❑	❑	❑		34.	❑	❑	❑	❑
17.	❑	❑	❑	❑		35.	❑	❑	❑	❑
18.	❑	❑	❑	❑						

CHAPTER 3

Medical, Legal, and Ethical Issues

1. The collective set of regulations and ethical considerations that defines the capacity of an EMT-B's job is referred to as:
   a. protocols.
   b. certification.
   c. scope of practice.
   d. improvement.

2. When writing a patient care report (PCR), the EMT-B should document _____ findings that have been observed during the time with the patient.
   a. objective
   b. subjective
   c. personal
   d. weighted

3. When operating an emergency vehicle, the general rule for EMT-Bs is to:
   a. assume that other drivers will yield to emergency traffic.
   b. let the most senior prehospital provider drive when using lights and sirens.
   c. always use both lights and sirens when responding to a call.
   d. exercise due regard for the safety of others.

4. Which of the following is most accurate regarding prehospital certification and licensing?
   a. EMT-Basic is a certification granted by a state.
   b. Before a state grants a license to an EMT-B, that EMT-B must obtain state certification.
   c. Most states allow EMT-Bs reciprocity for licensing only.
   d. Reciprocity is not applicable to EMT-Bs who are certified.

5. A do not resuscitate order (DNR) is a legal document, typically signed by the _____, that states the patient has a terminal illness and does not wish to prolong his life with resuscitative measures.
   a. patient
   b. patient and his physician
   c. patient's legal guardian
   d. patient and his spouse

6. A do not resuscitate order is called a/an _____, because it is drawn up and signed prior to an event when resuscitation might be initiated.
   a. declaration
   b. advance directive
   c. proximate decree
   d. expressed consent

7. A legal document that allows a person to designate an agent to make decisions as to the type of life-saving medical treatment the person wants or does not want, if he is terminally ill and unable to decide for himself, in a coma, or in a persistent vegetative state, is a/an:
   a. DNR.
   b. living will.
   c. expressed consent.
   d. health care proxy.

8. Living wills and health care proxies usually relate to situations that occur in:
   a. a nursing home.
   b. the residence.
   c. the hospital setting.
   d. the prehospital setting.

9. Permission to treat a patient, or *consent,* is required:
   a. only if the patient is conscious and sober.
   b. in writing, using a standard EMS consent form.
   c. for any treatment or action performed by the EMT-B.
   d. for every patient the EMT-B establishes contact with.

10. Which of the following methods is acceptable for the EMT-B to use to obtain consent from a patient?
    a. Tell the patient you are there to help him, and ask if it is okay.
    b. Introduce yourself and ask the patient if you may take his vital signs.
    c. Tell the patient that you are an EMT-B and that you are willing to treat him, and ask him to sign your agency's consent form.
    d. All of the above.

11. Prior to treating an adult patient with severe mental disability, legally the EMT-B must:

    a. obtain consent from a guardian.

    b. notify dispatch before transporting.

    c. use local law enforcement.

    d. obtain consent from the patient's physician.

12. The EMT-B must obtain expressed consent:

    a. from intoxicated adults of legal age.

    b. from all nursing home residents who do not have a DNR.

    c. from conscious and mentally competent adults.

    d. prior to treatment and transportation of the unconscious patient.

13. When care for a patient is begun under implied consent, this type of consent remains in effect as long as the patient is mentally impaired and:

    a. as long as the patient is in protective custody.

    b. as long as the patient requires life-saving treatment.

    c. until the patient arrives at the emergency department.

    d. until the patient is discharged from the hospital.

14. An EMT-B is caring for an unresponsive patient who was found alone, and who is wearing a Medic Alert® tag with "Diabetic" written on it. The EMT-B may treat this patient under which type of consent?

    a. expressed

    b. informed

    c. involuntary

    d. emergency doctrine

15. An EMT-B is attempting to assess and treat a patient who is reported to have a low blood sugar reading. Initially the patient was conscious, but refused any intervention. During the refusal, the patient became unconscious. Now the EMT-B may treat the patient under:

    a. medical control.

    b. implied consent.

    c. involuntary consent.

    d. protective custody.

16. You are called to care for a 22-year-old male who had openly stated that he wanted to harm himself, but now he has changed his mind. The patient is uninjured and is refusing care, so now you should:

    a. try to convince the patient to go to the hospital for evaluation.

    b. not leave the patient alone, but wait for family or a friend to arrive.

    c. transport the patient, as the threat to harm himself requires follow-up psychological care.

    d. allow the patient to refuse medical attention (RMA), as he is uninjured and has changed his mind about harming himself.

17. You have been called to a day care center for a 4-year-old child who is experiencing a severe allergic reaction after being stung by a bee. You may treat this child under which type of consent?

    a. implied

    b. informed

    c. expressed

    d. emergent

18. Under certain conditions, a minor may legally give consent for or refuse care. These minors are referred to as:

    a. liberated.

    b. adolescent.

    c. detached.

    d. emancipated.

19. Which of the following is considered an emancipated minor?

    a. a 17-year-old who lied about his age when he enlisted in the armed services

    b. two 17-year-olds who are parents themselves, but not married

    c. a 16-year-old with a notarized liberating contract signed by one parent

    d. a 16-year-old with a notarized liberating contract signed by both parents

20. After being dispatched to a grade school for a child with a hand laceration that will require sutures, what must occur before the EMT-B transports the child to the hospital?

    a. A parent or guardian must be contacted and give consent.

    b. The school nurse must provide consent for the EMT-B to treat the child.

    c. As the injury is minor, a parent or guardian must come to the school first.

    d. As the accident occurred on public property, the police must take a report.

21. You are treating a patient who sustained a possible spinal injury in a motor vehicle collision. The patient is willing to go to the hospital, but is adamantly refusing the application of a cervical collar. You should:

    a. carefully document the incident and refuse transport.

    b. tell the patient that without the cervical collar, he will become permanently crippled and have no recourse for a lawsuit.

    c. not transport the patient without the cervical collar and full spinal immobilization.

    d. document the refusal for the collar application, have the patient sign off on that matter, and then transport the patient to the hospital.

22. An EMT-B is assessing a 10-year-old child who has an ankle injury, but is refusing care and does not want to get into the ambulance. Which of the following statements is most accurate concerning this refusal of care?

    a. The EMT-B may treat the child under involuntary consent.
    b. Children may refuse care if they are given full disclosure by the EMT-B.
    c. The EMT-B may treat the child under expressed consent.
    d. Children cannot legally refuse care without a parent or guardian's agreement.

23. The EMT-B has the responsibility to be sure that all of the following conditions exist before allowing a patient to refuse care, except:

    a. the patient must be an adult.
    b. the patient must be mentally competent.
    c. all patients have a right to refuse care; no conditions can preclude that right.
    d. the patient must be fully informed and understand the risks of refusing care.

24. An EMT-B has responded to assist a 50-year-old male who has a deep laceration to the forearm. The wound was bandaged and bleeding has been controlled. Now the patient is refusing transport and states that he will drive himself to his doctor's office. It would now be appropriate for the EMT-B to:

    a. determine if the patient has a valid driver's license.
    b. try to get a family member or friend to take the patient to the doctor.
    c. ask the patient to take a breathalyzer test to reduce the liability for refusal of care.
    d. advise the patient not to call EMS again, as he cannot change his mind about help or transport once he has refused.

25. Which of the following statements regarding refusal of care is most accurate?

    a. A patient must sign a release-from-liability form.
    b. The patient cannot be left alone after refusing care.
    c. A competent adult patient can revoke consent at any time.
    d. An attempt to contact the patient's physician should be made before releasing the patient.

26. When harm occurs as a result of failure to exercise an acceptable degree of professional skill or competence while providing patient care, it is referred to as:

    a. negligence.
    b. consignment.
    c. discharge.
    d. obstruction.

27. An off-duty EMT-B stopped at the scene of a motor vehicle collision (MVC) to offer assistance, and began to triage patients. After several minutes the EMT-B heard the siren of the ambulance in the distance and realized that he was late for work. Knowing that the patient was stable and that the ambulance would soon arrive, the EMT-B left to go to work. This is an example of:

    a. neglect.
    b. indifference.
    c. abandonment.
    d. leaving the scene of an accident.

28. During the transport of a patient with an altered mental status, the patient punches the EMT-B. Which of the following has occurred?

    a. The patient assaulted the EMT-B.
    b. The EMT-B is responsible for contributory negligence.
    c. The EMT-B failed to act with due regard for the patient.
    d. The patient is protected under governmental immunity because of the altered mental status.

29. When the EMT-B does not obtain consent from an oriented, competent adult prior to treatment and transport, his actions may be considered:

    a. false imprisonment.
    b. negligence.
    c. slander.
    d. libel.

30. Touching a competent adult patient without the patient's consent may be construed as:

    a. battery.
    b. part of assessment.
    c. acceptable under the mental health laws.
    d. considered very serious if done in front of a child.

31. The EMT-B has a duty to act:

    a. only when he is paid to do so.
    b. when there is no threat to personal safety.
    c. only when his status is that of a volunteer.
    d. as soon as he receives state certification or licensure.

32. While on vacation in another state, you encounter a life-threatening medical emergency and quickly decide to help until the local EMS arrives at the patient's side. Legally, the safest approach is to:

    a. perform any actions necessary at the EMT-B level.
    b. identify yourself as a trained EMT-B and offer to ride to the hospital with the local EMS.
    c. stand by and intervene only if the patient requires CPR.
    d. limit your care to life-saving BLS treatment as a first responder.

33. The legal and primary responsibilities of an EMS provider concern the:
    a. patient and public only.
    b. agency's medical director only.
    c. patient and the agency's medical director.
    d. patient, the public, and the agency's medical director.

34. The EMT-B's duty to act is not always clear, because:
    a. there are no national standards for EMT-Bs.
    b. when an EMT-B is on duty he has an obligation to provide service.
    c. state and local laws can vary significantly.
    d. there are multiple definitions of *duty to act*.

35. Confidentiality is a professional and legal responsibility that pertains to:
    a. a patient's privacy.
    b. censoring a patient's medical information.
    c. your experience level.
    d. safeguarding a patient's medical identification tag.

36. In which of the following manners may information about your patient legally be released to someone other than a health care provider?
    a. the information may be given to a spouse without a release
    b. over the phone if the patient has given verbal permission
    c. with a written release signed by the patient
    d. by fax with permission from the patient's family

37. A health care professional who spreads rumors that may injure the reputation of another is guilty of:
    a. libel.
    b. slander.
    c. false compliment.
    d. damaging etiquette.

38. With respect to confidentiality, the EMT-B must report which of the following observations in a patient's residence?
    a. reserved untidiness
    b. suspected child abuse
    c. large sums of cash or coins
    d. excessive quantities of liquor bottles, both full and empty

39. Which of the following statements about organ donors is most correct?
    a. The EMS provider has no legal responsibility to resuscitate potential organ donors.
    b. The EMS provider has no ethical responsibility to resuscitate potential organ donors.
    c. The EMS provider has a legal and ethical responsibility to resuscitate any potential organ donor.
    d. The EMS provider has no legal or ethical responsibility to resuscitate any potential organ donor.

40. In which of the following ways could the EMT-B verify that a patient has consented to be an organ donor?
    a. A family member advises the EMT-B of the patient's wishes.
    b. The patient is carrying an organ donor card.
    c. The patient's driver's license indicates that the patient is an organ donor.
    d. All of the above.

41. When managing a critically injured patient who is a potential organ donor, the EMT-B should:
    a. provide comfort care only for the patient until arriving at the hospital.
    b. withhold treatment until the patient becomes pulseless, then begin CPR.
    c. care for the patient the same as for any other patient in need of emergency care.
    d. request police assistance, as the patient is now considered to be in protective custody.

42. The victim of a traumatic head injury is near death, and you are able to learn that he is an organ donor, but specifically for the eyes. During your assessment you discover that the patient's eyes are badly damaged. You should now:
    a. care for the patient the same as for any other patient.
    b. attempt to contact a relative for modified donor instructions.
    c. terminate your resuscitative efforts, because the eyes are not viable.
    d. call online medical control, report your findings, and inquire about advance directives.

43. You have been called to the scene of a hanging. The hanging is recent and you are going to attempt resuscitation. In helping to preserve the crime scene, you should avoid:
    a. untying the knot.
    b. cutting at least 6 inches above the knot.
    c. asking the police to manage the rope.
    d. using a sharp knife to make a clean cut in the rope.

44. Upon responding to a call for a cardiac arrest, you discover that the victim has been dead for hours; this appears to be an unattended death. To help preserve a possible crime scene, you should:
    a. leave the body in the position found.
    b. bag the victim's clothing in a brown paper bag for the police.
    c. wait for the police before touching the body to assess for signs of life.
    d. use the telephone at the victim's residence to call his doctor and ask about any advance directives.

45. While caring for the victim of a rape, the EMT-B can help to preserve evidence by:

    a. waiting for the police to arrive before talking to the patient.

    b. putting all the victim's clothing into one red bag and taking it along to the hospital.

    c. asking the victim not to change clothes or bathe.

    d. waiting for the police to interview the patient before treating any injuries.

46. Which of the following actions would be inappropriate for an EMT-B who is working at the scene of a call?

    a. assure scene safety

    b. provide patient care

    c. observe and document anything unusual at the scene

    d. document any suspicions based on prior calls to the scene

47. Which type of call is typically nonreportable by the EMT-B to a mandated reporter or legal authority?

    a. animal bite

    b. electrocution

    c. elder or spousal abuse

    d. gunshot or stab wound

48. An EMT-B is caring for a female who complains of abdominal pain. During the assessment and history taking, the patient reveals that she has been raped, but asks that this information not be disclosed to the police. Which of the following statements is most accurate regarding reporting of the rape?

    a. Failure to report this incident may actually be a crime.

    b. The EMT-B must keep the patient's information confidential upon her request.

    c. The patient has suffered a traumatic event and is not of sound mind to make such a request.

    d. The EMT-B can keep the information confidential from the hospital staff if the patient reports the crime on a hotline within 24 hours.

49. After responding to a call for an 80-year-old female who is unconscious, the EMT-B suspects that the patient may have taken too much of her medication, either accidentally or on purpose. The EMT-B should:

    a. consider this a crime scene and notify the police immediately.

    b. provide care for the patient, protect potential evidence, and notify the ED staff of his suspicions.

    c. provide care for the patient and wait to report the incident until the hospital can confirm an overdose.

    d. accurately document all suspicions and let the hospital make a report to the police.

50. While caring for an intoxicated patient who is uncooperative, the EMT-B is repeatedly grabbed by the patient, even after strongly urging to the patient to cease. The patient bruises the EMT-B's arm. The patient's actions may be considered:

    a. a civil offense.

    b. sexual harassment.

    c. a criminal offense.

    d. no crime because the patient had an altered mental status.

Chapter 3 Answer Form

	A	B	C	D			A	B	C	D
1.	❑	❑	❑	❑		26.	❑	❑	❑	❑
2.	❑	❑	❑	❑		27.	❑	❑	❑	❑
3.	❑	❑	❑	❑		28.	❑	❑	❑	❑
4.	❑	❑	❑	❑		29.	❑	❑	❑	❑
5.	❑	❑	❑	❑		30.	❑	❑	❑	❑
6.	❑	❑	❑	❑		31.	❑	❑	❑	❑
7.	❑	❑	❑	❑		32.	❑	❑	❑	❑
8.	❑	❑	❑	❑		33.	❑	❑	❑	❑
9.	❑	❑	❑	❑		34.	❑	❑	❑	❑
10.	❑	❑	❑	❑		35.	❑	❑	❑	❑
11.	❑	❑	❑	❑		36.	❑	❑	❑	❑
12.	❑	❑	❑	❑		37.	❑	❑	❑	❑
13.	❑	❑	❑	❑		38.	❑	❑	❑	❑
14.	❑	❑	❑	❑		39.	❑	❑	❑	❑
15.	❑	❑	❑	❑		40.	❑	❑	❑	❑
16.	❑	❑	❑	❑		41.	❑	❑	❑	❑
17.	❑	❑	❑	❑		42.	❑	❑	❑	❑
18.	❑	❑	❑	❑		43.	❑	❑	❑	❑
19.	❑	❑	❑	❑		44.	❑	❑	❑	❑
20.	❑	❑	❑	❑		45.	❑	❑	❑	❑
21.	❑	❑	❑	❑		46.	❑	❑	❑	❑
22.	❑	❑	❑	❑		47.	❑	❑	❑	❑
23.	❑	❑	❑	❑		48.	❑	❑	❑	❑
24.	❑	❑	❑	❑		49.	❑	❑	❑	❑
25.	❑	❑	❑	❑		50.	❑	❑	❑	❑

CHAPTER 4

The Human Body

1. The _____ position is the stance of the body when it is erect with the arms and hands to the side, palms facing forward.
   a. prone
   b. supine
   c. anatomical
   d. recumbent

2. Terms related to the surface and depth of body parts include all of the following *except:*
   a. plane.
   b. parietal.
   c. internal.
   d. superficial.

3. Which of the following posterior regions of the spine contains seven vertebrae?
   a. cervical
   b. thoracic
   c. lumbar
   d. sacral

4. When describing the location of an injury to the wrist, which of the following statements is correct?
   a. bilateral to the hand
   b. distal to the forearm
   c. proximal to the elbow
   d. superior to the forearm

5. The _____ position is the body lying in a horizontal position with the face up.
   a. prone
   b. lateral
   c. supine
   d. anatomical

6. The quadrants of the abdomen are named for the:
   a. underlying organs in each.
   b. technique used to assess the abdomen.
   c. position on the body they occupy.
   d. physician who discovered them.

7. Which of the following structures lies mostly in the midline of the body?
   a. stomach
   b. heart
   c. esophagus
   d. large intestine

8. You are caring for an 18-year-old male who fell while skateboarding and broke his forearm in the middle. How would you describe the location of the fracture?
   a. The fracture is proximal to the shoulder.
   b. The fracture is midshaft in the forearm.
   c. The fracture is superior to the elbow.
   d. The fracture is located on the inferior portion of the humerus.

9. The imaginary line that runs vertically from the armpit down to the ankle is the:
   a. midline.
   b. mid-clavicular line.
   c. bilateral line.
   d. mid-axillary line.

10. You have just finished palpating the cervical spine of a victim involved in a motor vehicle collision. This area is referred to as the _____ neck.
    a. lateral
    b. inferior
    c. posterior
    d. transverse

11. The _____ is the cavity connecting the nose and mouth with the esophagus and trachea.
    a. glottis
    b. nares
    c. sinus
    d. pharynx

12. The cavity that contains the vocal cords or "voice box" is the:
    a. larynx.
    b. pharynx.
    c. glottis.
    d. nasal.

13. The _____ prevents food from entering the larynx.
    a. tongue
    b. trachea
    c. glottis
    d. epiglottis

14. Oxygen and carbon dioxide exchange takes place in the:
    a. alveoli.
    b. bronchi.
    c. bronchioles.
    d. alveolar ducts.

15. Lungs are held in an inflated state by:
    a. ligaments.
    b. negative pressure.
    c. positive pressure.
    d. the mediastinum.

16. The primary muscles involved in breathing are the _____ and the _____ muscles.
    a. pleural, pulmonary
    b. diaphragm, glottis
    c. diaphragm, intercostal
    d. intercostal, extracostal

17. The prefix *pneumo* means:
    a. lung.
    b. air.
    c. breath.
    d. all of the above.

18. To increase the space in the thorax, the diaphragm _____ and pulls _____.
    a. contracts, upward
    b. relaxes, upward
    c. contracts, downward
    d. relaxes, downward

19. The pleural spaces in the thoracic cavity are filled with:
    a. lobes.
    b. alveoli.
    c. bronchus.
    d. serous fluid.

20. The respiratory system supplies oxygen to the cells of the body and:
    a. removes carbon dioxide.
    b. is a branch of the digestive process.
    c. operates in the senses of smell and taste.
    d. activates the constriction and relaxation of blood vessels.

21. Heart sounds are caused by:
    a. blood rushing through the heart.
    b. the contraction of the heart muscle.
    c. offloading of deoxygenated blood from the vena cava.
    d. the contraction of the aorta.

22. The reason you can feel a pulse is:
    a. because of the force of blood on the artery walls.
    b. because of the electrical impulse traveling through the vessels.
    c. because of the force of blood on the venous walls.
    d. because of the components of which the blood is made up.

23. Which of the following structures drains blood from the lower parts of the body?
    a. aorta
    b. inferior vena cava
    c. superior vena cava
    d. pulmonary artery

24. The _____ valve is the valve on the right side of the heart between the atrium and ventricle.
    a. aortic
    b. tricuspid
    c. bicuspid
    d. pulmonic

25. Which structure carries deoxygenated blood to the lungs?
    a. mitral valve
    b. pulmonary vein
    c. pulmonary artery
    d. superior vena cava

26. Plasma contains which of the following components?
    a. platelets
    b. red blood cells
    c. white blood cells
    d. minerals, salts, and proteins

27. As a baby matures into a child and then an adult, which structure of the heart enlarges to become the most muscular and strongest part of the heart?
    a. left atrium
    b. right atrium
    c. left ventricle
    d. right ventricle

28. Although the heart constantly has blood flowing through it, the heart receives its own blood supply from which vessel(s)?
    a. carotid artery
    b. coronary arteries
    c. pulmonary arteries
    d. superior vena cava

29. Blood is supplied to the extremities by _____ circulation.
    a. portal
    b. hepatic
    c. peripheral
    d. coronary

30. Necrosis, or death, of heart muscle is referred to as:
    a. myocardial infarction.
    b. cardiac tamponade.
    c. myocardial ischemia.
    d. coronary occlusion.

31. Which of the one-way valves of the heart is not work-ing properly when there is a backflow of blood in the right ventricle?
    a. aortic
    b. bicuspid
    c. tricuspid
    d. pulmonary

32. When you are searching for a pulse on the posterior aspect of the medial malleolus, you are palpating the posterior _____ artery.
    a. tibial
    b. femoral
    c. dorsalis pedis
    d. brachial

33. Blood is carried back to the heart by way of:
    a. veins.
    b. arteries.
    c. osmosis.
    d. dialysis.

34. A clot of blood, bubble of air, or other substance that creates an obstruction in a blood vessel is a/an:
    a. edema.
    b. embolism.
    c. varicose.
    d. palpation.

35. The term *conduction* refers to an action in which there is a transmission of _____ through the heart.
    a. pulses
    b. platelets
    c. epinephrine
    d. electrical impulses

36. _____ are a form of connective tissue that are hard-ened by calcium.
    a. Bones
    b. Tendons
    c. Ligaments
    d. Cartilage

37. _____ is/are a form of connective tissue covering the epiphysis that act(s) as a smooth surface for articulation.
    a. Bones
    b. Cartilage
    c. Tendons
    d. Ligaments

38. In an adult, a fracture of which of the following bones can potentially result in a 1,000-mL blood loss?
    a. tibia
    b. fibula
    c. femur
    d. humerus

39. A _____ is an injury to the ligaments around a joint.
    a. strain
    b. sprain
    c. fracture
    d. dislocation

40. Of the following areas for possible dislocations, select the two most potentially serious due to the possibility of complete disruption of blood supply to the distal body part.
    a. knee and elbow
    b. hip and knee
    c. elbow and wrist
    d. shoulder and knee

41. The 11th and 12th pairs of ribs are commonly referred to as "floating" ribs because:
    a. they are located below the lungs.
    b. they do not connect directly to the sternum.
    c. these two pair are covered (floating) in synovial fluid.
    d. when fractured, they tend to cause major bleeding.

42. _____ is the term for fractured bone ends that are grinding together.
    a. Crunch
    b. Masticate
    c. Machete
    d. Crepitation

43. _____ is the type of muscle found in the walls of ar-teries and veins.
    a. Cardiac
    b. Skeletal
    c. Voluntary
    d. Smooth

44. The _____ is the socket of the hip joint where the head or end of the proximal femur fits.
    a. ilium
    b. pubis
    c. ischium
    d. acetabulum

45. The sternum or breastbone is divided into _____ sections.
    a. 2
    b. 3
    c. 4
    d. 5

46. Which of the following is not considered a neurological event?
    a. stroke
    b. seizure
    c. heart attack
    d. spinal cord injury

47. The central nervous system (CNS) is comprised of the:
    a. cranial nerves and skin.
    b. nerves, skin, and electrons.
    c. muscle receptors and glands.
    d. brain, brain stem, and spinal cord.

48. A tract of communication unavailable to the peripheral nervous system is:
    a. from the brain to distal body parts.
    b. from the extremities back to the brain.
    c. through sensory and motor nerves.
    d. the release of hormones into the blood from glands.

49. The involuntary nervous system is known as the:
    a. meninges.
    b. control center.
    c. vegetative organism.
    d. autonomic nervous system.

50. While plugging a vacuum cleaner plug into a wall socket, you receive a shock and instinctively pull your hand away. Which structures are responsible for sending the message of pain to your brain?
    a. motor nerves
    b. sensory nerves
    c. sympathetic response
    d. parasympathetic response

51. While you are driving your car, another vehicle unexpectedly pulls into your path. You quickly step on the brake and avoid a collision; simultaneously, you take a deep breath and your heart races. What part of your nervous system has speeded up your heart rate in response to this situation?
    a. autonomic
    b. motor nerves
    c. voluntary
    d. sensory nerves

52. The largest organ of the human body is the:
    a. skin.
    b. intestines.
    c. stomach.
    d. nervous system.

53. Sweat glands are located in which layer(s) of the skin?
    a. dermis
    b. epidermis
    c. subcutaneous
    d. dermis and epidermis

54. Fat and soft tissue make the major function of the _____ layer(s) of skin shock absorption and insulation.
    a. dermis
    b. epidermis
    c. sebaceous
    d. subcutaneous

55. Except for the palms of the hands and the soles of the feet, the epidermis contains _____ layers.
    a. 2
    b. 3
    c. 4
    d. 5

56. The endocrine system is made up of _____ that produce _____, which help to regulate many body activities and functions.
    a. nerves, impulses
    b. vessels, platelets
    c. glands, hormones
    d. chemicals, plasma

57. The _____ produces insulin, a hormone that is critical in helping the body use glucose for fuel.
    a. thyroid
    b. pancreas
    c. adrenal glands
    d. gonads

58. The endocrine system includes which of the following reproductive organ(s)?
    a. ovaries and testes
    b. uterus
    c. mammary glands
    d. penis

59. The most common type of endocrine emergency that EMT-Bs respond to is:
    a. seizures.
    b. a diabetic emergency.
    c. a thyroid emergency.
    d. an allergic reaction.

60. Which of the following organs is *not* part of the endocrine system?
    a. kidneys
    b. pituitary gland
    c. thymus gland
    d. adrenal glands

Chapter 4 Answer Form

	A	B	C	D		A	B	C	D
1.	❑	❑	❑	❑	31.	❑	❑	❑	❑
2.	❑	❑	❑	❑	32.	❑	❑	❑	❑
3.	❑	❑	❑	❑	33.	❑	❑	❑	❑
4.	❑	❑	❑	❑	34.	❑	❑	❑	❑
5.	❑	❑	❑	❑	35.	❑	❑	❑	❑
6.	❑	❑	❑	❑	36.	❑	❑	❑	❑
7.	❑	❑	❑	❑	37.	❑	❑	❑	❑
8.	❑	❑	❑	❑	38.	❑	❑	❑	❑
9.	❑	❑	❑	❑	39.	❑	❑	❑	❑
10.	❑	❑	❑	❑	40.	❑	❑	❑	❑
11.	❑	❑	❑	❑	41.	❑	❑	❑	❑
12.	❑	❑	❑	❑	42.	❑	❑	❑	❑
13.	❑	❑	❑	❑	43.	❑	❑	❑	❑
14.	❑	❑	❑	❑	44.	❑	❑	❑	❑
15.	❑	❑	❑	❑	45.	❑	❑	❑	❑
16.	❑	❑	❑	❑	46.	❑	❑	❑	❑
17.	❑	❑	❑	❑	47.	❑	❑	❑	❑
18.	❑	❑	❑	❑	48.	❑	❑	❑	❑
19.	❑	❑	❑	❑	49.	❑	❑	❑	❑
20.	❑	❑	❑	❑	50.	❑	❑	❑	❑
21.	❑	❑	❑	❑	51.	❑	❑	❑	❑
22.	❑	❑	❑	❑	52.	❑	❑	❑	❑
23.	❑	❑	❑	❑	53.	❑	❑	❑	❑
24.	❑	❑	❑	❑	54.	❑	❑	❑	❑
25.	❑	❑	❑	❑	55.	❑	❑	❑	❑
26.	❑	❑	❑	❑	56.	❑	❑	❑	❑
27.	❑	❑	❑	❑	57.	❑	❑	❑	❑
28.	❑	❑	❑	❑	58.	❑	❑	❑	❑
29.	❑	❑	❑	❑	59.	❑	❑	❑	❑
30.	❑	❑	❑	❑	60.	❑	❑	❑	❑

CHAPTER 5

Baseline Vital Signs and SAMPLE History

1. The EMT-B uses which of the following senses to assess a patient's vital signs?
   a. sight and touch
   b. hearing and smell
   c. hearing and touch
   d. sight, hearing, and touch

2. The signs of life include respirations, heart rate, blood pressure, and:
   a. ECG.
   b. temperature.
   c. pulse oximetry.
   d. none of the above.

3. Assessing the breathing rate of an infant without disturbing the child can best be accomplished by:
   a. placing a hand on the chest to feel for rise and fall.
   b. placing a hand on the belly to feel for rise and fall.
   c. visualizing the belly and counting the breaths per minute.
   d. asking the parent to hold the child while listening to the chest with a stethoscope.

4. Because patients tend to change their breathing rate when they are being watched, the EMT-B should count the respirations:
   a. when the patient is not looking.
   b. while acting as if he is counting the pulse rate.
   c. while distracting the patient with SAMPLE questions.
   d. after assuring the patient that he is going to be fine.

5. Rate, quality, and effort are terms the EMT-B uses to:
   a. give report about a patient.
   b. describe the way a patient is breathing.
   c. document the way a patient is breathing.
   d. all of the above.

6. Which of the following terms is generally not used to describe the quality of a patient's breathing?
   a. thin
   b. labored
   c. shallow
   d. absent

7. Noisy breathing is usually a sign of respiratory distress. Which term is not used to describe noisy breathing?
   a. retractions
   b. wheezing
   c. snoring
   d. stridor

8. A patient with labored breathing is considered to be in severe respiratory distress when:
   a. there is a partial obstruction.
   b. wheezing becomes quiet, but the patient looks ill.
   c. the patient can speak only two words at a time.
   d. any of the findings listed above is consistent with severe respiratory distress.

9. In which of the following patients would you consider that something may be seriously wrong?
   a. a 3-year-old female with a heart rate of 120 bpm and a fever
   b. a 50-year-old male with a heart rate of 48 bpm who runs marathons
   c. a 2-week-old newborn with a heart rate of 160 bpm who is crying
   d. a 45-year-old female with a heart rate of 142 bpm who is moist and pale, but has no chest pain

10. After delivering a newly-born infant, the EMT-B should obtain the baby's pulse rate:
    a. every 15 minutes after birth.
    b. by palpating a distal pulse.
    c. by palpating the umbilical stump.
    d. only if the baby does not begin to cry.

11. While assessing for a radial pulse on an 18-month-old toddler, you palpate the:
    a. medial side of the forearm.
    b. proximal lateral side of the arm.
    c. distal lateral (thumb) side of the forearm.
    d. proximal lateral (thumb) side of the forearm.

12. The absence of peripheral pulses in a pediatric patient in warm ambient temperatures is usually an indication of:
    a. hyperthermia.
    b. hypoglycemia.
    c. poor perfusion.
    d. mild hypothermia.

13. An apical pulse is assessed by palpating:
    a. the umbilical stump of a newly born infant.
    b. the upper thigh on the medial side.
    c. both radial arteries simultaneously.
    d. or listening to the anterior chest with a stethoscope.

14. When you assess the pulse rate of an adult and find that the rhythm is irregular, the pulse should be:
    a. assessed on both sides.
    b. counted for one full minute.
    c. considered a sign of shock.
    d. considered a pulse deficit.

15. Constriction of the blood vessels causes the skin to become:
    a. pale in color.
    b. hot to the touch.
    c. flushed.
    d. jaundiced.

16. Which of the following mnemonics is used to remind the EMT-B what to assess on the skin?
    a. SAMPLE
    b. OPQRST
    c. HAZMAT
    d. D-CAP-BTLS

17. Skin color, temperature, and condition (CTC) can provide valuable information about:
    a. past medical history.
    b. a patient's overall physical health.
    c. a patient's circulatory status.
    d. the medication(s) a patient is taking.

18. Capillary refill is assessed by pressing down on the skin or nail bed, which should immediately:
    a. blanch or turn white.
    b. flush and redden.
    c. turn blue then pink.
    d. remained depressed for 2 seconds.

19. The lack of oxygen perfusion to blood cells and tissues would most likely make the skin look:
    a. flushed.
    b. cyanotic.
    c. jaundiced.
    d. hot and clammy.

20. Jaundiced or yellow skin is caused by abnormalities of the liver and is most visibly obvious in the:
    a. lips.
    b. eyes.
    c. palms.
    d. nail beds.

21. While assessing the skin temperature of a 65-year-old female with a history of diabetes, you note that her lower left leg is red and feels hot compared to the rest of her body. You suspect:
    a. an infection.
    b. poor circulation.
    c. heat exposure.
    d. vascular disease.

22. You are assessing a 24-year-old male with symptoms of the flu. He tells you he has been running a fever for the past couple of hours. His skin temperature and condition will most likely be:
    a. cool and clammy.
    b. cold and moist.
    c. warm and pink.
    d. hot and dry, or hot and moist.

23. When distal circulation to an injured extremity is impaired, you would expect the skin that is distal to the injury to feel:
    a. hot.
    b. cool.
    c. moist.
    d. warm.

24. The local ski patrol found a hiker who wandered around in the woods in very cold weather for several hours. They tell you that the hiker has suffered deep frostbite on the toes of his right foot. What skin color, temperature, and condition would you expect the affected toes to have?
    a. pale, moist, and normal tone
    b. black, cool, and hard to the touch
    c. red, cold, and limp to the touch
    d. white or waxy, cold, and hard to the touch

25. You are assessing a 12-year-old female who is experiencing a severe anaphylactic reaction to a bee sting. What skin color, temperature, and condition would you expect to find on this patient?

    a. cool, pale, and moist
    b. hot, flushed, and moist
    c. warm with generalized flushing
    d. warm, raised, and red itchy blotches

26. A capillary refill time of more than _____ second(s) is considered an abnormal finding in infants.

    a. 1
    b. 2
    c. 3
    d. 4

27. Capillary refill in infants is considered a very reliable indicator of the:

    a. perfusion status.
    b. distal sensory status.
    c. neurological status.
    d. accurate pulse rate.

28. When the ambient light is so bright that your patient's pupils are fully constricted, you can stimulate a pupillary response by:

    a. shining a really large flashlight into both eyes.
    b. asking the patient to hold his breath for 30 seconds.
    c. shading both eyes for 30 seconds, while watching for dilation.
    d. there is no way to stimulate a pupillary response under these conditions.

29. Examination of the head includes assessment of the pupils. Which of the following includes an accurate measurement of the pupil?

    a. diameter in millimeters
    b. diameter in centimeters
    c. circumference in centimeters
    d. circumference in millimeters

30. When a light is shined into the right pupil in an effort to get it to constrict, which of the following would be considered a normal response?

    a. Both pupils react equally.
    b. The left pupil gets large.
    c. The right pupil gets large.
    d. Only the right pupil constricts.

31. In bright ambient light, you would expect a patient's pupils to be:

    a. fixed.
    b. constricted.
    c. dilated.
    d. nonreactive.

32. During an initial assessment of an 18-year-old female with an isolated cut on her arm from a utility knife, you notice that her pupils are unequal. She denies any loss of consciousness or any other injury. What is the appropriate action to take regarding your abnormal finding?

    a. Ask her if this is normal for her.
    b. Consider the possibility of a head injury and immobilize her.
    c. Consider the possibility of a stroke and perform a stroke exam.
    d. Just ignore the finding, because the present problem is totally unrelated.

33. While assessing a 62-year-old male who had fallen and injured his hip, you note that he has unequal pupils. His wife tells you that this is not normal for him, so one of the first things you consider as the cause for the abnormal finding is:

    a. shock.
    b. stroke.
    c. hypotension.
    d. hypoglycemia.

34. You are assessing an alert, 40-year-old male who struck his head after falling from a standing position. He did not lose consciousness and denies any significant pain or injury. When you assess his pupils, you find that his right pupil is nonreactive to light. You consider _____ to be the possible cause for the abnormal finding.

    a. fright
    b. pink eye
    c. a concussion
    d. an artificial eye

35. Taking a blood pressure by palpation would be most reasonable in which situation?

    a. when the patient has no distal pulse
    b. when auscultation is taking too long
    c. when the BP cuff gauge is not calibrated
    d. the sirens are turned on en route to the hospital

36. You are obtaining a blood pressure on a patient by auscultation. As you release the pressure in the cuff, the first sound you hear indicates the:

    a. systolic reading.
    b. diastolic reading.
    c. cardiac output.
    d. stroke volume.

37. The systolic blood pressure relates to the:

    a. contraction of the ventricles.
    b. relaxation of the ventricles.
    c. contraction of the atria.
    d. none of the above.

38. During the normal heart cycle, the pressure created within the arteries is known as the _____ blood pressure.
    a. atrial
    b. systolic
    c. diastolic
    d. ventricular

39. The diastolic blood pressure relates to the:
    a. contraction of the heart.
    b. atria refilling with blood.
    c. relaxation phase of the heart cycle.
    d. conduction phase of the heart cycle.

40. The unit of measure "mm Hg" refers to the:
    a. ancient Greek formula of liquid measure.
    b. Latin measure of liquid under hydrostatic pressure.
    c. apothecary unit of measure for liquid mercury hydraulic pressure.
    d. height of mercury in millimeters to which the blood pressure elevates a column of liquid mercury in a glass tube.

41. Which of the following statements about blood pressure readings is false?
    a. Over the brachial artery is the only proper location for a BP cuff.
    b. Improper size and placement of the BP cuff can result in false readings.
    c. The diastolic pressure cannot be obtained by the palpation method.
    d. The first blood pressure reading on a patient is usually higher than rapidly repeated assessments.

42. Which of the following statements about blood pressure readings is most accurate?
    a. The method of obtaining a BP by auscultation is more accurate than by palpation.
    b. Obtaining a BP by palpation is more accurate than by auscultation.
    c. It is easier to obtain a BP by palpation than by auscultation.
    d. Both auscultation and palpation are equally accurate.

43. The "E" in the mnemonic SAMPLE represents:
    a. episodes of a similar nature.
    b. evidence of the mechanism of injury.
    c. events that have been previously diagnosed for the patient.
    d. events that led up to what the patient was doing when the current episode began.

44. When a patient is unconscious or has an altered mental status, obtaining the SAMPLE history:
    a. is not going to matter.
    b. can be completed by the police.
    c. can wait until the patient becomes alert.
    d. may be attempted with family or a caretaker.

45. Which of the following is considered a symptom rather than a sign?
    a. edema
    b. dizziness
    c. fainting
    d. wheezing

46. Which of the following is considered a sign rather than a symptom?
    a. headache
    b. crepitus
    c. numbness
    d. blurred vision

47. Recording a baseline set of vital signs, followed by a reassessment of vital signs during the ongoing assessment, is:
    a. helpful to establish or recognize a pattern.
    b. referred to as *trending*.
    c. the standard of care.
    d. all of the above.

48. Ideally, vital signs should be taken and recorded every _____ minutes on a stable patient.
    a. 5
    b. 10
    c. 15
    d. 20

49. Some patients keep a written record of their medical information and place it in a container called a Vial of Life®. This container is typically stored:
    a. by the telephone.
    b. in the refrigerator.
    c. with the closest relative.
    d. with the next-door neighbor.

50. An example of critical but nonemergent medical information the EMT-B should record and relay to the next health care provider receiving the patient is:
    a. the name and address of the patient's closest relative.
    b. any evidence of neglected yard work and a sloppy garage.
    c. the number and type of pets found in the patient's residence.
    d. any evidence of the patient's inability to perform activities of daily living.

Chapter 5 Answer Form

	A	B	C	D		A	B	C	D
1.	❏	❏	❏	❏	26.	❏	❏	❏	❏
2.	❏	❏	❏	❏	27.	❏	❏	❏	❏
3.	❏	❏	❏	❏	28.	❏	❏	❏	❏
4.	❏	❏	❏	❏	29.	❏	❏	❏	❏
5.	❏	❏	❏	❏	30.	❏	❏	❏	❏
6.	❏	❏	❏	❏	31.	❏	❏	❏	❏
7.	❏	❏	❏	❏	32.	❏	❏	❏	❏
8.	❏	❏	❏	❏	33.	❏	❏	❏	❏
9.	❏	❏	❏	❏	34.	❏	❏	❏	❏
10.	❏	❏	❏	❏	35.	❏	❏	❏	❏
11.	❏	❏	❏	❏	36.	❏	❏	❏	❏
12.	❏	❏	❏	❏	37.	❏	❏	❏	❏
13.	❏	❏	❏	❏	38.	❏	❏	❏	❏
14.	❏	❏	❏	❏	39.	❏	❏	❏	❏
15.	❏	❏	❏	❏	40.	❏	❏	❏	❏
16.	❏	❏	❏	❏	41.	❏	❏	❏	❏
17.	❏	❏	❏	❏	42.	❏	❏	❏	❏
18.	❏	❏	❏	❏	43.	❏	❏	❏	❏
19.	❏	❏	❏	❏	44.	❏	❏	❏	❏
20.	❏	❏	❏	❏	45.	❏	❏	❏	❏
21.	❏	❏	❏	❏	46.	❏	❏	❏	❏
22.	❏	❏	❏	❏	47.	❏	❏	❏	❏
23.	❏	❏	❏	❏	48.	❏	❏	❏	❏
24.	❏	❏	❏	❏	49.	❏	❏	❏	❏
25.	❏	❏	❏	❏	50.	❏	❏	❏	❏

Lifting and Moving Patients

1. The EMT-B should practice the principles and techniques of proper lifting and moving:
   a. daily.
   b. annually.
   c. semi-annually.
   d. in a monthly continuing education program.

2. _____ refers to safe lifting and moving techniques that help prevent personal injury.
   a. Supination
   b. Body mechanics
   c. Proprioception
   d. Hydraulics

3. To help avoid a back injury when lifting any patient, the EMT-B should:
   a. keep her back straight and locked.
   b. call the fire department and wait for assistance.
   c. never lift a patient who weighs more than 200 pounds.
   d. only lift with another EMT-B of the same size and weight.

4. Which of the following is not considered proper form for the EMT-B who is about to lift and carry a patient who weighs more than 150 pounds?
   a. Lift with the legs, not the back.
   b. Avoid keeping the weight close to one's body.
   c. Avoid lifting on uneven surfaces whenever possible.
   d. Avoid leaning to the left or right to compensate for the weight.

5. To keep a stretcher from becoming unbalanced and possibly tipping, the EMT-B should:
   a. keep the center of gravity close to the ground.
   b. always use four people to lift the stretcher while moving on stairs.
   c. only raise and lower from the ends of the stretcher, not the sides.
   d. never place a patient weighing more than 250 pounds in the sitting position.

6. The _____ is/are most commonly utilized by EMT-Bs during safe lifting of a stretcher.
   a. four-person method
   b. power lift and power grip
   c. method with one EMT-B on each side
   d. none of the above

7. Of the following, the most critical factor in selecting the type of patient carrying device is:
   a. the age of the patient.
   b. the gender of the patient.
   c. the weight of the patient.
   d. a suspected spinal injury.

8. The extremity lift, direct ground lift, and firefighter's carry are all moving techniques that would be appropriate for moving patients:
   a. who are apneic and pulseless.
   b. with suspected spinal injury.
   c. with no suspected spinal injury.
   d. who are contaminated with hazardous materials.

9. To avoid injury while carrying a single piece of equipment with only the right hand, it is necessary to:
   a. carry the object in front of the body.
   b. avoid leaning to the left.
   c. lean to the loaded side of the body.
   d. carry another item of equal weight in the other hand to balance the load.

10. _____ is an example of when the one-handed carrying technique is used.
    a. Moving a patient using a power lift
    b. Rescuing a patient using a firefighter's drag
    c. Lifting an AED out of a cabinet and walking it over to a patient
    d. Raising a stretcher from the lowest position to the highest by yourself

11. Which of the following carrying methods or devices is the least safe for getting a patient down a flight of stairs?
    a. stair chair
    b. long backboard
    c. extremity carry
    d. scoop stretcher

12. The _____ is the ideal lifting device for getting a conscious patient safely out of a basement.
    a. Reeves
    b. stretcher
    c. stair chair
    d. long backboard

13. The only moving technique in which twisting is helpful and not potentially harmful to the EMT-B is:
    a. lifting.
    b. lowering.
    c. when reaching.
    d. none of the above.

14. Reaching for a piece of equipment or for a patient increases the risk of injury for the EMT-B and can be avoided by:
    a. moving closer to the object.
    b. leaning forward from the waist.
    c. keeping the knees locked.
    d. extending and locking the elbows.

15. The ideal arm positioning for reaching while logrolling a patient to assess for any injuries to the back is to:
    a. keep the elbows locked.
    b. keep the elbows bent.
    c. lock the wrists and flex the elbows.
    d. keep the arms aligned and avoid overreaching.

16. When performing a logroll to get a patient onto a long spine board, the proper reaching technique includes:
    a. reaching with the low back arched.
    b. keeping your head as low as possible.
    c. leaning from the hips with your back locked.
    d. extending and locking the elbows.

17. While pushing and pulling a stretcher from the ambulance, the guidelines recommend:
    a. always push and never pull.
    b. tucking your chin into your chest and locking your back.
    c. keeping your elbows bent and your arms close to your torso.
    d. asking the patient her weight so you can make the proper adjustment.

18. Pushing or pulling equipment and other objects is routine for the EMT-B. To significantly help decrease the risk of injury, she should avoid pushing or pulling:
    a. overhead.
    b. backward.
    c. a wheeled stair chair.
    d. anything that has wheels.

19. You are treating the victim of a motor vehicle collision (MVC) who has an altered mental status and suspected cervical injury. Her condition is deteriorating rapidly. Which of the following moves is most appropriate for this patient?
    a. direct
    b. urgent
    c. emergency
    d. nonurgent

20. For moving the patient with no suspected spinal injury, which of the following considerations is most commonly utilized by the EMT-B?
    a. the age of the patient
    b. ease of lifting for the EMT-B
    c. distance to the hospital
    d. position of comfort for the patient

21. After responding to a call for a respiratory arrest, you find the patient lying on the floor between her bed and the wall. You and your partner move her out into the middle of the room where there is space to work. This move is considered:
    a. an urgent move.
    b. a nonurgent move.
    c. inappropriate without the use of a cervical collar and backboard.
    d. foolish because of the potential for a back injury to the EMT-Bs.

22. In which of the following situations would it be appropriate to use an urgent move?
    a. 43-year-old driver complaining of neck pain entrapped in the driver's side of a stable vehicle
    b. a female in her thirties who is having a seizure while lying on the floor in a department store
    c. a 50-year-old female who collapsed while working outside on a very hot day
    d. a crying 18-month old infant who is in a car seat at the scene of a minor MVC

23. The _____ stretcher is typically made of canvas and has wooden slats for stability and carrying handles on the sides.
    a. scoop
    b. wheeled
    c. basket
    d. flexible or Reeves

24. A _____ is a carrying device consisting of an aluminum frame and a rectangular tube with shovel-type side flaps for sliding underneath the patient.
    a. stair chair
    b. scoop stretcher
    c. basket stretcher
    d. Stokes® basket

25. When moving a patient who has a suspected spinal injury, which of the following methods or devices would not be appropriate?
    a. logroll
    b. extremity lift
    c. basket stretcher
    d. short spine board

Chapter 6 Answer Form

	A	B	C	D
1.	❏	❏	❏	❏
2.	❏	❏	❏	❏
3.	❏	❏	❏	❏
4.	❏	❏	❏	❏
5.	❏	❏	❏	❏
6.	❏	❏	❏	❏
7.	❏	❏	❏	❏
8.	❏	❏	❏	❏
9.	❏	❏	❏	❏
10.	❏	❏	❏	❏
11.	❏	❏	❏	❏
12.	❏	❏	❏	❏
13.	❏	❏	❏	❏

	A	B	C	D
14.	❏	❏	❏	❏
15.	❏	❏	❏	❏
16.	❏	❏	❏	❏
17.	❏	❏	❏	❏
18.	❏	❏	❏	❏
19.	❏	❏	❏	❏
20.	❏	❏	❏	❏
21.	❏	❏	❏	❏
22.	❏	❏	❏	❏
23.	❏	❏	❏	❏
24.	❏	❏	❏	❏
25.	❏	❏	❏	❏

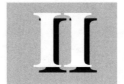

SECTION

II

Airway

CHAPTER

7

Airway

1. The upper airway consists of the:
   a. mouth, uvula, and carina.
   b. nose, mouth, and bronchioles.
   c. mouth, nasopharynx, and oropharynx.
   d. oropharynx, nasopharynx, and bronchi.

2. The potential space between the visceral and parietal pleura is known as the:
   a. epiglottis.
   b. alveoli sac.
   c. diaphragm.
   d. pleural space.

3. Oxygenated blood from the lungs enters the _____ of the heart and is pumped to the tissues of the body.
   a. left atrium
   b. left ventricle
   c. right atrium
   d. right ventricle

4. The lower airway begins at which of the following structures?
   a. carina
   b. bronchi
   c. larynx
   d. diaphragm

5. Which of the following is a sign of inadequate breathing?
   a. skin color that is pink or flushed
   b. air movement out of the mouth and nose
   c. equal and prolonged exhalations with grunting
   d. equal expansion of both sides of the chest during inhalation

6. To properly assess a pediatric patient for adequate breathing, the EMT-B will need to:
   a. position the patient upright.
   b. expose the torso to perform a complete exam.
   c. reposition the patient in semi-Fowler's position.
   d. assess by looking, listening, and feeling for signs of adequate breathing.

7. Which of the following is most likely an indication of inadequate breathing?
   a. a pulse oximetry reading of 90 percent
   b. slow and deep respirations while sleeping
   c. snoring respirations while sleeping
   d. wheezing sounds that can be heard without a stethoscope

8. When a patient is showing signs of inadequate breathing, the first step the EMT-B should take is:
   a. apply high-flow oxygen.
   b. assure that the airway is open and will remain open.
   c. expose the chest and stabilize any holes or fractures.
   d. insert an airway adjunct and suction as necessary.

9. _____ is a condition characterized by blue or gray skin color as a result of hypoxia.
   a. COPD
   b. Cyanosis
   c. Epistaxis
   d. Diaphoresis

10. One of the easiest and least invasive methods of correcting airway obstruction caused by the tongue is:
    a. the head-tilt chin-lift maneuver.
    b. to suction the oropharynx as needed.
    c. to awaken the patient as soon as possible.
    d. to insert a nasopharyngeal airway into one or both nostrils.

11. When performing the head-tilt chin-lift maneuver, the EMT-B should begin by:
    a. moving the patient onto a long backboard.
    b. placing the patient in a supine position.
    c. moving the patient into the recovery position.
    d. turning the patient over into the prone position.

12. The head-tilt chin-lift maneuver is helpful in all of the following situations, except for a/an:
    a. unresponsive diabetic who is drooling.
    b. postictal seizure patient who is alert to painful stimuli.
    c. 75-year-old male found in cardiac arrest on the floor at home.
    d. basketball player who was knocked unconscious and has not awakened.

13. A 2-year-old child was reported to have been choking on a foreign body while in his highchair, and became unresponsive just prior to your arrival. The first step you take to open and maintain his airway is to:
    a. use a jaw-thrust maneuver.
    b. measure and insert an oral airway.
    c. perform a head-tilt chin-lift maneuver.
    d. roll him into the recovery position and perform back blows.

14. You have been called to care for a patient with an altered mental status, whom you suspect has a head injury as a result of a traumatic injury. While you are immobilizing the patient, he becomes unresponsive. Which method is the recommended procedure to open and maintain this patient's airway?
    a. Place the patient supine and use a jaw-thrust maneuver.
    b. Place the patient supine and use a head-tilt chin-lift maneuver.
    c. Roll the patient into the recovery position, allowing secretions to drain from the mouth.
    d. Finish immobilizing the patient on a long board and hold the mouth open with your thumb and forefinger.

15. Your patient is the driver of a vehicle that was hit head on. He is still belted into the driver's seat and there is evidence that his neck struck the steering wheel. He is having difficulty breathing and is becoming unresponsive. The first step you take to open and maintain his airway is to:
    a. suction the mouth and nose, then insert an oral airway.
    b. hold cervical stabilization while your partner applies a non-rebreather mask with high flow.
    c. quickly place a cervical collar on the patient and perform a rapid extrication.
    d. hold cervical stabilization while you sit him up and open his airway using the jaw-thrust maneuver.

16. When performing the jaw-thrust maneuver, the EMT-B places his fingers on:
    a. the patient's chin and bridge of the nose.
    b. each side of the patient's head just above the ears.
    c. the patient's chin and upper jaw just below the nose.
    d. each side of the patient's lower jaw just below the ears.

17. The primary objective of the jaw thrust maneuver is to:
    a. not stimulate a gag reflex.
    b. open the airway as soon as possible.
    c. open the airway without moving the head or neck.
    d. clear any obstructions or secretions as soon as possible.

18. The optimal position for the EMT-B while performing a jaw-thrust maneuver is:
    a. over the patient's torso with one hand on each side of the patient's lower jaw.
    b. beside the patient's head with one hand on each side of the patient's upper jaw.
    c. beside the patient's torso with one hand on each side of the patient's head.
    d. at the top of the patient's head with elbows resting on the same surface as the patient's head.

19. Suction units with rigid-tip catheters are designed for removal of:
    a. big chunks of food.
    b. blood and broken teeth.
    c. blood, fluid, and secretions.
    d. foreign body airway obstructions (FBAOs).

20. The danger of aspirating vomitus into the lungs is that:
    a. stomach acids can easily destroy lung tissue.
    b. it creates an obstruction in the airway.
    c. it decreases the ability to ventilate.
    d. all of the above.

21. When suctioning the oropharynx of an adult, the _____ device is preferred because you can direct where the tip is going.
    a. rigid-tip
    b. soft-tip
    c. semi-rigid
    d. French catheter

22. As a general rule for suctioning the upper airway of a patient, the suction is applied:

    a. before, during, and on the way out of the oropharynx.

    b. while guiding the catheter around the airway adjunct.

    c. after insertion of the catheter tip into the oropharynx and on the way out.

    d. after measuring the catheter and during insertion of the catheter into the oropharynx.

23. Suctioning a patient carries a high risk of exposure for the EMT-B. The recommended PPE includes:

    a. mask, gloves, and gown.

    b. eye protection and gloves.

    c. gloves, gown, and eye protection.

    d. gloves, eye protection, and mask.

24. While suctioning a patient with a soft or flexible catheter, oxygen delivery is:

    a. discontinued only while suctioning.

    b. reduced until suction is completed.

    c. discontinued only during insertion of the catheter.

    d. never discontinued, as oxygen delivery is very important.

25. Ventilating a patient with a pocket mask requires that the EMT-B to be able to do all of the following, except:

    a. maintain a good mask seal over the patient's mouth only.

    b. maintain a good mask seal over the patient's mouth and nose.

    c. suction and properly insert an airway adjunct prior to ventilating.

    d. hold the mask firmly in place while maintaining the proper head tilt.

26. Pocket face masks are made of clear plastic so that the EMT-B can:

    a. protect himself from exposure to vomitus.

    b. see if the mask is properly placed on the face.

    c. recognize when the patient needs to be suctioned.

    d. observe the mouth and nose for signs of spontaneous breathing.

27. Which of the following statements is most correct about ventilations provided with a pocket face mask?

    a. Pocket face masks are one-size-fits-all patients.

    b. When used properly, the face mask will deliver higher volumes of air than a bag-valve mask (BVM).

    c. All pocket face masks protect the rescuer from exposure to patient secretions.

    d. When used with supplemental oxygen, the face mask will deliver an oxygen concentration of 90 percent.

28. You need to ventilate a child patient with a BVM while using the jaw-thrust maneuver. Ventilations will be delivered:

    a. over 1 to 1½ seconds.

    b. over 1½ to 2 seconds.

    c. before securing the pop-off valve.

    d. after you have confirmed that there is no suspected spinal injury.

29. Ventilating a patient with a BVM while using the jaw-thrust maneuver requires a minimum of _____ rescuer(s).

    a. one

    b. two

    c. three

    d. four

30. Using the jaw-thrust maneuver while ventilating with a BVM is indicated:

    a. on a patient with a suspected neck, spine, or head injury.

    b. on an adult patient who is experiencing status epilepticus.

    c. for the patient who is entrapped and awaiting extrication.

    d. when the head-tilt chin-lift maneuver is not adequate for opening the airway.

31. One of the primary advantages of a BMV is that the:

    a. BVM can be used with one hand.

    b. EMT-B can easily decontaminate the device for reuse on another patient.

    c. BVM provides an infection control barrier between the EMT-B and the patient.

    d. EMT-B can deliver higher volumes of air than ventilations with a pocket face mask.

32. Bag-valve mask systems are available in _____ sizes.

    a. one-size-fits-all

    b. adult and child

    c. adult, child, and infant

    d. obese adult, adult, and child

33. Which of the following items is not a part of a bag-valve mask system?

    a. nasal prongs

    b. oxygen tubing

    c. reservoir bag

    d. clear face mask

34. The greatest disadvantage for one rescuer ventilating a patient with a BVM is:

    a. not squeezing the bag fast enough.

    b. not squeezing the bag hard enough.

    c. obtaining a proper mask seal on the face.

    d. there is no disadvantage for one rescuer ventilating with a BVM.

35. When two EMT-Bs are ventilating an adult patient using a BVM, one EMT-B will squeeze the bag:
    a. once every 5 seconds.
    b. enough to assure that the patient is hyperventilated.
    c. to produce a minimum ventilation of 1,500 mL.
    d. to produce a minimum ventilation of 1,000 mL.

36. Before beginning two-rescuer ventilations with a BVM, one EMT-B should:
    a. call for backup assistance.
    b. immobilize the patient's head and neck.
    c. check the patient's wallet for identification.
    d. suction as needed and insert an airway adjunct.

37. Several minutes after you use a BVM to ventilate a patient who is in respiratory distress, you reassess the patient and find that your ventilations are adequate. Which of the following signs have you found?
    a. improved skin color
    b. rapid spontaneous breathing
    c. resistance to your ventilations
    d. air is moving out of the mouth and nose

38. Which of the following is an indication that your ventilations with a BVM are adequate?
    a. equal chest expansion and rise
    b. a heart rate that increases from 40 to 60 bpm
    c. the bag has good compliance during squeezing
    d. all of the above

39. Which of the following methods is most reliable for assessing the adequacy of ventilations with a BVM?
    a. getting a pulse oximetry reading over 95 percent
    b. noting good compliance while squeezing the bag
    c. auscultating both sides of the chest with a stethoscope
    d. noting that the reservoir bag is filling completely between ventilations

40. Using a BVM, you are ventilating an unresponsive patient who initially was breathing too slowly. Squeezing the bag is difficult and after a couple of minutes you see no improvement. Which of the following is most likely the problem?
    a. No airway adjunct is in place.
    b. The patient is having a heart attack.
    c. You are not squeezing the bag fast enough.
    d. You are not allowing the bag enough time to refill with oxygen.

41. Which of the following conditions will most likely be the cause of inadequate ventilation with the use of a BVM?
    a. poor mask seal
    b. ventilating with one rescuer
    c. no oxygen supply to the reservoir
    d. squeezing the bag with two hands

42. No chest rise, difficulty squeezing the bag, and decreased breath sounds are all:
    a. signs that the patient requires suction.
    b. indications that the patient is in shock.
    c. signs of inadequate ventilation using a BVM.
    d. indications that oxygen is not attached to the BVM.

43. When the relief valve is activated on a flow-restricted, oxygen-powered ventilation device (FROPVD) it will cause:
    a. an audible alarm.
    b. a pneumothorax.
    c. gastric distention.
    d. the device to shut off.

44. A primary advantage of using a FROPVD is that:
    a. it never has to be decontaminated.
    b. the trigger is an inexpensive, disposable item.
    c. this device does not need a lot of oxygen as a power source.
    d. one rescuer can use both hands to maintain a seal while triggering the device.

45. A major disadvantage of using a FROPVD is that:
    a. it can be used only on adult patients.
    b. there is no disadvantage with the use of this device.
    c. it cannot be used on a patient with a suspected spinal injury.
    d. gastric distention is a common problem when using this device.

46. When providing mouth-to-mask ventilations with no oxygen source, each ventilation should be delivered over:
    a. 1½ to 2 seconds in children.
    b. 1½ to 2 seconds in adults.
    c. 1½ to 2 seconds in infants.
    d. 1½ to 2 seconds in all patients.

47. To obtain to good seal while ventilating a patient with a partial stoma, the EMT-B must:
    a. use a water-soluble jelly.
    b. cover the mouth and nose.
    c. ventilate with a minimum of 800 mL.
    d. insert an oropharyngeal airway prior to ventilating.

48. A very common problem associated with ventilation through a stoma is:
    a. using the wrong size BVM.
    b. not squeezing the bag hard enough.
    c. not being able to properly attach a BVM.
    d. that mucus and secretions create an obstruction.

49. When measuring an oropharyngeal airway for insertion into a patient, the EMT-B measures:

    a. from the tip of the nose to the angle of the jaw.

    b. from the center of the chin to the earlobe.

    c. the length of the patient's pinky (fifth digit or little) finger.

    d. the distance from the center of the lips to the angle of the jaw.

50. Oropharyngeal airways (OPAs) are made of hard plastic and are designed to:

    a. prevent the tongue from obstructing the glottis.

    b. keep the patient from choking on secretions.

    c. prevent the patient from aspirating vomit.

    d. prevent the patient from gagging.

51. The use of an OPA is indicated when a patient:

    a. is experiencing a seizure.

    b. is unconscious without a gag reflex.

    c. has an altered mental status and is choking.

    d. has broken teeth as a result of trauma to the face.

52. Before inserting a nasopharyngeal airway (NPA) into a patient, the EMT-B must:

    a. lubricate the tube with petroleum jelly.

    b. perform a head-tilt chin-lift maneuver.

    c. lubricate the tube with a water-soluble jelly.

    d. hyperventilate the patient using high-flow oxygen.

53. Which of the following is a disadvantage for use of an NPA?

    a. The NPA will not fit into every patient.

    b. The NPA can be suctioned through; there is no need to remove it.

    c. The NPA protects the airway without stimulating a gag reflex.

    d. The NPA can be placed blindly, without the patient's mouth being opened.

54. When measuring an nasopharyngeal airway for insertion into a patient, the EMT-B:

    a. measures from the tip of the nose to the angle of the jaw.

    b. measures from the tip of the patient's earlobe to the tip of the nose.

    c. measures the distance from the center of the nose to the Adam's apple.

    d. uses an airway that is the same diameter as the patient's pinky (fifth digit or little) finger.

55. Which of the following components of an oxygen delivery system must be hydrostatically tested on a regular schedule?

    a. oxygen cylinder

    b. pressure regulator

    c. the cascade system

    d. positive pressure ventilator

56. When a patient is not breathing adequately on his own, which of the following devices cannot be used to ventilate oxygen into the lungs?

    a. BVM

    b. pocket face mask

    c. oxygen cylinder

    d. positive pressure regulator

57. The basic components of an oxygen delivery system used in the prehospital setting by EMT-Bs include a/an:

    a. pocket mask, suction, and humidifier.

    b. BVM, airway adjunct, and non-rebreather mask.

    c. suction, airway adjunct, and pressure regulator.

    d. oxygen cylinder, pressure regulator, and delivery device.

58. When a patient who is wearing a non-rebreather mask inhales, he receives oxygen-enriched gas from the:

    a. reservoir bag.

    b. partial-rebreather bag.

    c. two-way valve on a supplied line.

    d. none of the above.

59. A non-rebreather mask is indicated whenever a patient needs oxygen and:

    a. is apneic.

    b. is in respiratory arrest.

    c. is in cardiac arrest.

    d. can maintain the airway.

60. Of the following devices, the _____ is the oxygen delivery device that can provide the highest oxygen concentration enrichment.

    a. humidifier

    b. nasal cannula

    c. non-rebreather mask

    d. pocket mask with an oxygen port

61. To enrich the oxygen of a stoma patient with mild respiratory distress, the preferred oxygen delivery device is a:

    a. nasal cannula.

    b. bag-valve mask.

    c. non-rebreather mask.

    d. flow-restricted, oxygen-powered ventilation device.

62. The use of a nasal cannula for a hypoxic patient is preferred over a non-rebreather mask in which of the following cases?

    a. facial injury

    b. infants and children

    c. a patient who refuses to wear a mask

    d. foreign body airway obstruction

63. In which of the following cases would an NRB be indicated rather than a nasal cannula?
    a. a preschool child with a croupy cough who is crying
    b. a newly born infant with poor respiratory effort after 1 minute
    c. the patient in the second stage of active labor who feels nauseated
    d. a COPD patient who fainted, but is now awake with no respiratory distress

64. In the prehospital setting, the EMT-B occasionally responds to a patient who is wearing a cannula and is not in respiratory distress. When transporting this patient, the EMT-B should:
    a. change the cannula to an NRB on 10 liters.
    b. leave the cannula in place, but adjust the liter flow to 6.
    c. leave the cannula in place using the same liter flow as found.
    d. begin transport without the cannula and request advice from Medical Control while en route.

65. Which of the following is an indication for use of a nasal cannula?
    a. severe hypoxia
    b. mouth breathing
    c. poor respiratory effort
    d. moderate oxygen enrichment for long periods

66. A common problem associated with the use of a nasal cannula is:
    a. that prolonged use causes nausea.
    b. drying of the nasal mucous membranes.
    c. the device is difficult to use and uncomfortable to adjust.
    d. the patient has to be weaned off after long periods of use.

67. Your unit was the first to arrive at a residence for a difficulty-breathing call; ALS is also en route. You discover an elderly male in bed, unresponsive and gasping for breath. His airway is open and clear. With auscultation, you find that there is no air movement, the distal pulse is weak and fast, and his skin CTC is pale, warm, and dry. You begin assisting ventilations with a BVM. Your partner attempts to insert an OPA and the patient gags, but does not vomit. ALS notifies you on the radio that they are 5 minutes away. What steps do you take next?
    a. Insert an NPA and place a non-rebreather mask on the patient.
    b. Insert an NPA and continue ventilations with the BVM once every 5 seconds.
    c. Continue ventilations with the BVM and hyperventilate the patient in preparation for intubation.
    d. Attempt to reinsert the OPA again and be prepared to suction if the patient vomits.

68. (Continuing with the preceding question) Five minutes later a paramedic arrives and you give report. The paramedic rapidly assesses the patient, asks you to continue with your interventions, and decides to intubate the patient. The paramedic quickly assembles the necessary equipment and is ready to intubate. Now she asks you to stop what you are doing and prepare to assister her to visualize the vocal cords by:
    a. lifting the patient's tongue.
    b. turning on every light in the room.
    c. placing cricoid pressure on the patient.
    d. holding the patient's head in a neutral position.

69. A local nursing home has called EMS this morning for an elderly patient who fell out of bed during the night. Staff reports that the patient denied any injury at the time of the fall, so they put her back to bed. This morning the patient has a decreased mental status, and the following vital signs: respiratory rate 12 and shallow, with decreased lung sounds on both sides; pulse 58 and regular; BP 100/60; skin CTC is cyanotic, warm, and dry. The patient opens her eyes when touched and spoken to. She denies any neck or back pain, but points to her chest. You discover a bruise and tenderness on her left chest. What do you suspect is the patient's immediate problem?
    a. inadequate ventilations due to injured ribs
    b. decompensated shock due to tension pneumothorax
    c. compensated hypovolemic shock due to intraabdominal bleeding
    d. inadequate breathing due to an acute myocardial infarction (AMI)

70. (Continuing with the preceding question) You begin treatment by administering high-flow oxygen and observe that the patient has pain in the left lateral chest with movement. Based on your assessment of the patient's immediate problem, what is your initial management plan for this patient?
    a. Lay the patient on her back, elevate her legs, provide warmth, and provide rapid transport to the ED.
    b. Splint the left arm to the chest using a sling and swathe and coach the patient to take deeper breaths.
    c. Assist the patient with the administration of nitroglycerin for chest pain and call for an ALS intercept.
    d. Treat the patient for shock and call for an ALS intercept for a possible chest decompression due to tension pneumothorax.

71. Early in the evening, you are dispatched to a call for a sick patient. After arriving at a residence, you discover that a 30-year-old female, her husband, and their two sons are experiencing flu-like symptoms. You suspect carbon monoxide poisoning, request the fire department to the scene, and evacuate the family out to your ambulance. The female's symptoms are the worst, with headache, nausea, and vomiting. While you administer oxygen to each family member and obtain vital signs, your partner talks to the firefighters and confirms that there is an elevated CO reading in the home. In addition to obtaining vital signs, you obtain pulse oximetry readings while the patients are on oxygen. What would you expect for an SpO2 reading for the female in this case?

    a. The SpO2 reading will be low, but inaccurate.
    b. The SpO2 reading will be low and accurate.
    c. The SpO2 reading will be high, but inaccurate.
    d. The SpO2 reading will be high and accurate.

72. (Continuing with the previous question) What is the most likely reason for the female to be experiencing more severe symptoms than other members of the household?

    a. The female had the longest exposure to CO.
    b. All females are more susceptible to CO poisoning.
    c. Females do not recover from hypoxic states as easily as males.
    d. The affinity for hemoglobin to bind to CO is greater in females of childbearing age.

73. Dispatch has sent your unit to a fast-food restaurant for a choking victim. Arrival time was very short since you were returning from another call. When you arrive, bystanders summon you to a 16-year-old male who is in the men's room. The patient is responsive, cyanotic, and working hard to breathe. When you get closer, you hear faint stridor when he tries to breathe in. What do these findings indicate?

    a. complete airway obstruction
    b. partial airway obstruction with poor air exchange
    c. partial airway obstruction with adequate air exchange
    d. partial airway obstruction requiring immediate suctioning

74. (Continuing with the previous question) What immediate intervention is appropriate?

    a. Perform abdominal thrusts.
    b. Suction the patient's oropharynx.
    c. Administer high-flow oxygen and transport him.
    d. Assist ventilations with a BVM and high-flow oxygen.

75. Your unit has been dispatched to a call for an unresponsive patient. The mother of a 12-year-old female anxiously awaits you and takes you to her daughter's bedside. The child appears unresponsive. She is breathing deeply and rapidly as if she is hyperventilating. The airway is open and clear, lung sounds are clear, and skin CTC is pink and red, warm, and dry. The mother tells you that the patient is diabetic and that her glucose readings have been a little high. She has been sick for 3 days with abdominal pain and flu symptoms. What do these findings indicate?

    a. hypoglycemia
    b. respiratory distress
    c. Kussmaul's respirations
    d. partial airway obstruction

Chapter 7 Answer Form

	A	B	C	D		A	B	C	D
1.	❏	❏	❏	❏	33.	❏	❏	❏	❏
2.	❏	❏	❏	❏	34.	❏	❏	❏	❏
3.	❏	❏	❏	❏	35.	❏	❏	❏	❏
4.	❏	❏	❏	❏	36.	❏	❏	❏	❏
5.	❏	❏	❏	❏	37.	❏	❏	❏	❏
6.	❏	❏	❏	❏	38.	❏	❏	❏	❏
7.	❏	❏	❏	❏	39.	❏	❏	❏	❏
8.	❏	❏	❏	❏	40.	❏	❏	❏	❏
9.	❏	❏	❏	❏	41.	❏	❏	❏	❏
10.	❏	❏	❏	❏	42.	❏	❏	❏	❏
11.	❏	❏	❏	❏	43.	❏	❏	❏	❏
12.	❏	❏	❏	❏	44.	❏	❏	❏	❏
13.	❏	❏	❏	❏	45.	❏	❏	❏	❏
14.	❏	❏	❏	❏	46.	❏	❏	❏	❏
15.	❏	❏	❏	❏	47.	❏	❏	❏	❏
16.	❏	❏	❏	❏	48.	❏	❏	❏	❏
17.	❏	❏	❏	❏	49.	❏	❏	❏	❏
18.	❏	❏	❏	❏	50.	❏	❏	❏	❏
19.	❏	❏	❏	❏	51.	❏	❏	❏	❏
20.	❏	❏	❏	❏	52.	❏	❏	❏	❏
21.	❏	❏	❏	❏	53.	❏	❏	❏	❏
22.	❏	❏	❏	❏	54.	❏	❏	❏	❏
23.	❏	❏	❏	❏	55.	❏	❏	❏	❏
24.	❏	❏	❏	❏	56.	❏	❏	❏	❏
25.	❏	❏	❏	❏	57.	❏	❏	❏	❏
26.	❏	❏	❏	❏	58.	❏	❏	❏	❏
27.	❏	❏	❏	❏	59.	❏	❏	❏	❏
28.	❏	❏	❏	❏	60.	❏	❏	❏	❏
29.	❏	❏	❏	❏	61.	❏	❏	❏	❏
30.	❏	❏	❏	❏	62.	❏	❏	❏	❏
31.	❏	❏	❏	❏	63.	❏	❏	❏	❏
32.	❏	❏	❏	❏	64.	❏	❏	❏	❏

	A	B	C	D		A	B	C	D
65.	❏	❏	❏	❏	71.	❏	❏	❏	❏
66.	❏	❏	❏	❏	72.	❏	❏	❏	❏
67.	❏	❏	❏	❏	73.	❏	❏	❏	❏
68.	❏	❏	❏	❏	74.	❏	❏	❏	❏
69.	❏	❏	❏	❏	75.	❏	❏	❏	❏
70.	❏	❏	❏	❏					

Patient Assessment

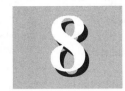
Scene Size-Up

1. The EMT-B performs a scene size-up to obtain valuable information about the:
   a. need for BSI.
   b. safety issues at the scene.
   c. mechanism of injury (MOI) or nature of illness (NOI).
   d. all of the above.

2. It is late at night and you have responded to a residence that appears to have no lights on. What should you do next?
   a. Put on your BSI equipment.
   b. Suspect a potentially threatening environment.
   c. Bring your flashlight, because the power might be out.
   d. Begin forming your general impression of the patient.

3. After responding to a private residence for a 42-year-old female with a severe headache and nausea, you discover that other family members in the house have the same symptoms, but not as severe. What action should you take first?
   a. Transport the entire family because of flu symptoms.
   b. Put a face mask on the patient and each family member.
   c. Put on a face mask and have your crew members do the same.
   d. Evacuate the house and call the fire department to have the residence checked for a gas leak.

4. While sizing up the scene of a two-car motor vehicle collision, which of the following hazards would be more dangerous for you than for any of the vehicle occupants?
   a. undeployed airbags
   b. downed power lines
   c. a vehicle occupant using a cell phone
   d. broken glass on the vehicle and ground

5. When you are dispatched to a scene for a traumatic injury with hemorrhage, what is the minimum personal protective equipment (PPE) you will need?
   a. gloves
   b. gown
   c. turnout gear
   d. HEPA mask

6. You are entering a single-family residence for an elderly woman who lives alone. Her chief complaint is chest pain. Which of the following could present as a hazard for you and your crew, but probably not the patient?
   a. pet poodle
   b. small doorways
   c. family member
   d. expired nitroglycerin prescription

7. Which of the following scenes would be the least dangerous to enter prior to the arrival of any other support such as police or fire department?
   a. vehicle engine fire
   b. patient struck by lightning
   c. yelling and fighting inside a first-floor apartment
   d. hazardous materials incident from a leaking 55-gallon drum

8. Before entering a motor vehicle that was involved in a collision, to care for an injured passenger, which of the following actions should the EMT-B take first to quickly stabilize the vehicle?
   a. Let the air out of two of the tires.
   b. Turn off the engine and set the parking brake.
   c. Instruct the occupants to keep their seat belts on.
   d. Check to see if the doors are unlocked before breaking any glass.

9. How can the EMT-B stabilize a vehicle that has been turned on its side, in order to gain access to a patient?
   a. Do not do anything until the fire department arrives.
   b. With help from your crew, push the vehicle right side up.
   c. Place cribbing around the vehicle to keep it from tipping.
   d. With help from your crew, push the vehicle onto its roof.

10. Which of the following conditions is not a common nature of illness (NOI) found in the prehospital setting?
    a. seizure
    b. thermal burn
    c. asthma attack
    d. hypoglycemia

11. During the scene size-up of a motor vehicle collision, it becomes obvious to you that the driver of the vehicle involved was unrestrained and went up and over the steering column. In which of the following areas would you expect to find primary injuries?
    a. head, face, and neck
    b. head, chest, and knees
    c. face, chest, and femurs
    d. neck, back, and abdomen

12. A common injury pattern seen when a/an _____ pedestrian is struck by a vehicle is called *Waddell's triad*. This pattern consists of injuries to the torso, legs, and then head.
    a. infant
    b. child
    c. adult
    d. pregnant woman

13. The police are on the scene of a domestic violence call. A husband and wife were fighting and both were injured during the altercation. One has minor injuries and the other is potentially unstable. How many ambulances will be needed?
    a. For safety reasons, one ambulance for each patient.
    b. Both can go in one ambulance, because neither is a high-priority patient.
    c. None; both have been charged with assault and can be transported by the police to the hospital after processing at the police station.
    d. Two: one for the couple and one for their children, as the children cannot be left unattended.

14. Upon arrival at a scene where a vehicle is off the road in the woods, you find that the windshield is broken out and is lying on the hood. The driver is behind the wheel and appears to be unrestrained and unconscious. While you begin your approach to the vehicle, your partner does a perimeter sweep for:
    a. snakes.
    b. signs of any hunters in the area.
    c. other occupants who may have been ejected.
    d. any personal items that may have been tossed from the vehicle.

15. Your ambulance is the second to arrive at the scene of a potentially large multiple casualty incident (MCI). You are directed to make a quick count of all the patients. You have been asked to do this because the:
    a. transport officer has to make room for incoming fire apparatus.
    b. incident commander needs to assess for appropriate resources.
    c. triage officer needs to know how many triage tags will be needed.
    d. incident commander does not trust the triage officer to make the count.

16. The last component of scene size-up is determining:
    a. which level of PPE to don.
    b. the need for additional resources.
    c. when it is safe for your crew members to proceed into the scene.
    d. none of the above.

17. During your assessment of an elderly patient, whom you are going to transport to the hospital for evaluation of a minor laceration that requires sutures, it becomes apparent that the patient's disabled spouse cannot be left alone. What action would you take?
    a. Take the spouse along to the hospital.
    b. Call a friend or relative to come over after you leave.
    c. Notify adult protective services before leaving the scene.
    d. Ask dispatch to send a police unit over to handle the matter.

18. You are the incident commander at the scene of an MCI. There are two critical and two stable patients. With adequate resources and a two-person crew for each ambulance, what is the minimum number of ambulances you need to effectively transport all the patients?
    a. one
    b. two
    c. three
    d. four

19. While walking up to a residence where dispatch sent you for a medical emergency, your partner states that he forgot a piece of equipment; he returns to the ambulance to retrieve it. Which of the following actions is most appropriate for you and your partner now?

    a. You wait until your partner returns and enter the residence together.
    b. Your partner conducts a scene size-up as he enters the residence.
    c. You enter the residence and conduct a scene size-up and advise your partner when he enters.
    d. You wait for your partner to return and allow him to perform the scene size-up, as he is the senior crew member.

20. Which of the following statements is most correct about the scene size-up?

    a. The scene size-up is completed only one time for each EMS call.
    b. The scene size-up is the responsibility of the most senior EMT-B on the call.
    c. The most junior EMT-B on the call is never responsible for completing the scene size-up.
    d. The elements of the scene size-up should be reconsidered throughout the entire time on the scene.

21. The police have advised you that the scene is safe to enter at the residence of a patient who is experiencing a behavioral emergency. The patient is agitated after failing to complete a suicide attempt. You approach the patient to begin your initial assessment and ask your partner to _____ as an additional safety measure.

    a. call another ambulance to assist
    b. have the police handcuff the patient
    c. keep the exit accessible at all times
    d. tie the patient's wrists with a cravat

22. While sizing up the scene of an accidental injury to a child, you get the impression that the MOI does not fit the injuries you discover. Your plan of action now includes:

    a. confronting the caregiver with your suspicions.
    b. transporting the child, but not telling anyone of your suspicions.
    c. immediately calling for the police while you wait on scene.
    d. not confronting the caregiver or calling the police, but notifying the ED staff.

23. After being dispatched to a residence for an elderly gentleman who is unable to get out of bed, it quickly becomes obvious to you that his living conditions are unhealthy and possibly dangerous. This information is:

    a. necessary to report to the ED staff.
    b. irrelevant to your care of the patient.
    c. reportable to the health department once you notify the police.
    d. reportable to the health department once you notify your supervisor.

24. Your crew has just loaded the only patient involved in a MVC into the ambulance and you are ready to transport him. The EMS supervisor who was on scene hands you a Polaroid snapshot of the patient's vehicle to take with you. The photograph was taken so that:

    a. you can add it to your EMS photo collection.
    b. the patient can use it later for the insurance claim.
    c. the ED staff may appreciate the MOI better when they have a photograph for reference.
    d. your crew will be protected in litigation, because the patient mentioned getting a lawyer.

25. Which of the following hazards poses the highest risk for EMT-Bs working at the scene of an auto accident?

    a. traffic
    b. broken glass
    c. loaded bumper
    d. undeployed airbag

Chapter 8 Answer Form

	A	B	C	D		A	B	C	D
1.	❑	❑	❑	❑	14.	❑	❑	❑	❑
2.	❑	❑	❑	❑	15.	❑	❑	❑	❑
3.	❑	❑	❑	❑	16.	❑	❑	❑	❑
4.	❑	❑	❑	❑	17.	❑	❑	❑	❑
5.	❑	❑	❑	❑	18.	❑	❑	❑	❑
6.	❑	❑	❑	❑	19.	❑	❑	❑	❑
7.	❑	❑	❑	❑	20.	❑	❑	❑	❑
8.	❑	❑	❑	❑	21.	❑	❑	❑	❑
9.	❑	❑	❑	❑	22.	❑	❑	❑	❑
10.	❑	❑	❑	❑	23.	❑	❑	❑	❑
11.	❑	❑	❑	❑	24.	❑	❑	❑	❑
12.	❑	❑	❑	❑	25.	❑	❑	❑	❑
13.	❑	❑	❑	❑					

CHAPTER

Initial Assessment

1. Your general or first impression of a patient helps you to:
   a. ensure that the scene is safe.
   b. rapidly identify all threats to life.
   c. fully appreciate the mechanism of injury or illness.
   d. get a sense of how serious the patient's condition is.

2. When forming a general impression of a patient, which of the following components is usually not a factor?
   a. allergies
   b. the environment
   c. patient's age
   d. patient's level of distress

3. When using the mnemonic AVPU to assess a patient's mental status, a rating of "V" relates to:
   a. how well the patient speaks.
   b. the inability of the patient to speak.
   c. the tone of the patient's voice.
   d. how the patient responds to your voice.

4. After physically stimulating a patient who initially appeared unresponsive, the patient moaned loudly and pushed your hand away. Using the mnemonic AVPU, rate this patient's mental status.
   a. alert
   b. verbal
   c. painful
   d. unresponsive

5. You are assessing an elderly patient who is not answering your questions appropriately. How can you determine if this is normal for the patient or a new onset?
   a. Obtain a Glasgow Coma Score (GCS).
   b. Test the patient's blood sugar level.
   c. Wait to check the patient's medical records at the hospital.
   d. Discuss your findings with the patient's spouse or caregiver.

6. A reliable way of determining the mental status of a child or infant is to:
   a. ask the caregiver if the patient has ingested any poisons.
   b. keep the patient with the caregiver when you perform your examination.
   c. use a favorite toy to distract the patient while you assess reflexes.
   d. ask the caregiver if the patient is acting different today and if so, how.

7. Which of the following conditions would lead you to suspect that a conscious patient has a potentially serious airway problem?
   a. epistaxis
   b. broken jaw and nose
   c. patient with active tuberculosis
   d. drooling as a result of a dental procedure

8. The primary method for assessing the airway in a patient of any age is:
   a. palpation.
   b. auscultation.
   c. visual inspection.
   d. talking to the patient.

9. On the scene of a construction site accident, witnesses state that the patient fell to the ground from a height of 25 feet. The patient is alert, oriented, and denies any pain or injury. Which of the following statements is least accurate?
   a. If the patient has no pain, there is no cervical injury.
   b. The MOI is reason enough to take cervical precautions.
   c. It is possible to have a broken neck without having any pain.
   d. Anyone who falls from a height of 25 feet is likely to have a cervical injury.

10. In most cases, the _____ is/are the most reliable evidence that a patient experienced a significant MOI.
    a. environment
    b. patient's report
    c. witnesses on scene
    d. police on scene

11. _____ is/are a reliable indication that an adult patient's breathing is not adequate.
    a. Retractions
    b. Slow speech
    c. Delayed capillary refill
    d. A low pulse oximeter reading

12. In the unresponsive patient, the EMT-B initially assesses _____ by looking for rise and fall of the chest.
    a. breathing
    b. oxygenation
    c. airway patency
    d. perfusion status

13. An 18-month-old infant is postictal after experiencing febrile seizure. She is sleepy, her airway is clear, respiratory rate is 28, and her skin is pink, warm, and moist. How would you characterize her breathing and state the initial care to be given?
    a. Breathing is adequate: do nothing at this point.
    b. Breathing is inadequate: assist with positive pressure ventilations.
    c. Breathing is adequate: administer high-flow oxygen with a non-rebreather mask.
    d. Breathing is inadequate: administer high-flow oxygen with a non-rebreather mask.

14. You have completed an initial assessment on an unresponsive medical patient and have determined that the airway is clear and breathing and circulation are adequate. You initial care would now include:
    a. suction the airway and apply a nasal cannula at 4 to 6 liters per minute.
    b. attempted to insert an airway adjunct and begin ventilations with a BVM.
    c. insert an oral airway and administer high-flow oxygen with a non-rebreather mask.
    d. position the patient on his side and administer high-flow oxygen with a non-rebreather mask.

15. You are called to care for a 2-year-old male who is wheezing and has been sick for 3 days. The patient's mental status is alert to his mother's presence, respiratory rate of 36 with nasal flaring, and the skin is pale, warm, and dry. What would you do next?
    a. Keep the child calm, reassess, and transport.
    b. Keep the child calm and administer blow-by oxygen.
    c. Administer high-flow oxygen with a non-rebreather mask.
    d. Ask the child's mother to help you assist ventilations with positive pressure.

16. A 30-year-old male fell approximately 20 feet off a ladder and landed on his side. His chief complaint is left-side rib pain. His respirations are shallow and he has guarding over his rib cage. No deformities or external bleeding are apparent. Initial interventions for this patient are cervical stabilization and:
    a. rapid packaging and transport.
    b. assist the patient with positive pressure ventilations.
    c. keep the patient calm and administer oxygen by nasal cannula.
    d. encourage the patient to take deeper breaths and administer high-flow oxygen by non-rebreather mask.

17. Which skin finding distinctly indicates decreased oxygenation associated with inadequate breathing?
    a. pale
    b. moist
    c. yellow
    d. cyanosis

18. _____ is a term for the sensation of labored breathing that may be characterized by noisy respirations or increased work of breathing.
    a. Apnea
    b. Dyspnea
    c. Tachypnea
    d. Tachycardia

19. In which age group is the impact of a stuffy nose from a cold the most significant?
    a. ages 2 to 4
    b. first 4 weeks of life
    c. last 4 months of life
    d. under 5 years of age

20. _____ and nasal flaring are indications that an infant is having difficulty breathing.
    a. Coughing
    b. Flushed skin
    c. Grunting
    d. An elevated temperature

21. You are assisting a small child with positive pressure ventilations. You know the ventilations are adequate when:
    a. there are equal breath sounds.
    b. the skin color improves.
    c. there is a good mask seal and the chest rises.
    d. all of the above.

22. The lower airways are softer and more flexible than in any other age group in:
    a. infants up to 1 year old.
    b. adolescents.
    c. elderly patients older than 75 years.
    d. elderly patients older than 90 years.

23. The two attributes that are used to determine quality of the pulse are:
    a. age and gender.
    b. rate and strength.
    c. rhythm and regularity.
    d. weakness and strength.

24. To assess a central pulse on a patient, the EMT-B should _____ pulse.
    a. palpate a femoral
    b. palpate a brachial
    c. auscultate for an apical
    d. use a Doppler to locate a femoral

25. In infants, the pulse is assessed in the brachial artery in the:
    a. medial aspect of the upper arm.
    b. medial aspect of the lower arm.
    c. thumb side of the lower arm near the wrist.
    d. left side of the chest near the sternal margin.

26. As part of the initial assessment of an unresponsive 8-year-old child, the EMT-B performs the American Heart Association's "quick check" by assessing the _____ pulse.
    a. apical
    b. carotid
    c. radial
    d. brachial

27. During the initial assessment of a patient with a deep laceration of the forearm, you recognize that the bleeding is arterial. Your next step is to:
    a. call for ALS.
    b. prioritize the patient as critical.
    c. prioritize the patient as unstable.
    d. manage the bleeding immediately.

28. When a patient has life-threatening external bleeding, the EMT-B should _____ during the initial assessment.
    a. attempt to control the bleeding
    b. estimate the rate of blood loss
    c. report to the emergency department
    d. classify the stage of shock as grade I, II, or III.

29. A patient suffering from acute hepatitis or renal failure may exhibit skin color that is:
    a. blue.
    b. yellow.
    c. anemic.
    d. dark around the eyes.

30. Skin color is best assessed by looking at the:
    a. eyes, ears, and nose.
    b. eyes, lips, and nail beds.
    c. palms and soles of the feet.
    d. tongue and mucous membranes.

31. You have been called to assess a toddler who might have swallowed a small amount of shampoo. Which of the following skin signs or conditions is the child most likely to have?
    a. pink, warm, and dry
    b. pale, cold, and dry
    c. blue lips and pale skin
    d. mottled, hot, and dry

32. An ill patient who has been lying in bed all day in a room with a comfortable ambient temperature has skin that appears flushed, hot, and moist. This patient is most likely experiencing:
    a. a high fever.
    b. dehydration.
    c. a medication overdose.
    d. a mild allergic reaction.

33. Tenting of the skin is a condition associated with:
    a. alcoholism.
    b. dehydration.
    c. congestive heart failure.
    d. a communicable disease.

34. Goose pimples, chattering teeth, and pale skin suggests that the patient has:
    a. been exposed to cold temperatures.
    b. an infection.
    c. pain or fever.
    d. all of the above.

35. A capillary refill time of less than _____ seconds is considered normal in a healthy 3-year-old child.
    a. 2
    b. 3
    c. 4
    d. 5

36. A delayed capillary refill time in an infant is:
    a. a finding that suggests a circulation problem.
    b. not a problem unless it exceeds 5 seconds.
    c. a finding that suggests there are no peripheral pulses.
    d. normal in children with dark skin.

37. As the team leader on a crew, you may be the provider who will prioritize a patient as part of the initial assessment. Completing this task:
    a. sets the tone for a management plan.
    b. lets the crew know you are clearly in charge of the call.
    c. allows you to gain permission to treat the patient.
    d. is reassuring to the patient and the patient's family.

38. The primary reason for prioritizing a patient for treatment and transport is:
   a. to know when to stabilize a patient on the scene or call for ALS.
   b. to determine the need for rapid transport for definitive care.
   c. that no other task is as important in the first phase of patient contact.
   d. to be able to locate and manage life-threatening conditions affecting the airway, breathing, and circulation.

39. You have arrived at the side of an unconscious adult patient who is breathing. You are unable to locate a radial pulse, and find the carotid pulse to be present and weak. What does this finding suggest about the patient's blood pressure?
   a. The patient will have a low blood pressure.
   b. The diastolic can be estimated as at least 70 mm Hg.
   c. The patient will have a systolic but no diastolic pressure.
   d. This finding is not associated with the patient's blood pressure.

40. A construction worker has fallen from a height of 10 feet. When you arrive, he is conscious, but confused about how the fall occurred. He tells you that he is having difficulty breathing and cannot feel his legs. What is the first priority in the initial assessment of this patient?
   a. Open the airway.
   b. Take spinal precautions.
   c. Obtain a blood pressure.
   d. Check for distal pulses, motor function, and sensation.

41. Your ambulance is dispatched to an office building for a 24-year-old male who is having difficulty breathing. As you approach the patient, he appears anxious and is talking fast and in long sentences. He looks well and skin color is good, yet he tells you that he is having trouble catching his breath. What is your priority consideration for this patient?
   a. Provide high-flow oxygen.
   b. Do nothing and observe for a while.
   c. Consider that he is faking being sick to get out of work.
   d. Have him breathe into a paper bag for one minute, then reevaluate.

42. A patient tells you "I feel bloated and my stomach hurts." This is referred to as the:
   a. field diagnosis.
   b. chief complaint.
   c. objective finding.
   d. general impression.

43. The family of an elderly patient tells you that they have been unable to wake her up this morning. You approach and shake her arm gently; as you speak to her, she awakens and is able to tell you her name, day of the week, and where she is. She cannot tell you the date. You classify her mental status as:
   a. alert.
   b. verbal.
   c. painful.
   d. unresponsive.

44. Which of the following statements is most correct with regard to making a priority decision about a patient's condition?
   a. Every patient will need definitive care within the "Golden Hour."
   b. When a presenting problem could be either more or less serious, consider it to be more serious.
   c. When a presenting problem could be either more or less serious, consider it to be less serious.
   d. When a presenting problem could be either more or less serious, let the crew chief make the priority decision.

45. The Glasgow Coma Scale is useful for assessing mental status and for making a priority decision about a patient. It does not, however, provide you with information about the best _____ response.
   a. verbal
   b. motor
   c. sensation
   d. eye-opening

Chapter 9 Answer Form

	A	B	C	D			A	B	C	D
1.	❏	❏	❏	❏		24.	❏	❏	❏	❏
2.	❏	❏	❏	❏		25.	❏	❏	❏	❏
3.	❏	❏	❏	❏		26.	❏	❏	❏	❏
4.	❏	❏	❏	❏		27.	❏	❏	❏	❏
5.	❏	❏	❏	❏		28.	❏	❏	❏	❏
6.	❏	❏	❏	❏		29.	❏	❏	❏	❏
7.	❏	❏	❏	❏		30.	❏	❏	❏	❏
8.	❏	❏	❏	❏		31.	❏	❏	❏	❏
9.	❏	❏	❏	❏		32.	❏	❏	❏	❏
10.	❏	❏	❏	❏		33.	❏	❏	❏	❏
11.	❏	❏	❏	❏		34.	❏	❏	❏	❏
12.	❏	❏	❏	❏		35.	❏	❏	❏	❏
13.	❏	❏	❏	❏		36.	❏	❏	❏	❏
14.	❏	❏	❏	❏		37.	❏	❏	❏	❏
15.	❏	❏	❏	❏		38.	❏	❏	❏	❏
16.	❏	❏	❏	❏		39.	❏	❏	❏	❏
17.	❏	❏	❏	❏		40.	❏	❏	❏	❏
18.	❏	❏	❏	❏		41.	❏	❏	❏	❏
19.	❏	❏	❏	❏		42.	❏	❏	❏	❏
20.	❏	❏	❏	❏		43.	❏	❏	❏	❏
21.	❏	❏	❏	❏		44.	❏	❏	❏	❏
22.	❏	❏	❏	❏		45.	❏	❏	❏	❏
23.	❏	❏	❏	❏						

CHAPTER 10

Focused History and Physical Exam—Trauma Patient

1. While sizing up the scene at a trauma incident, you determine that the mechanism of injury (MOI) is potentially life-threatening. However, the patient appears to be in stable condition. You should now:
   a. get the patient's SAMPLE history.
   b. provide care appropriate for the stable condition.
   c. begin treatment and transport based on the MOI.
   d. treat the patient only if she begins to become unstable.

2. When determining the severity of the MOI, the EMT-B will:
   a. recognize all potential injuries.
   b. identify when a patient is in shock.
   c. relate the forces of energy to the pathology of injury.
   d. recognize which patients will make it through to hospital discharge.

3. The most important aspect of trauma assessment is the:
   a. MOI.
   b. age of the patient.
   c. most obvious injury.
   d. patient's chief complaint.

4. The EMT-B is trained to perform the rapid trauma assessment:
   a. on all trauma patients.
   b. on all unconscious patients.
   c. only on conscious trauma patients.
   d. on all patients with a significant MOI.

5. On which of the following patients should the EMT-B perform a rapid trauma assessment on the scene?
   a. a teenager who stepped on a two-inch nail
   b. an unconscious child who is lying next to a fallen ladder
   c. an adult with a swollen ankle injury from stepping into a pothole
   d. an adult with an isolated burn on the hand from cooking grease

6. While performing the rapid trauma assessment, the EMT-B:
   a. may discover injuries that could become life-threatening later.
   b. may discover life-threatening injuries not found in the initial assessment.
   c. will examine each body area briefly for actual or potential life-threatening injuries.
   d. all of the above.

7. After performing a rapid trauma assessment on a patient who was involved in a serious motor vehicle collision, your partner obtains a second set of vital signs. You find that the patient's rapid heart rate is persisting despite her having no apparent injuries. Your next step is to:
   a. complete a detailed physical exam.
   b. calm her down and the heart rate will slow.
   c. treat her as a high-priority patient with possible internal bleeding.
   d. repeat the rapid trauma assessment, as you have probably missed an injury.

8. In which of the following cases would a rapid trauma assessment be most appropriate?
   a. a patient with a significant MOI
   b. a trauma patient who is a low priority for transport
   c. a trauma patient who is conscious with a neck injury
   d. a patient involved in a MVC 2 days ago and today is unable to get out of bed due to low back pain

9. The findings obtained from a rapid trauma assessment:
   a. come from observation only.
   b. can help you determine the patient's final outcome.
   c. will help you determine what care to provide on the way to the hospital.
   d. will help you stabilize the patient on the scene prior to beginning transport.

10. Crepitation is an abnormal finding of the _____ and will typically be discovered during the rapid trauma assessment.

    a. flank
    b. skull
    c. scalp
    d. abdomen

11. _____ is a mnemonic that is helpful in remembering what should be evaluated about the patient in the rapid trauma assessment.

    a. MOI
    b. SAMPLE
    c. OPQRST
    d. D-CAP-BTLS

12. Paradoxical motion is an abnormal finding of the _____, which may be discovered in a rapid trauma assessment.

    a. neck
    b. eyes
    c. chest
    d. abdomen

13. While conducting a rapid trauma assessment on an unconscious patient, you discover a medical alert device that identifies the patient as a diabetic. What action should you take next?

    a. Administer oral glucose.
    b. Finish conducting the rapid trauma assessment.
    c. Look for the patient's glucometer and obtain a reading.
    d. Skip the RTA and go right to a detailed physical examination.

14. You are performing a rapid trauma assessment of a conscious patient who had a witnessed seizure. During your assessment of the head and neck, the patient begins to seize again. Your next action is to:

    a. suction the airway.
    b. administer high-flow oxygen.
    c. gently lay the patient supine, protecting the head.
    d. pry open the airway with an OPA.

15. The rapid trauma assessment is generally performed in a head-to-toe manner, except when:

    a. the patient is unconscious.
    b. there are multiple patients.
    c. there is a suspected spinal injury.
    d. a life-threatening injury is discovered.

16. After completing a scene size-up and performing an initial assessment, on which of the following trauma patients would you perform a focused physical exam?

    a. ankle injury with no significant MOI
    b. minor injuries with a loss of consciousness
    c. no spinal tenderness or deformity but a significant MOI
    d. seizure patient who is conscious with an altered mental status

17. After completing the initial assessment, in which of the following situations would a focused physical exam be most appropriate?

    a. unconscious elderly patient with no apparent injuries
    b. 34-year-old female with multiple bee stings on her right hand
    c. 16-year-old male with possible multiple fractured toes on the same foot
    d. unrestrained 21-year-old female with chest pain from striking the steering wheel

18. For the trauma patient in the preceding question, the EMT-B would proceed with the focused history and physical exam based on the:

    a. MOI only.
    b. MOI and the chief complaint.
    c. chief complaint of the patient.
    d. age and findings in the initial assessment.

19. The driver involved in a serious MVC is uncooperative and quarrelsome. There is no evidence of intoxication, and you consider _____ to be a possible reason for his behavior.

    a. hypoxia
    b. head injury
    c. hypovolemia
    d. any of the above

20. During the physical exam of a trauma patient, in which of the following areas or regions would you be least likely to find crepitus?

    a. back
    b. face
    c. sternum
    d. abdomen

21. You are caring for a victim who has a gunshot wound (GSW) through the leg. In the initial assessment the patient is alert, is breathing adequately, has a strong distal pulse, and has minimal external bleeding from a wound in his upper thigh. After completing a rapid trauma assessment, you find no other holes and you bandage his leg wound. What should you do next?

    a. Obtain vital signs.
    b. Transport immediately.
    c. Perform a detailed physical exam.
    d. Repeat the initial assessment.

22. For the patient in the previous question, which of the following factors can best help you determine if the wound is an entry or exit GSW?

    a. the caliber of the gun
    b. the gender of the shooter
    c. the shell type of ammunition used
    d. presence of powder residue at the injury site

23. Asymmetry, crepitus, and paradoxical motion are abnormal findings consistent with traumatic injury to the:
    a. pelvis.
    b. skull.
    c. chest.
    d. abdomen.

24. You have discovered signs and symptoms of a pelvic injury during a rapid trauma assessment of a patient who was involved in a motorcycle collision. Your next step should be to:
    a. stabilize the pelvis.
    b. obtain a blood pressure.
    c. not move the patient until ALS arrives.
    d. finish the remainder of the rapid trauma assessment.

25. When assessing an alert trauma patient without a significant MOI, your examination should:
    a. follow a head-to-toe pattern.
    b. be the same as for a patient with a significant MOI.
    c. take no more than 30 seconds to complete.
    d. be directed where the patient indicates there is a problem.

26. You have responded to a residence for a 34-year-old woman complaining of neck pain. She appears to be guarding her neck muscles as she tells you that she was involved in a minor motor vehicle collision yesterday. She was evaluated at an emergency department and the x-rays were clear. The pain and guarding are most likely associated with:
    a. arthritis.
    b. muscle strain.
    c. osteoporosis.
    d. a new case of meningitis.

27. The driver of a snowmobile struck a tree and was thrown from the sled. A witness confirms that there was a brief loss of consciousness; that was why he called 9-1-1. The patient is awake when you reach him. Which of the following is the most significant finding concerning the MOI?
    a. the condition of the rider's helmet
    b. the amount of damage to the snowmobile
    c. the number of years experience riding a snowmobile
    d. the amount of time the patient has been out in the cold

28. Injury patterns associated with specific MOIs, from which the EMT-B can anticipate the potential for shock or other problems, are referred to as:
    a. nature of illness.
    b. predictable shock.
    c. index of suspicion.
    d. history of traumatic impression.

29. The police have called you to evaluate 11-year-old twins who were seat-belted into the back seat of a minivan that was involved in a moderate-speed collision. The children deny any injury, but after 15 minutes on the scene one has a rapid heart rate and appears pale. Which of the following is the likely cause of the persistent rapid heart rate?
    a. anxiety
    b. head injury
    c. hypoglycemia
    d. internal bleeding

30. While you were obtaining equipment from the ambulance, your partner performed an initial assessment on an unconscious male who had been struck by a car. You take over and conduct the rapid trauma exam and discover a life-threatening injury that was missed in the initial assessment. What should you do?
    a. Immediately manage the life threat.
    b. Have a discussion with your partner.
    c. Call the EMS supervisor to the scene.
    d. Complete the rapid trauma exam and begin the detailed physical exam.

Chapter 10 Answer Form

	A	B	C	D			A	B	C	D
1.	❏	❏	❏	❏		16.	❏	❏	❏	❏
2.	❏	❏	❏	❏		17.	❏	❏	❏	❏
3.	❏	❏	❏	❏		18.	❏	❏	❏	❏
4.	❏	❏	❏	❏		19.	❏	❏	❏	❏
5.	❏	❏	❏	❏		20.	❏	❏	❏	❏
6.	❏	❏	❏	❏		21.	❏	❏	❏	❏
7.	❏	❏	❏	❏		22.	❏	❏	❏	❏
8.	❏	❏	❏	❏		23.	❏	❏	❏	❏
9.	❏	❏	❏	❏		24.	❏	❏	❏	❏
10.	❏	❏	❏	❏		25.	❏	❏	❏	❏
11.	❏	❏	❏	❏		26.	❏	❏	❏	❏
12.	❏	❏	❏	❏		27.	❏	❏	❏	❏
13.	❏	❏	❏	❏		28.	❏	❏	❏	❏
14.	❏	❏	❏	❏		29.	❏	❏	❏	❏
15.	❏	❏	❏	❏		30.	❏	❏	❏	❏

CHAPTER

Focused History and Physical Exam—Medical Patient

1. You arrive at the residence of a 23-year-old male, who called because he had a sudden onset of severe chest pain "like no other pain he has ever had before." Now he states that the pain is completely gone, and is refusing transportation for evaluation. With no prior history and the quick resolution of pain, what should you do now?
    a. Let the patient refuse.
    b. Convince the patient to get evaluated at the hospital.
    c. Ask the patient to call his own physician and follow up.
    d. Convince the patient to drive to the hospital if the pain comes back.

2. You are about to interview a patient about her chief complaint of "nausea and vomiting." Which mnemonic can you use to remember which questions to ask about the chief complaint?
    a. AVPU
    b. OPQRST
    c. SAMPLE
    d. D-CAP-BTLS

3. While obtaining a focused history from an elderly patient, it becomes obvious that he is having trouble remembering certain things. Except for your crew, the patient is alone in his residence. What can you use at the residence to help discover the patient's past medical history?
    a. Call a family member or friend.
    b. Locate any medications prescribed for the patient.
    c. Ask your dispatcher for information on any prior calls to the residence.
    d. Any of the above.

4. Which of the following patient complaints would make you suspect that the patient is most likely experiencing a new onset of diabetes?
    a. fainting twice in a month
    b. increased thirst and urination
    c. feeling sweaty for no apparent reason
    d. feeling short of breath with exertion

5. Which of the following clues may indicate that a patient has a cardiac history?
    a. a midline scar on the chest
    b. aspirin in the medicine cabinet
    c. a bottle of medication in the refrigerator
    d. a prescribed inhaler on the bedside table

6. You obtain a medication list from a patient, but you do not recognize two of the medication names, and the patient cannot tell you why he is taking them. Which of the following questions may provide a clue about the unfamiliar medications?
    a. Are you allergic to anything?
    b. What was your last oral intake?
    c. What were you doing when this episode began?
    d. What type of medical problems have you had in the past?

7. You have been called to care for a diabetic patient who was found unresponsive, on the floor, by strangers. She remains unresponsive upon scene size-up. Your next action is to:
    a. assess the SpO2.
    b. check for a pulse.
    c. ensure cervical stabilization.
    d. back off and wait for the police.

8. After performing an initial assessment of an unresponsive patient, you determine that the ABCs are adequate. What do you do next?
    a. Obtain a set of vital signs.
    b. Perform a rapid physical exam.
    c. Perform a focused physical exam.
    d. Look for a diabetic Medic Alert tag.

9. Your primary concern for the unresponsive medical patient is:
    a. airway patency.
    b. administering oxygen.
    c. completing a physical exam.
    d. getting a history of the present illness.

10. A 23-year-old female shows you a rash on both arms and tells you that this rash is new and is occurring for the first time. She has no other symptoms, but is very upset about the rash. You suspect that she is:

   a. poisoned.

   b. contagious.

   c. trying to get attention.

   d. going into anaphylaxis.

11. For the medical patient complaining of dizziness, the focused history and physical exam are performed:

   a. en route to the hospital.

   b. after placing the patient on the stretcher.

   c. immediately after the rapid physical exam.

   d. simultaneously after the initial assessment.

12. The SAMPLE history for a medical patient does not include the patient's:

   a. age.

   b. primary symptom.

   c. history of smoking.

   d. history of the last trip to the hospital.

13. The police have requested transport for a male in his twenties who appears to be intoxicated. The patient does not appear to be injured, but is not very alert. Your approach to this patient is to:

   a. let him sleep it off during the transport.

   b. assume there is a head injury until proven otherwise.

   c. complete an examination and keep an open mind about the intoxication.

   d. restrain him so he does not become violent or a threat to you and your crew.

14. When caring for a medical patient, whether the patient is conscious or unconscious, the highest priority is:

   a. airway maintenance.

   b. positioning the patient.

   c. getting a SAMPLE history.

   d. making a transportation decision.

15. After being dispatched for a cardiac arrest, you arrive to find that the patient is unconscious, is breathing, and has a pulse. Once the initial assessment is completed, you _____ and obtain a baseline set of vital signs.

   a. contact medical control

   b. complete a rapid physical exam

   c. call the dispatcher and cancel the police

   d. obtain a SAMPLE history from the patient's physician

16. The adult patient you are caring for is experiencing an asthma attack, with severe difficulty breathing and speaking. How would you proceed with the focused history?

   a. Call medical control for advice.

   b. Phrase your questions for yes-or-no answers.

   c. Wait to ask any questions until the patient is stable.

   d. Wait to ask questions until after you have assisted the patient with her inhaler.

17. During your interview, a patient complains of chest pain. Which of the following pieces of information is least helpful for the presenting problem?

   a. There is a family history of cardiac disease.

   b. The spouse and children are currently out of town.

   c. The patient has no known allergies to medications.

   d. The patient took his own nitroglycerin with no relief of pain.

18. You suspect that your patient with an altered mental status may be diabetic. One way to verify this is to direct a crew member to look _____ for an insulin bottle.

   a. in the refrigerator

   b. in the nightstand

   c. under the pillow

   d. in the medicine cabinet

19. When your general impression is that a patient appears to have an altered mental status, the first person from whom you try to get patient information is:

   a. the patient.

   b. a friend or neighbor.

   c. the caretaker or parent.

   d. the patient's physician.

20. The _____ is/are the information obtained from the patient or bystanders about the current event and what led up to it.

   a. baseline data

   b. demographics

   c. focused history

   d. chief complaint

21. A baseline set of vital signs taken during a patient assessment is:

   a. the most important set of vital signs.

   b. the first set of vital signs used to establish a trend.

   c. completed on scene only if a life-threatening condition exists.

   d. the responsibility of the most senior EMS provider on scene.

22. When your patient says that she is having multiple symptoms, which one do you consider to be the chief complaint?

    a. the symptom that worries her the most
    b. the first symptom the patient describes
    c. the last symptom the patient describes
    d. all of the symptoms are considered part of the chief complaint

23. You are treating a 60-year-old female who fainted, but is now alert. She denies difficulty breathing, chest pain, or any injuries, yet she feels weak and is unable to stand and walk. Her vital signs are: respiratory rate 16, nonlabored, with clear lung sounds; pulse rate 70, strong and regular; BP 180/110; skin is pink, warm, and dry. Which of the following conditions do you suspect?

    a. stroke or TIA
    b. hypoglycemic event
    c. hyperglycemic event
    d. acute myocardial infarction

24. After assisting a patient who was complaining of chest pain to take his prescribed nitroglycerin, the patient tells you that the pain is gone. What do you do now?

    a. Transport the patient to the hospital.
    b. Wait 15 minutes before releasing the patient.
    c. Transport the patient to his doctor's office for follow-up.
    d. Release the patient and tell him to call 9-1-1 if the pain returns.

25. While transporting a patient who has generalized weakness, your patient's eyes roll back and he begins to have a seizure. Which of the following actions should you take first?

    a. Prepare for vomiting.
    b. Call for ALS to meet you en route.
    c. Tell the driver to turn on the lights and siren.
    d. Make sure the patient is securely strapped in.

26. During your interview of a 61-year-old patient, you learn that she has a pacemaker. Where would you expect to see the scar associated with the implantation of such a device?

    a. in the upper left thigh area
    b. in the midline of the chest
    c. in the upper right or left chest
    d. below the left armpit (midaxillary line)

27. While assessing a 48-year-old male with a complaint of chest pain, you obtain a focused history including SAMPLE and OPQRST questions. Which of the following is considered to be a pertinent negative when managing a patient with chest pain?

    a. The patient denies having a pacemaker.
    b. The patient has no shortness of breath or difficulty breathing.
    c. The patient feels better after taking nitroglycerin and now refuses transportation for evaluation at the hospital.
    d. All of the above.

28. You have arrived at the apartment of an elderly couple with a report of a fainting episode. When you ask for information about the patient, the spouse tells you they have a Vial of Life. What is this?

    a. a prescription vitality medication
    b. an over-the-counter vitality medication
    c. a subscription service with an 800 number that provides patient information
    d. a small plastic container that holds a rolled piece of paper with patient information

29. You are transporting a cancer patient who complains of generalized weakness. From your first impression, it is obvious that the patient has yellow in the normally white part of the eyes. He tells you that he has had jaundice before, and this is not bad. What precautions do you need to take with this patient?

    a. none, jaundice is not contagious
    b. gloves, eyewear, and handwashing
    c. place a mask on the patient and yourself
    d. notify the hospital that you are bringing in a highly infectious patient

30. While assessing a patient who has flu symptoms, you quickly notice that the patient has a persistent cough. Now your first priority is to:

    a. provide high-flow oxygen immediately.
    b. be prepared for nausea and vomiting.
    c. ask the patient if she is contagious.
    d. take precautions for yourself and put on a mask.

Chapter 11 Answer Form

	A	B	C	D			A	B	C	D
1.	❏	❏	❏	❏		16.	❏	❏	❏	❏
2.	❏	❏	❏	❏		17.	❏	❏	❏	❏
3.	❏	❏	❏	❏		18.	❏	❏	❏	❏
4.	❏	❏	❏	❏		19.	❏	❏	❏	❏
5.	❏	❏	❏	❏		20.	❏	❏	❏	❏
6.	❏	❏	❏	❏		21.	❏	❏	❏	❏
7.	❏	❏	❏	❏		22.	❏	❏	❏	❏
8.	❏	❏	❏	❏		23.	❏	❏	❏	❏
9.	❏	❏	❏	❏		24.	❏	❏	❏	❏
10.	❏	❏	❏	❏		25.	❏	❏	❏	❏
11.	❏	❏	❏	❏		26.	❏	❏	❏	❏
12.	❏	❏	❏	❏		27.	❏	❏	❏	❏
13.	❏	❏	❏	❏		28.	❏	❏	❏	❏
14.	❏	❏	❏	❏		29.	❏	❏	❏	❏
15.	❏	❏	❏	❏		30.	❏	❏	❏	❏

CHAPTER
12

Detailed Physical Exam

1. Which of the following is an example of nondiagnostic information obtained in the detailed physical exam?
   a. allergies
   b. temperature
   c. blood glucose
   d. pulse oximetry

2. The _____ is considered part of the detailed physical exam.
   a. scene size-up
   b. administration of oxygen
   c. neurological status
   d. age of the patient

3. The detailed physical exam is typically performed on:
   a. trauma patients with a significant mechanism of injury.
   b. trauma patients without a significant mechanism of injury.
   c. responsive medical patients.
   d. responsive medical patients with an isolated extremity injury.

4. During the detailed physical exam, you discover pain and swelling on the humerus, which is located in the:
   a. lower arm.
   b. upper arm.
   c. pelvic girdle.
   d. lower extremity.

5. While performing a detailed physical exam of the _____, you have discovered pulsing, guarding, and distention.
   a. neck
   b. pelvis
   c. abdomen
   d. lower extremity

6. HEENT is a mnemonic used to help remember the items to examine on the:
   a. back.
   b. extremities.
   c. head and face.
   d. hips and pelvis.

7. During the detailed physical exam of your patient's chest, you discover a clear patch adhering to the upper left side just below the collarbone. You do not recognize the name written on the patch. What should you do first?
   a. Call medical control for advice.
   b. Ask the patient what the patch is for.
   c. Leave the patch on and forget about it.
   d. Remove the patch and wipe the skin clean.

8. All of the injuries listed below were discovered during a detailed physical exam. Which injury should be treated first?
   a. broken tooth
   b. scalp abrasion
   c. dislocated thumb
   d. foreign body in the eye

9. During your assessment of your patient's pupils, you note that they both respond to light but are unequal in size. Your next action should be to:
   a. call medical control for advice.
   b. do nothing and reassess in five minutes.
   c. ask the patient if this is normal for her.
   d. provide high-flow oxygen and rapid transport.

10. A patient sustained a back injury during a motor vehicle collision. He is awake and was immobilized on a long backboard at the scene by first responders. During transport, you attempt to perform a detailed physical exam of the back. How should you proceed?
    a. It is too late to check the back, as the patient is immobilized.
    b. Reach under the back from both sides of the patient as far as you can.
    c. Roll the patient on his side and reach down to the low back from the side.
    d. Loosen the straps and ask the patient to bend his knees and arch his back while you reach under him.

11. Your ambulance was dispatched for a "fainting episode." When you arrive, the patient is awake and complaining of neck and back pain. After the initial assessment, your plan of action should be to:
    a. assess the neck and back pain first.
    b. assess for a medical cause for the fainting first.
    c. call for ALS, as the patient is too unstable for BLS.
    d. perform a rapid trauma exam followed by a detailed physical exam.

12. You have arrived on scene at a supermarket on a call for an unconscious checkout clerk, who is lying on the floor beneath the register. Who would likely provide the best information about what has just happened to the patient?
    a. the patient
    b. the patient's boss
    c. the customer at the checkout who witnessed the episode
    d. the police officer on the scene

13. The detailed physical exam is not performed on every patient because:
    a. there is not enough time.
    b. often transport time is short.
    c. the patient's condition makes treatment a higher priority.
    d. all of the above.

14. The detailed physical exam is typically performed:
    a. en route to the hospital.
    b. after the ABCs are assessed and managed.
    c. right after the patient tells you his chief complaint.
    d. none of the above.

15. You are performing a detailed physical examination of the scalp. Which of the following is considered an abnormal finding for this area of the body?
    a. paradoxical motion
    b. jugular vein distention
    c. dry mucous membranes
    d. depression on palpation

16. What is the value of a detailed physical exam?
    a. Performing a detailed physical exam will really impress the ED staff.
    b. The EMT-B may discover information not obtained in the rapid physical exam.
    c. Completing a detailed physical exam will keep the EMT-B from becoming involved in a lawsuit.
    d. Completion of a detailed physical exam helps to establish a better rapport with the patient.

17. The detailed physical exam is typically performed in a head-to-toe order because:
    a. this order is the quickest method.
    b. most local protocols mandate this order.
    c. the patient is usually most cooperative with this order of assessment.
    d. using this same order every time helps to minimize missing any pertinent findings.

18. Which of the following statements about trauma patients with significant MOIs is most correct?
    a. The baseline vital signs appear better than they actually are.
    b. The MOI will help the EMT-B decide when to obtain baseline vital signs.
    c. Baseline vital signs should be obtained prior to performing a detailed physical exam.
    d. The patient's level of consciousness will determine when to perform a detailed physical exam.

19. How often should the detailed physical exam be performed?
    a. every 15 minutes
    b. every 5 minutes for a high-priority patient
    c. typically once while en route to the hospital
    d. repeat only when there is a change in mental status

20. Which of the following statements about the detailed physical exam is incorrect?
    a. The abdominal cavity can hide significant blood loss.
    b. The back is often overlooked during the physical exam.
    c. The detailed physical exam is not performed on children under 8 years of age.
    d. Special considerations may be necessary when performing a detailed physical exam on the elderly.

21. Which of the following is an open soft tissue injury?
    a. degloving
    b. contusion
    c. hematoma
    d. crushing injury

22. A detailed physical exam of the eyes would include checking the response of the pupils, eye movement, and:
    a. discoloration in the eyes.
    b. ability to open the eyelids.
    c. ability to close the eyelids.
    d. ability to read one line on an eye chart.

23. During a detailed physical exam, where would you expect to find drainage of cerebral spinal fluid (CSF)?
    a. ears only
    b. fractured pelvis
    c. ears, mouth, and nose
    d. laceration to the cervical spine

24. As you perform a detailed physical exam of the neck on a patient who is immobilized to a long backboard, you observe the presence of jugular vein distention (JVD). This finding:
    a. indicates hypertension.
    b. is normal in a supine patient.
    c. is an abnormal finding in a supine patient.
    d. indicates a possible life-threatening condition.

25. In the initial assessment of a patient with chest trauma, you discovered a flail segment and immediately stabilized it. During the detailed physical exam of the patient, you:
    a. reassess the injury for stability.
    b. reassess the injury only if there is significant bleeding.
    c. skip over the stabilized injury, but listen to lung sounds.
    d. reassess the injury only if the patient's breathing becomes worse.

Chapter 12 Answer Form

	A	B	C	D			A	B	C	D
1.	❏	❏	❏	❏		14.	❏	❏	❏	❏
2.	❏	❏	❏	❏		15.	❏	❏	❏	❏
3.	❏	❏	❏	❏		16.	❏	❏	❏	❏
4.	❏	❏	❏	❏		17.	❏	❏	❏	❏
5.	❏	❏	❏	❏		18.	❏	❏	❏	❏
6.	❏	❏	❏	❏		19.	❏	❏	❏	❏
7.	❏	❏	❏	❏		20.	❏	❏	❏	❏
8.	❏	❏	❏	❏		21.	❏	❏	❏	❏
9.	❏	❏	❏	❏		22.	❏	❏	❏	❏
10.	❏	❏	❏	❏		23.	❏	❏	❏	❏
11.	❏	❏	❏	❏		24.	❏	❏	❏	❏
12.	❏	❏	❏	❏		25.	❏	❏	❏	❏
13.	❏	❏	❏	❏						

CHAPTER

13

Ongoing Assessment

1. Your initial assessment of a 55-year-old male complaining of abdominal pain revealed that he has tachycardia and that his skin is pale, warm, and moist. In your ongoing assessment you found that there was increased tachycardia, he still looks pale, and is now hypotensive. These findings may indicate:
   a. shock.
   b. anxiety.
   c. hypoglycemia.
   d. intracranial bleeding.

2. Repeating the initial assessment as part of the ongoing assessment en route to the hospital is necessary to:
   a. reevaluate the treatment priorities for the patient.
   b. predict all possible trends before arriving at the ED.
   c. have all information documented before arriving at the ED.
   d. provide any needed definite care prior to arriving at the ED.

3. The primary reason for conducting an ongoing assessment on all patients is to:
   a. correct any life-threatening conditions.
   b. identify changes in a patient's condition.
   c. determine if the patient is competent to give consent.
   d. be able to complete the patient care report accurately.

4. It is time for you to document the ongoing assessment findings for a patient you have brought to the hospital. Each of the following components should be documented as part of the ongoing assessment, except:
   a. serial vital signs.
   b. response to interventions.
   c. pertinent past medical history.
   d. findings from the repeat focused assessment.

5. Which of the following is most often repeated first in the ongoing assessment?
   a. vital signs
   b. initial assessment
   c. checking interventions
   d. status of chief complaint

6. _____ is the primary focus of the ongoing assessment.
   a. Assessing interventions
   b. Providing definitive care
   c. Reconsidering the MOI or NOI
   d. Early notification of the patient's status to the ED

7. In addition to vital signs, which of the following assessment components is used to establish a trend?
   a. pulse oximetry
   b. compliance with medications
   c. events leading up to the current episode
   d. all of the above

8. On the way to the hospital, you take repeated sets of vital signs on a conscious medical patient and compare them to the baseline set of vital signs. This skill is known as:
   a. trending.
   b. reporting.
   c. appraising.
   d. reassuring.

9. You are en route to the hospital with a trauma patient whom you are treating for internal bleeding and head injury. While conducting the ongoing assessment, you find that the systolic blood pressure has decreased from 110 to 100, and is now 92. What is the significance of this finding?
   a. The patient is in irreversible shock.
   b. The patient is in compensated shock.
   c. The patient is in decompensated shock.
   d. The patient has lost approximately 55 percent of his blood volume.

10. You are caring for a 30-year-old male who suspects that he has cracked or fractured a rib after falling. He has had broken ribs before and tells you that it hurts to take a deep breath. During your ongoing assessment, you recognize that the patient is guarding his chest and his breathing seems much shallower. The emergency care for this patient includes:

    a. placing the patient on a pulse oximeter.
    b. providing high-flow oxygen and keeping the patient still.
    c. encouraging the patient to take deeper breaths and providing high-flow oxygen.
    d. encouraging the patient to take deeper breaths despite the increase in pain; no oxygen is necessary.

11. The ongoing assessment of a patient with an isolated extremity injury includes reassessing:

    a. lung sounds and adequacy of the splint.
    b. pulse, blood pressure, and pulse oximetry.
    c. mental status and vital signs every 5 minutes.
    d. distal pulse, motor and sensation (PMS), and the adequacy of the splint.

12. When providing high-flow oxygen to a patient with a history of COPD, reassessment of this intervention includes assessing the skin color, checking the tank pressure and flow rate, and:

    a. documenting the procedure.
    b. removing nail polish to observe the nail beds.
    c. watching the patient for decreased respiratory effort.
    d. assessing for the development of congestive heart failure.

13. You have delivered three shocks with an AED to a pulseless and nonbreathing patient. Reassessment of this intervention will include each of the following, except:

    a. checking for pulses.
    b. assessing the need to continue CPR.
    c. assuring that the electrodes are properly attached.
    d. assessing the need to shave the patient's chest.

14. When assisting a patient who has chest pain to take his nitroglycerin, the EMT-B should reassess the _____ 3 to 5 minutes after the administration and before any additional medication is taken.

    a. pulse rate
    b. mental status
    c. blood pressure
    d. position of comfort

15. The driver of a mid-sized vehicle that was involved in a low-speed collision initially complained of cervical tenderness, with no other injuries. Your crew put on a cervical collar and immobilized her to a long backboard. En route to the hospital, the patient tells you that she is now experiencing low back spasms. This finding:

    a. is a pertinent negative.
    b. is not uncommon for this situation.
    c. indicates that the patient was improperly immobilized.
    d. indicates that the injury was missed during the physical exam.

16. Which of the following is the earliest indication that a patient's condition is worsening?

    a. a drop in blood pressure
    b. changes in lung sounds
    c. subtle changes in mental status
    d. change in skin color from pink to cyanotic

17. En route to the hospital, the ongoing assessment will often guide the EMT-B to:

    a. provide additional interventions.
    b. revise the plan of care for a patient.
    c. make the patient more comfortable.
    d. all of the above.

18. Which of the following statements about repeating an ongoing assessment is most correct?

    a. The ongoing assessment for trauma patients with a significant MOI should be performed only by a paramedic.
    b. The ongoing assessment for really sick patients should be performed by the most senior EMT-B on the call.
    c. Anyone who is trained as an EMT-B may perform an ongoing assessment on any patient.
    d. The time interval for repeating the ongoing assessment for an unstable trauma patient is the same as for an unstable medical patient.

19. When reassessing _____, the EMT-B will determine if a pressure bandage or elevation is needed.

    a. head injury
    b. femur fracture
    c. bleeding control
    d. blood pressure

20. You are assessing a conscious patient who was reported to have passed out briefly. As you are talking to him and getting ready to move him onto your stretcher, you see his face get very pale and he starts sweating. What should you do next?

   a. Check to see if he has a pacemaker.
   b. Take off the oxygen mask and prepare for him to vomit.
   c. Elevate the patient's legs and reassess the blood pressure.
   d. Increase the flow of oxygen and sit him up in case he vomits.

21. When attempting to establish a trend, the EMT-B must obtain at least _____ set(s) of vital signs.

   a. one
   b. two
   c. three
   d. four

22. Before documenting any trends observed during the time spent with the patient, the EMT-B should:

   a. reconsider the MOI.
   b. reassess the need for BSI.
   c. reassess the need for ALS.
   d. perform serial assessments.

23. Which of the following is one of the only times during the care of a patient that the EMT-B may omit the ongoing assessment?

   a. short transport time
   b. treating a life-threatening condition
   c. when the patient is faking the complaint
   d. when a patient is too scared or embarrassed to be touched

24. You are transporting a conscious 34-year-old male who was hit by a car while walking in a parking lot. He has a broken right lower leg, which is splinted, and he is fully immobilized to a long backboard. His last set of vital signs was: pulse 94, regular; respirations 26, adequate, and BP 130/74. During the ride to the hospital, you repeat the ongoing assessment:

   a. every 5 minutes.
   b. every 15 minutes.
   c. after every intervention.
   d. only if there is a change in his condition.

25. (Continuing with the preceding question) The ongoing assessment of the injured extremity should include:

   a. assessing for loss of range of motion.
   b. alternating cold and heat packs to the injured site.
   c. rechecking the distal pulse, motor function, and sensation (PMS).
   d. rechecking the proximal pulse and skin color, temperature, and condition (CTC).

Chapter 13 Answer Form

	A	B	C	D		A	B	C	D
1.	❏	❏	❏	❏	14.	❏	❏	❏	❏
2.	❏	❏	❏	❏	15.	❏	❏	❏	❏
3.	❏	❏	❏	❏	16.	❏	❏	❏	❏
4.	❏	❏	❏	❏	17.	❏	❏	❏	❏
5.	❏	❏	❏	❏	18.	❏	❏	❏	❏
6.	❏	❏	❏	❏	19.	❏	❏	❏	❏
7.	❏	❏	❏	❏	20.	❏	❏	❏	❏
8.	❏	❏	❏	❏	21.	❏	❏	❏	❏
9.	❏	❏	❏	❏	22.	❏	❏	❏	❏
10.	❏	❏	❏	❏	23.	❏	❏	❏	❏
11.	❏	❏	❏	❏	24.	❏	❏	❏	❏
12.	❏	❏	❏	❏	25.	❏	❏	❏	❏
13.	❏	❏	❏	❏					

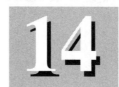

Communications

1. Select the inappropriate method for dispatch to acknowledge receiving your radio transmission.
   a. repeating part of your message
   b. saying your unit name or number
   c. providing the time in military hours
   d. using your first name as an identifier

2. The proper method of establishing radio contact between two units is to:
   a. push the PTT button and wait to be acknowledged.
   b. speak with your upper lip touching the microphone.
   c. say the name of the unit being called followed by the name of your unit.
   d. say the name of your unit followed by the name of the unit being called.

3. To effectively initiate a radio call, the EMT-B must first:
   a. learn all the radio codes.
   b. anticipate what the unit being called is going to say next.
   c. monitor the channel for a clear frequency before beginning the transmission.
   d. all of the above.

4. One thing to avoid when presenting patient information over the radio is:
   a. speaking slowly and clearly.
   b. planning what you will say before transmitting.
   c. deviating from the standard medical radio format.
   d. keeping the microphone about two inches from your mouth.

5. The ambulance-to-hospital communication should:
   a. be less than 30 seconds long.
   b. never be more than 90 seconds long.
   c. follow the standard medical case presentation.
   d. begin with the estimated time of arrival at the hospital.

6. A typical medical radio report is presented in which order?
   a. vital signs, chief complaint, allergies, mental status, and ETA
   b. patient's age, sex, chief complaint, severity, treatment, and ETA
   c. ETA, patient's name, chief complaint, and social security number
   d. chief complaint, past medical history, date of birth, and health insurance number

7. An EMT-B's inability to communicate effectively about the patient may lead to:
   a. delayed care and transfer of the patient.
   b. a possible better outcome for the patient.
   c. practice of professional patient advocacy.
   d. a smoother transition of the patient between health care providers.

8. Standard radio operating procedures are created and designed to:
   a. reduce the number of misunderstood messages.
   b. get the units back in service as soon as possible.
   c. allow dispatch to know where all units are at all times.
   d. keep users from using complicated codes in their transmissions.

9. Which of the following factors directly interferes with effective radio communication of patient information to the hospital?
   a. background noise
   b. patient's condition
   c. training level of EMS provider
   d. the EMS provider's years of experience

10. Which of the following is considered an essential component of the verbal report for patient registration?
    a. SAMPLE history
    b. patient's address and telephone number
    c. pertinent positive and negative findings
    d. emergency care provided to the patient

11. Upon arrival at the hospital, the EMT-B will first provide the staff with a _____ report about the patient.

    a. rapid
    b. verbal
    c. written
    d. controlled

12. The _____ is responsible for giving report of the patient to the hospital staff.

    a. ambulance driver
    b. most senior crew member
    c. EMT-B in charge of the patient
    d. highest-ranking crew member

13. You are taking report from a registered nurse (RN) in a nursing home about an elderly patient who has dementia and hearing deficit. What can you do to increase the effectiveness of your communication with this type of patient?

    a. Look into the patient's eyes when you speak.
    b. Speak in a clear tone and at a normal rate.
    c. Touch her hand and smile as you speak.
    d. All of the above.

14. In an effort to become more skillful at verbal communication, the EMT-B should consider each of the following techniques, except:

    a. listen and acknowledge what the patient has to say.
    b. watch the patient's facial expression to see if she understands.
    c. use layman's terms and avoid complicated medical terminology.
    d. stand over the patient while speaking, whenever possible, to show confidence.

15. You are caring for a 4-year-old who seems to be frightened of you and your crew. How can you appear less threatening and begin effective communication with the patient?

    a. Let the parent be the liaison for you.
    b. Tell the patient that you are not the police and promise her a toy.
    c. Use an authoritative tone and tell the child you will not give her any shots.
    d. Keep a friendly smile on your face and kneel down to her height as you speak.

16. When two units transmit at the same time:

    a. only one unit will be heard.
    b. both units' transmissions will be heard.
    c. neither unit's transmission will be heard.
    d. both units can be subject to a fine for improper communications.

17. The _____ is the agency that assigns and licenses radio frequencies.

    a. Homeland Security Agency
    b. Federal Telecommunications Commission
    c. Federal Corrections Commission
    d. Federal Communications Commission

18. Slang terms and vulgarity should be avoided when making radio transmissions using a:

    a. repeater.
    b. base station.
    c. mobile or portable.
    d. all of the above.

19. Which of the following is an inappropriate form of communication that should be avoided when interacting with a patient?

    a. Use the patient's surname when making an introduction with a patient.
    b. Take off your glove to shake hands when making an introduction with a patient.
    c. Allow the patient to describe his concerns before asking the SAMPLE questions.
    d. Use the patient's first name or nickname to put the patient at ease when making an introduction with a patient.

20. How can the EMT-B best communicate with an elderly patient who cannot hear without his hearing aids?

    a. Shout into the ear that has the best hearing.
    b. Use sign language to communicate your questions.
    c. Make sure that the patient is wearing his hearing aids and that they are turned on.
    d. Look into the patient's face and exaggerate your lip movement when speaking.

21. You are caring for a patient who speaks a foreign language and does not appear to understand English. Which of the following methods of communications will be most useful in this situation?

    a. Make eye contact and maintain friendly facial expressions.
    b. Avoid talking to the patient; instead, draw pictures to communicate.
    c. Call the hospital and advise them that the patient is in need of an interpreter.
    d. Avoid talking to or touching the patient unless he becomes unresponsive.

22. You have just loaded your patient into the ambulance when a neighbor runs over to you and asks what is going on. You tell the neighbor:

    a. that the patient is going to be fine and not to worry.
    b. that you are taking the patient to the hospital and nothing else.
    c. to call the patient's family if she wants to know what is happening.
    d. everything that has happened on the scene and to meet you at the hospital if she wishes.

23. You are treating a 55-year-old female for symptoms of chest pain and dizziness. As you are getting ready to move the patient to the ambulance, the family asks you how she is doing. You should tell the patient's family:
    a. that the patient is going to be fine and not to worry at this point.
    b. nothing and let the emergency department physician explain.
    c. what you suspect is happening and what you are going to do en route to the hospital.
    d. that the patient has a 50/50 chance of going into cardiac arrest and that you need to get going.

24. Using medical terminology when discussing a patient's present condition or past medical history is not appropriate when:
    a. documenting your patient care report.
    b. presenting your patient in case review.
    c. giving report to the next health care provider.
    d. demonstrating your expertise to the patient's family.

25. You are contacting medical control to obtain an order to assist a patient with a medication. The typical request should be stated by:
    a. describing the patient's condition, requesting the order, and confirming the order.
    b. requesting the order, describing the patient's condition, and asking questions if you do not understand the order.
    c. requesting the order, confirming the order, describing the patient's condition, and never questioning the order.
    d. describing the patient's condition, requesting the order, repeating the order, confirming the order, and never asking questions about the order.

26. In which order does the communication between dispatch and a transporting ambulance occur?
    a. The ambulance notifies dispatch, when leaving the scene, of the destination and when they will arrive; dispatch acknowledges with a time check.
    b. Dispatch assigns the destination hospital; the ambulance acknowledges and calls out upon arrival at that hospital.
    c. The ambulance advises of ETA at the hospital; dispatch acknowledges and approves transport; the ambulance calls out when arriving.
    d. The ambulance calls dispatch after arriving at the hospital, relaying with the time it left the scene, time of arrival at the hospital, and time back in service; dispatch acknowledges.

27. Which of the following practices is appropriate when talking to dispatch on an approved radio frequency?
    a. using clear and brief communication
    b. including personal patient information
    c. using "please" and "thank you"
    d. using a tone of voice that implies anger, frustration, or extreme emotion

28. Safety hazards, patient condition, number of patients, and confirmation of the number of ambulances needed are all pieces of information that should be provided:
    a. while at the scene.
    b. en route to the scene.
    c. en route to the hospital.
    d. upon returning to service.

29. You need to contact medical control for an order to assist a patient with his medication. Ideally, the contact should be made by:
    a. getting dispatch to call the hospital and make the request.
    b. radio, so that the entire request is recorded for quality assurance.
    c. cell phone, as it is the quickest way to make contact and obtain an order.
    d. land line from the patient's residence, as it is the clearest form of communication.

30. When you are unable to acknowledge a long incoming radio message promptly, you should:
    a. acknowledge by saying "Stand by."
    b. ignore the transmission and pretend that you did not hear it.
    c. not answer the radio until you are free to accept the entire message.
    d. acknowledge by saying "I acknowledge the message and will get back in a minute."

Chapter 14 Answer Form

	A	B	C	D		A	B	C	D
1.	❑	❑	❑	❑	16.	❑	❑	❑	❑
2.	❑	❑	❑	❑	17.	❑	❑	❑	❑
3.	❑	❑	❑	❑	18.	❑	❑	❑	❑
4.	❑	❑	❑	❑	19.	❑	❑	❑	❑
5.	❑	❑	❑	❑	20.	❑	❑	❑	❑
6.	❑	❑	❑	❑	21.	❑	❑	❑	❑
7.	❑	❑	❑	❑	22.	❑	❑	❑	❑
8.	❑	❑	❑	❑	23.	❑	❑	❑	❑
9.	❑	❑	❑	❑	24.	❑	❑	❑	❑
10.	❑	❑	❑	❑	25.	❑	❑	❑	❑
11.	❑	❑	❑	❑	26.	❑	❑	❑	❑
12.	❑	❑	❑	❑	27.	❑	❑	❑	❑
13.	❑	❑	❑	❑	28.	❑	❑	❑	❑
14.	❑	❑	❑	❑	29.	❑	❑	❑	❑
15.	❑	❑	❑	❑	30.	❑	❑	❑	❑

CHAPTER

Documentation

1. When reporting time data on a patient care report (PCR), which of the following are typically included?
   a. date, time the report was written, time back in service
   b. time of dispatch, arrival at the scene, leaving the scene, and arrival at the hospital
   c. time initial call for help was received, time of dispatch, time arrived at and left the scene, time the report was written
   d. time of call received, time of acknowledgment of call received, on-scene time, time of end of shift when the shift end occurs during a call

2. When tracking the times on a written report, the EMT-B should use:
   a. the time provided by dispatch.
   b. universal Greenwich Mean Time.
   c. his watch and convert to military time.
   d. the clock in the ambulance and convert to military time.

3. The typical patient prehospital care report contains three copies. A copy is reserved for each of the following purposes, except:
   a. EMS agency tracking.
   b. hospital patient records.
   c. patient discharge instructions.
   d. statistical research or education.

4. Patient information that includes age, date of birth, gender, address, and telephone number is considered:
   a. universal statistics.
   b. assessment findings.
   c. patient demographics.
   d. all of the above.

5. The _____ portion of the written prehospital care report includes information that is most useful to the next health care provider to care for the patient.
   a. narrative
   b. run-times
   c. insurance
   d. administrative

6. When completing a written report, the emergency care provided to a patient by the EMT-B should be documented:
   a. in the narrative.
   b. on the billing form.
   c. in check boxes provided.
   d. any of the above.

7. In the EMS profession, times are recorded in military time because:
   a. fire departments and police agencies use it.
   b. it helps to minimize documentation and recording errors.
   c. the government has ultimate oversight over such matters.
   d. compliance is mandated by the American Medical Association.

8. Many prehospital care reports include use of the Glasgow Coma Scale, which provides information about a patient's mental status in the form of a:
   a. trend.
   b. number.
   c. disposition.
   d. brief narrative.

9. During the scene size-up and general impression of a trauma patient, you discovered that your unconscious patient has no identification. This information should be documented in which portion of the patient care report?
   a. administrative
   b. chief complaint
   c. demographics
   d. statistics and research

10. Which of the following patients should the EMT-B allow to refuse treatment or transport?
    a. a competent 12-year-old with a minor abrasion from a skateboard accident
    b. a 17-year-old married female with a black eye and several fresh cuts and bruises on her body
    c. a 30-year-old with a possible sprained ankle who admits to having had two beers
    d. a 32-year-old mother of three who is home without transportation and has a child that choked, but appears fine upon your initial assessment

11. When a patient refuses care or transport, the EMT-B should disclose and document what information to the patient?
    a. billing information
    b. dispatch information
    c. treatment recommendations
    d. transportation considerations

12. You are assessing a patient who was involved in a MVC. He complains of neck pain as a result of the collision. The patient has requested transport to the hospital for evaluation, but is refusing to be immobilized because he fears being confined. You should:
    a. refuse to transport without immobilization.
    b. transport the patient without any immobilization.
    c. request police intervention to get the patient to comply with standard immobilization practices.
    d. document the refusal of care, have the patient sign the refusal, and transport the patient.

13. After completing your written report on a patient, you realize that you forgot to document an important assessment finding from the initial assessment. How should you correct this error?
    a. Verbally report the omitted finding to the patient's nurse.
    b. Make the change on your copy only, then initial and date it.
    c. Make the change on all copies of the written report, then initial and date it.
    d. Make the change on your copy and have your supervisor initial and date it.

14. A written patient care report that is _____ may give rise to a presumption that the proper care was omitted or lacking.
    a. legible
    b. intelligible
    c. incomplete
    d. comprehensible

15. A written report is considered to be credible when the EMT-B completes it accurately, objectively, promptly, and:
    a. upholds stereotyping.
    b. preserves judgmental biases.
    c. maintains patient confidentiality.
    d. includes extraneous statements.

16. Reporting suspected abuse of an elderly patient by a family member:
    a. is mandated by AARP.
    b. varies from state to state.
    c. is mandatory in all 50 states.
    d. is optional and not required in all 50 states.

17. While inside the home of a patient, you notice some unusual findings. Which of the following are you mandated to report?
    a. suspected child abuse
    b. calendars with nudity
    c. whips and restraining devices
    d. a couple hundred full and empty liquor bottles

18. _____ are often used as the first form of documentation at a multiple casualty incident (MCI).
    a. Triage tags
    b. Colored tape
    c. Patient care reports
    d. Special incident reports

19. Using medical terminology when completing a written patient care report is appropriate in which of the following cases?
    a. when the term is spelled incorrectly
    b. when the medical terms are used suitably
    c. only when the report is one page long
    d. only when the report is two or more pages long

20. Which of the following commonly used medical terms is spelled incorrectly?
    a. apnea
    b. pnuemonia
    c. hypovolemia
    d. musculoskeletal

21. You have successfully assisted a diabetic who has an altered mental status to take oral glucose. Which of the following should you document on your written report?
    a. time of absorption
    b. time of medication administration
    c. contraindications for oral glucose
    d. date of expiration on the oral glucose

22. Which of the following is an example of something that should be documented on the patient care report?
    a. radio failure
    b. route of transport
    c. exposure to blood
    d. standard operating procedures

23. In a court of law, poor documentation is often characterized as:
    a. forgetfulness.
    b. poor assessment.
    c. improper training.
    d. delegation of authority.

24. Which of the following would be considered a pertinent negatives on your written report?
    a. the MOI
    b. trending vital signs
    c. the position in which the patient was found
    d. head injury without a loss of consciousness

25. The _____ has standardized a minimum data set to be included in all prehospital care reports.
    a. Surgeon General
    b. American Ambulance Association
    c. National Highway Traffic Safety Administration
    d. Occupational Safety and Health Administration

Chapter 15 Answer Form

	A	B	C	D
1.	❏	❏	❏	❏
2.	❏	❏	❏	❏
3.	❏	❏	❏	❏
4.	❏	❏	❏	❏
5.	❏	❏	❏	❏
6.	❏	❏	❏	❏
7.	❏	❏	❏	❏
8.	❏	❏	❏	❏
9.	❏	❏	❏	❏
10.	❏	❏	❏	❏
11.	❏	❏	❏	❏
12.	❏	❏	❏	❏
13.	❏	❏	❏	❏

	A	B	C	D
14.	❏	❏	❏	❏
15.	❏	❏	❏	❏
16.	❏	❏	❏	❏
17.	❏	❏	❏	❏
18.	❏	❏	❏	❏
19.	❏	❏	❏	❏
20.	❏	❏	❏	❏
21.	❏	❏	❏	❏
22.	❏	❏	❏	❏
23.	❏	❏	❏	❏
24.	❏	❏	❏	❏
25.	❏	❏	❏	❏

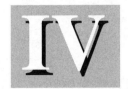

SECTION

IV

Medical/Behavioral Emergencies and Obstetrical/Gynecology

CHAPTER

16

General Pharmacology

1. The DOT National Standard Curriculum states that the EMT-B may administer or use medical control to assist a patient with taking which of the following medications?
   a. aspirin and oral glucose
   b. Benadryl, oxygen, and oral glucose
   c. activated charcoal, oral glucose, and oxygen
   d. epinephrine auto-injectors and atropine inhalers

2. Which of the following medications does not require a written prescription from a physician?
   a. oxygen
   b. Atrovent
   c. Benadryl
   d. nitroglycerin

3. Which of the following medications requires a prescription and therefore is not typically carried on a BLS unit?
   a. oxygen
   b. nitroglycerin
   c. oral glucose
   d. activated charcoal

4. What is the trade name for activated charcoal?
   a. Actidose-Aqua
   b. CharcoAid
   c. EZ-Char
   d. all of the above

5. The official name of a drug is the _____ name followed by the initials USP or NF.
   a. brand
   b. product
   c. generic
   d. chemical

6. The EMT-B is responsible for knowing the generic and _____ names of the medications carried on the unit.
   a. trade
   b. slang
   c. official
   d. chemical

7. You have been dispatched on a seizure call. When you arrive, the patient is unresponsive, breathing, and has a pulse. A family member reports that the patient has diabetes and just finished having a second seizure, with a brief period of alertness between the two seizures. Which medication should you assist the patient with?
   a. oxygen
   b. oral glucose
   c. activated charcoal
   d. prescribed nitroglycerin

8. A 30-year-old female with a history of asthma is complaining of difficulty breathing and chest tightness. She appears anxious and slightly confused, yet you can hear her wheezing. Which of the following medications will you assist her with?
   a. albuterol
   b. oral glucose
   c. nitroglycerin
   d. epinephrine auto-injector

9. The EMT-B may assist a patient with _____ when the patient is exhibiting signs of wheezing, airway swelling, tachycardia, and hives.
   a. prescribed nitroglycerin
   b. over-the-counter Benadryl
   c. prescribed bronchodilator inhaler
   d. prescribed epinephrine auto-injector

10. _____ is the trade name for a common preparation of oral glucose that EMT-Bs can give as a treatment if authorized by medical control.
    a. Glutose
    b. Oragel
    c. Fructose
    d. Maltose

11. Epi-Pen is the _____ name for an epinephrine auto-injector.
    a. brand
    b. official
    c. generic
    d. street

12. You are going to be assisting an asthma patient with her medication. Your partner brings you several of her metered dose inhalers. Of the following medication names, which is the generic form?

    a. ventolin
    b. albuterol
    c. proventil
    d. combivent

13. Liquids that contain dissolved drugs are called:

    a. solutions.
    b. suspensions.
    c. suppositories.
    d. transdermals.

14. A _____ is a single dose of medication that is shaped like a disc and can be chewed or swallowed whole.

    a. tablet
    b. capsule
    c. suppository
    d. suspension

15. _____ are a form of medication consisting of liquids with solid particles mixed within them, but not dissolved.

    a. Syrups
    b. Tinctures
    c. Solutions
    d. Suspensions

16. For the patient who is experiencing an asthma attack, the EMT-B should first assist the patient with _____ followed by:

    a. oxygen and the patient's inhaler.
    b. the patient's inhaler and a position of comfort.
    c. a position of comfort and the patient's inhaler.
    d. oxygen and an epinephrine auto-injector.

17. Epinephrine works on a patient who is experiencing anaphylaxis by:

    a. blocking the release of histamines.
    b. dilating coronary vessels and improving oxygenation.
    c. dilating peripheral vessels to relieve itching and hives.
    d. relaxing airway passages and constricting the blood vessels.

18. Activated charcoal works with poisons that have been:

    a. inhaled.
    b. injected.
    c. ingested.
    d. all of the above.

19. Epinephrine is a powerful vasoconstrictor that causes:

    a. increased blood pressure.
    b. decreased blood pressure.
    c. no change in blood pressure.
    d. increased bronchoconstriction.

20. Which of the following is not a "right" of medication administration?

    a. right drug
    b. right dose
    c. right patient
    d. right PPE precautions

21. Bronchodilators, antihistamines, and antihypertensives are all examples of:

    a. forms of medications.
    b. routes of medications.
    c. classifications of medications.
    d. medications the EMT-B can assist a patient with.

22. A/an _____ warns that something is inappropriate as a treatment.

    a. side effect
    b. classification
    c. adverse effect
    d. contraindication

23. _____ is/are derived from both animal and human sources.

    a. Benadryl
    b. Oral glucose
    c. Activated charcoal
    d. Epinephrine and insulin

24. _____ is not a route of drug administration.

    a. Inhalation
    b. Intravenous
    c. Immunization
    d. Intramuscular

25. Which of the following is a route for administering medication?

    a. gas
    b. syrup
    c. sublingual
    d. suspension

26. A/an _____ is a response to a drug that is not the principal intent for giving that drug.

    a. defect
    b. side effect
    c. additive effect
    d. contraindication

27. The most significant side effect of epinephrine is:

    a. anxiety.
    b. increased heart rate.
    c. decreased blood pressure.
    d. decreased respiratory rate.

28. Nitroglycerin works to decrease chest pain by:
    a. constricting coronary vessels and increasing the blood pressure.
    b. dilating coronary vessels, thus increasing blood supply to the heart.
    c. constricting coronary vessels, thus improving oxygenation to the heart.
    d. dilating coronary vessels, thus decreasing the muscle spasm of the heart.

29. _____ is a side effect of bronchodilators.
    a. Increased heart rate
    b. Decreased heart rate
    c. Altered mental status
    d. Increased respiratory rate

30. In the patient with poisoning (whether intentional or unintentional), activated charcoal works by:
    a. absorbing most of the poison.
    b. inactivating the chemical composite.
    c. causing the patient to vomit the poison.
    d. allowing the poison to be reabsorbed, causing dilution.

31. Your unit has been dispatched to the high school for an allergic reaction to a bee sting. In the school nurse's office, a 16-year-old female is sitting up and appears very ill. She is working hard to breathe, is pale and moist, one side of her face is swollen, and she has hives on her neck and arms. The nurse reports that the patient's pulse is 130, weak and regular, and that her BP is 78/40. The patient has a history of allergies to bee stings and used her epinephrine auto-injector shortly after being stung on the face approximately 20 minutes ago. What is the patient's present condition?
    a. She is potentially unstable.
    b. She is in anaphylactic shock.
    c. She is experiencing hypotension as a side effect of the epinephrine.
    d. She has signs and symptoms of a possible reaction to epinephrine as well as the bee sting.

32. (Continuing with the preceding question) You administer high-flow oxygen and confirm that ALS is en route. Further examination findings include wheezing, hives on the front and back torso, and new patient complaints of a swollen tongue, dizziness, and chest tightness. The nurse has additional epinephrine auto-injectors, as well as a few over-the-counter medications, on hand. Which treatment or medication would be the most appropriate for the patient now?
    a. Benadryl
    b. contact medical control for another dose of epinephrine
    c. do not administer any more epinephrine, but treat for shock
    d. provide only high-flow oxygen and wait for ALS to arrive

33. The aunt of a 4-year-old male called EMS when the child developed shortness of breath and wheezing while the child was in her care. She tells you that the child does have a history of asthma and that she has his metered dose inhaler (MDI). However, she has never had to give it until today and she is not sure that she did it correctly. You assess the child and find him to be very anxious; he has audible wheezing, and his skin CTC is pale, warm, and moist. Respiratory rate is 40 and labored, and his pulse is 120, strong and regular. You verify that the MDI is the patient's and obtain permission from medical control to assist the patient with the MDI. You attempt to assist with the MDI, but cannot be sure that any medication was inhaled. The child begins to exhibit tremors and has a significant decrease in mental status. What do you suspect is the cause of the sudden change in the patient's condition?
    a. The medication is beginning to work.
    b. The patient has received a lethal dose of medication.
    c. The tremors and decreased mental status indicate that the patient has received too much medication.
    d. Tremors are a side effect of the medication and the child's decreased mental status is a sign of inadequate breathing.

34. (Continuing with the preceding question) What is the appropriate action to take next?
    a. Rapidly administer an additional dose.
    b. Stop giving the medication and assist ventilations with a BVM.
    c. Request ALS for a possible overdose of medication from the MDI.
    d. Stop giving the medication and administer high-flow oxygen by non-rebreather mask.

35. An elderly male is experiencing respiratory distress from recently diagnosed pneumonia. The patient has a history of COPD, specifically emphysema, and for most of the day and night uses a nasal cannula. Since being discharged from the hospital 2 days ago for the pneumonia, the patient has had progressively worsening dyspnea. He is cyanotic, warm, and dry; lung sounds are diminished on the right; respiratory rate is 28 and labored, pulse is 110 and irregular, and BP is 144/90. You administer high-flow oxygen by non-rebreather mask and prepare the patient for transport. En route to the ED, you see the patient become sleepy, and his respiratory rate and effort decrease. What action is appropriate for this patient now?
    a. Assist the patient's ventilations using a BVM.
    b. Gently wake the patient and encourage him to stay awake.
    c. Replace the non-rebreather mask with a nasal cannula turned on at 2 lpm.
    d. Remove the oxygen and observe the patient for the duration of the transport.

Chapter 16 Answer Form

	A	B	C	D
1.	❑	❑	❑	❑
2.	❑	❑	❑	❑
3.	❑	❑	❑	❑
4.	❑	❑	❑	❑
5.	❑	❑	❑	❑
6.	❑	❑	❑	❑
7.	❑	❑	❑	❑
8.	❑	❑	❑	❑
9.	❑	❑	❑	❑
10.	❑	❑	❑	❑
11.	❑	❑	❑	❑
12.	❑	❑	❑	❑
13.	❑	❑	❑	❑
14.	❑	❑	❑	❑
15.	❑	❑	❑	❑
16.	❑	❑	❑	❑
17.	❑	❑	❑	❑
18.	❑	❑	❑	❑

	A	B	C	D
19.	❑	❑	❑	❑
20.	❑	❑	❑	❑
21.	❑	❑	❑	❑
22.	❑	❑	❑	❑
23.	❑	❑	❑	❑
24.	❑	❑	❑	❑
25.	❑	❑	❑	❑
26.	❑	❑	❑	❑
27.	❑	❑	❑	❑
28.	❑	❑	❑	❑
29.	❑	❑	❑	❑
30.	❑	❑	❑	❑
31.	❑	❑	❑	❑
32.	❑	❑	❑	❑
33.	❑	❑	❑	❑
34.	❑	❑	❑	❑
35.	❑	❑	❑	❑

CHAPTER

17

Respiratory Emergencies

1. The _____ is/are a strong, dome-shaped muscle(s) required for normal respirations.
   a. lungs
   b. tongue
   c. epiglottis
   d. diaphragm

2. The _____ is the pipe-shaped structure through which air moves from the larynx to the lungs.
   a. bronchi
   b. trachea
   c. epiglottis
   d. cricoid cartilage

3. The lower airways are comprised of _____ muscles.
   a. skeletal
   b. cardiac
   c. smooth
   d. voluntary

4. A 26-year-old female with a history of asthma is wheezing, and complaining of breathing difficulty and chest tightness. She also complains of dizziness and tingling in her hands. You should:
   a. provide high-flow oxygen and assist her with her inhaler.
   b. lay her down to relieve the dizziness and assist her with her inhaler.
   c. provide high-flow oxygen for the breathing difficulty and assist her with nitroglycerin for the chest tightness.
   d. get her to slow her breathing to relieve the dizziness and tingling; then, after those symptoms are relieved, administer high-flow oxygen.

5. Which of the following is a symptom rather than a sign of breathing difficulty?
   a. The patient is coughing.
   b. The patient has an altered mental status.
   c. The patient has a sustained increased heart rate.
   d. The patient tells you that it is hard to take a deep breath.

6. You are assessing a patient who is complaining of difficulty breathing. She is speaking in full sentences with no trouble, her skin signs are good, and her lung sounds are clear in all fields. You should:
   a. consider that she may be faking the complaint.
   b. believe her complaint and provide her with high-flow oxygen.
   c. tell her that she is okay for now and have her go to her own doctor.
   d. believe her complaint and withhold oxygen until signs of respiratory distress are present.

7. During a routine return transport of an elderly nursing home resident, from his dental appointment back to the nursing home, you notice that he has fallen asleep. Suddenly the patient has snoring and gurgling respirations. The first action you should take is to:
   a. check for a pulse.
   b. assess responsiveness.
   c. lay the patient supine and suction his airway.
   d. do nothing, as the snoring will stop without intervention.

8. For the patient who is having breathing difficulty, a _____ is indicated whenever the patient needs oxygen, has a good respiratory effort, and is not apneic.
   a. nasal cannula
   b. bag-valve mask
   c. simple face mask
   d. non-rebreather mask

9. Oxygen delivery by nasal cannula is usually tolerated well by most patients, but is contraindicated when a:
   a. patient is a mouth breather.
   b. hypoxic patient will not tolerate a mask.
   c. child with respiratory distress pushes away a non-rebreather mask.
   d. patient with no distress is receiving low to moderate oxygen enrichment for long periods.

10. All of the following patients are having breathing difficulty. For which one would you need medical direction to assist in emergency medical care?

    a. a 14-year-old female with asthma, who is wheezing after gym class
    b. a 30-year-old female with a respiratory rate of 30 after a near-fainting event
    c. an 18-month-old infant who choked on a hot dog and is breathing without distress upon initial assessment
    d. a postictal seizure patient who is awake but confused, with a respiratory rate of 16 breaths per minute

11. A 65-year-old female who is having difficulty breathing tells you that she has history of COPD, hypertension, and diabetes. You listen to her breath sounds and hear faint wheezing. Vital signs are: respiratory rate 26, pulse 78, regular; BP 150/100. Her skin signs are good. Which of the following would you consider assisting her with?

    a. her home nebulizer
    b. her metered dose inhaler
    c. the scheduled insulin dose she is late with
    d. increasing the flow rate on her home oxygen unit

12. Your ambulance has been dispatched for a 16-year-old male who is having difficulty breathing. Upon your initial assessment, you find that he is alert, gasping for air, and has hives on his neck, arms, and chest. Your partner quickly administers high-flow oxygen and you:

    a. look for a possible poisoning agent.
    b. look into the airway for a possible foreign body airway obstruction.
    c. contact medical control for an order to assist with a bronchodilator inhaler.
    d. assist the patient with an epinephrine auto-injector, after obtaining permission from medical control.

13. An elderly man with a history of chronic bronchitis wears a nasal cannula delivering 2 to 4 lpm of oxygen most of the time. He appears distressed and complains of having had increased difficulty breathing since he was recently discharged from the hospital with pneumonia. Initial management of this patient will include:

    a. gentle handling, position of comfort, warmth, and high-flow oxygen by NRB mask if tolerated.
    b. high-flow oxygen by non-rebreather mask, and being prepared with assist with bag-valve ventilations.
    c. sitting the patient upright, giving high-flow oxygen by non-rebreather mask, and assisting with a bronchodilator inhaler.
    d. keeping the patient calm, turning up the oxygen flow on the cannula to 8 lpm, and providing warmth and gentle transport.

14. After responding to a call for a cardiac arrest, you find an unresponsive elderly male who is breathing at a rate of 6 breaths per minute and has a pulse of 60. You attempt to place an OPA, but the patient gags. Now you should:

    a. suction the patient and provide blow-by oxygen.
    b. administer high-flow oxygen via non-rebreather mask.
    c. insert an NPA and provide bag-valve mask ventilations once every 5 seconds.
    d. insert an NPA and provide bag-valve mask ventilations once every 3 seconds.

15. You are attempting to coach an asthmatic patient, who is in respiratory distress, to use her inhaler. You tell her to:

    a. exhale, then inhale while spraying and then hold her breath.
    b. take a deep breath while spraying and hold her breath; then repeat.
    c. slow her breathing, lean forward, spray, inhale, exhale deeply, and repeat.
    d. put her head back, exhale, inhale while spraying, swallow, and hold her breath.

16. You have decided to assist ventilations with a bag-valve mask for a patient with severe breathing difficulty. You know you are providing effective ventilations when:

    a. the chest rises with each ventilation.
    b. the pulse oximetry reading is above 95%.
    c. the patient begins to fight or pushes you away.
    d. there is little or no resistance squeezing the bag.

17. You are assessing and treating a patient who is in respiratory distress. Which of the following signs would give you the indication to assist the patient with bag-valve ventilations?

    a. decreased wheezing respirations and increased retractions
    b. a slowing pulse rate and a decrease in mental status
    c. respiratory rate of 10 and change in pulse rate from 68 to 48 bpm
    d. all of the above

18. In which of the following patients would a nasal pharyngeal airway be most appropriate?

    a. an 80-year-old male in cardiac arrest
    b. a 2-year-old with stridor and drooling
    c. an 18-year-old male who is experiencing a seizure
    d. an alert 24-year-old female who is having an asthma attack

19. In forming a general impression of the patient, the EMT-B can rapidly assess for adequate air exchange by:
    a. noting the skin color.
    b. getting a pulse oximetry reading.
    c. assuring an open and patent airway.
    d. observing movement of the diaphragm.

20. When a patient is receiving ventilations with a BVM, the EMT-B should assess for adequate ventilations by:
    a. assuring a tight mask seal.
    b. assessing for pupillary reactions.
    c. relying on pulse oximeter readings.
    d. assuring that the oxygen flow rate is high.

21. The three signs of adequate air exchange are:
    a. regular rhythm, inability to speak, and warm and pink skin.
    b. alert mental state, equal breath sounds, and a regular rhythm.
    c. high pulse oximetry reading, unilateral breath sounds, and no wheezing.
    d. a rate of 12 to 20 breaths per minute in an adult, pink and dry skin, and unequal chest rise and fall.

22. Before assisting a patient who has respiratory difficulty to administer a dose of his prescribed inhaler, the EMT-B must assure all of the following "rights," except right:
    a. dose.
    b. vital signs.
    c. medication.
    d. prescription for the patient.

23. Which of the following conditions is not an indication for the EMT-B to assist a patient with difficult breathing to use her own prescribed inhaler?
    a. The patient has two different prescribed inhalers.
    b. The patient is experiencing anxiety and a fast pulse rate.
    c. Vital signs and a focused history have yet to be obtained.
    d. An asthma patient has severe breathing difficulty, but no wheezing.

24. A prescribed inhaler containing albuterol has which of the following actions?
    a. dilates coronary vessels
    b. reduces airway constriction
    c. increases mucus production
    d. decreases mucus production

25. You are using a BVM to assist ventilations for a 7-year-old child who has severe breathing distress. You squeeze the bag once every _____ seconds.
    a. 3
    b. 4
    c. 5
    d. 6

26. For the child who is experiencing respiratory distress due to asthma or bronchiolitis, _____ is the most important treatment the EMT-B can provide.
    a. oxygen
    b. rapid transport
    c. a bronchodilator
    d. a prescribed inhaler

27. A 12-month-old infant is suspected of having swallowed a marble and is now unresponsive. The correct sequence for treating a foreign body airway obstruction (FBAO) when no foreign body is visible in the airway is to:
    a. open the airway, do a finger sweep, and give a breath and back blows.
    b. open the airway, give a breath, administer abdominal thrusts, and repeat.
    c. open the airway and give a breath, back blows, and chest thrusts. Repeat as needed.
    d. perform back blows, chest thrusts, and a finger sweep, and give a breath.

28. Signs and symptoms of _____ include pain and difficulty swallowing, profound drooling, a sore throat, and difficulty breathing.
    a. croup
    b. epiglottitis
    c. bronchitis
    d. pneumonia

29. _____ is swelling in the upper airways caused by an infection and is marked by a mild or severe seal-like bark; it usually occurs in children in the 3-month to 3-year age group.
    a. Croup
    b. Asthma
    c. Epiglottitis
    d. Bronchiolitis

30. _____ is an infection that results in a swelling of the lower airways and typically occurs in children less than 2 years of age during the winter and spring seasons.
    a. Croup
    b. Epiglottitis
    c. Bronchiolitis
    d. Emphysema

31. Respiratory exchange between the lung and blood vessels occurs in the:
    a. alveoli.
    b. bronchi.
    c. bronchioles.
    d. coronary vessels.

32. The _____ closes during swallowing to prevent food or liquids from entering the lower airways.
    a. larynx
    b. mouth
    c. trachea
    d. epiglottis

33. The primary respiratory center, which controls the stimulus to breathe, is located in the:
   a. brain.
   b. lungs.
   c. heart.
   d. diaphragm.

34. During exhalation, carbon dioxide is:
   a. converted to energy.
   b. eliminated from the body.
   c. dissolved into the bloodstream.
   d. retained as needed in asthmatics.

35. Hypoxia is defined as a:
   a. total absence of oxygen.
   b. lack of oxygen in the blood.
   c. deficit of red blood cells in the blood.
   d. lack of oxygen in the tissues of the body.

36. _____ is a whistling sound caused by constriction of the lower airways, and is most often heard at the end of exhalation.
   a. Stridor
   b. Croup
   c. Grunting
   d. Wheezing

37. A person with breathing distress may be found in a tripod position because this position:
   a. prevents air trapping in the upper airways.
   b. reduces pressure in the pulmonary vessels.
   c. allows more expansion of the rib cage and lungs.
   d. helps to prevent excessive use of accessory muscles to breathe.

38. _____ occurs with exhalation against a partially opened epiglottis, and is an abnormal sound heard primarily in infants and small toddlers. It is usually a sign of breathing distress.
   a. Stridor
   b. Grunting
   c. Gasping
   d. Whooping cough

39. An irregular breathing pattern associated with diabetic acidosis is referred to as:
   a. hyperventilation.
   b. agonal respirations.
   c. Kussmaul's respirations.
   d. Cheyne-Stokes respirations.

40. When a patient with breathing distress tells you that she has been coughing up green sputum, this is a sign of:
   a. hypoxia.
   b. a respiratory infection.
   c. a chronic breathing disorder.
   d. impending respiratory failure.

41. For a patient with breathing difficulty, what is the significance of a history of cigarette smoking?
   a. Smoking may set off an asthma attack.
   b. Smoking may exacerbate a recent pneumonia.
   c. Smoking may have caused a chronic lung disease or worsened it.
   d. All of the above.

42. When listening to breath sounds with a stethoscope, the _____ sounds are louder and clearer than _____ sounds.
   a. posterior, anterior
   b. anterior, posterior
   c. wheezing, stridorous
   d. rales, wheezing

43. When connecting a BVM to an oxygen source, which piece attaches to the regulator?
   a. the bag
   b. the reservoir
   c. the pop-off valve
   d. oxygen tubing

44. _____ is a technique used to measure the percentage of hemoglobin saturated with oxygen.
   a. Capnography
   b. Capillary refill
   c. Hypoxic drive
   d. Pulse oximetry

45. _____ is an abnormal condition that results in a collection of air in the pleural space of the chest; it can cause one or both lungs to collapse.
   a. Pleurisy
   b. Pneumonia
   c. Pneumothorax
   d. Tension pneumothorax

46. COPD is a progressive and irreversible lung disease that is prevalent in which age group?
   a. the elderly
   b. young adults
   c. the middle-aged
   d. persons more than 90 years of age

47. A person experiencing an asthma attack may also be described as having:
   a. COPD.
   b. bronchospasm.
   c. Kussmaul's respirations.
   d. foreign body airway obstruction.

48. Hyperventilation results in too much intake of _____ and an excessive elimination of _____.
   a. oxygen, glucose
   b. oxygen, carbon dioxide
   c. carbon dioxide, oxygen
   d. oxygen, carbon monoxide

49. Which of the following traumatic injuries is associated with breathing distress?
   a. broken rib
   b. spinal fracture
   c. bruised heart
   d. all of the above

50. During the physical examination of a child who has severe breathing distress, where would you expect to see retractions?
   a. nares
   b. mouth
   c. neck and chest
   d. chest and back

Chapter 17 Answer Form

	A	B	C	D			A	B	C	D
1.	❏	❏	❏	❏		26.	❏	❏	❏	❏
2.	❏	❏	❏	❏		27.	❏	❏	❏	❏
3.	❏	❏	❏	❏		28.	❏	❏	❏	❏
4.	❏	❏	❏	❏		29.	❏	❏	❏	❏
5.	❏	❏	❏	❏		30.	❏	❏	❏	❏
6.	❏	❏	❏	❏		31.	❏	❏	❏	❏
7.	❏	❏	❏	❏		32.	❏	❏	❏	❏
8.	❏	❏	❏	❏		33.	❏	❏	❏	❏
9.	❏	❏	❏	❏		34.	❏	❏	❏	❏
10.	❏	❏	❏	❏		35.	❏	❏	❏	❏
11.	❏	❏	❏	❏		36.	❏	❏	❏	❏
12.	❏	❏	❏	❏		37.	❏	❏	❏	❏
13.	❏	❏	❏	❏		38.	❏	❏	❏	❏
14.	❏	❏	❏	❏		39.	❏	❏	❏	❏
15.	❏	❏	❏	❏		40.	❏	❏	❏	❏
16.	❏	❏	❏	❏		41.	❏	❏	❏	❏
17.	❏	❏	❏	❏		42.	❏	❏	❏	❏
18.	❏	❏	❏	❏		43.	❏	❏	❏	❏
19.	❏	❏	❏	❏		44.	❏	❏	❏	❏
20.	❏	❏	❏	❏		45.	❏	❏	❏	❏
21.	❏	❏	❏	❏		46.	❏	❏	❏	❏
22.	❏	❏	❏	❏		47.	❏	❏	❏	❏
23.	❏	❏	❏	❏		48.	❏	❏	❏	❏
24.	❏	❏	❏	❏		49.	❏	❏	❏	❏
25.	❏	❏	❏	❏		50.	❏	❏	❏	❏

CHAPTER

18

Cardiovascular Emergencies

1. The _____ is the largest artery in the cardiovascular system.
   a. aorta
   b. superior vena cava
   c. left pulmonary artery
   d. right pulmonary artery

2. The _____ pumps blood into the pulmonary circulation.
   a. left ventricle of the heart
   b. right ventricle of the heart
   c. diaphragm
   d. coronary arteries

3. Which of the following statements is most correct regarding the function of the heart?
   a. Contraction and relaxation of the heart normally occur simultaneously.
   b. The four valves of the heart normally open and close at the same time.
   c. Heart sounds are generated by the sound of contracting coronary blood vessels.
   d. The four valves of the heart normally open and close to carry the flow of blood forward.

4. When a patient is experiencing chest pain or discomfort, place the patient:
   a. in a position of comfort.
   b. lying down with legs elevated, after assisting with nitroglycerin.
   c. supine, because this is the best position if CPR becomes necessary.
   d. on the side, because nausea and vomiting are common with chest pain.

5. When the EMT-B is assessing a patient who is experiencing acute chest discomfort, she should:
   a. assess for a possible pneumothorax.
   b. call medical control before transporting the patient.
   c. look for signs of trauma before starting any treatment.
   d. treat the patient as if he is having a life-threatening event.

6. When treating a patient who has chest pain, the goal for the EMT-B is to:
   a. help increase the workload on the heart.
   b. relax skeletal muscle with nitroglycerin if possible.
   c. reduce the patient's blood pressure with nitroglycerin.
   d. provide high-flow oxygen and transport quickly without increasing the patient's anxiety.

7. The EMT-B should attach an AED to a patient who is unresponsive:
   a. with no signs of circulation, and is apneic.
   b. and is under the supervision of hospice care.
   c. seizing, and is breathing at a rate of six breaths per minute.
   d. and was witnessed to be choking prior to becoming unresponsive.

8. Which of the following situations indicates a need to use an AED?
   a. a 60-year-old cancer patient who is unresponsive, is not breathing, and has no pulse
   b. an 8-year-old who is unresponsive after being hit in the chest with a soccer ball, but has a pulse
   c. a 54-year-old male who is complaining of severe chest pain, and has profuse sweating and no distal pulse
   d. an unresponsive elderly patient in a nursing home who was found in bed and who is not breathing, but has a pulse

9. You are treating a patient whom you suspect is having a heart attack. For which of the following reasons would you attach an AED?
   a. You witness an arrest en route to the hospital.
   b. The patient has taken his nitroglycerin three times with no relief.
   c. The patient tells you he has had two heart attacks in the last 10 years.
   d. The patient is responsive but has an implanted defibrillator that is firing.

10. Which of the following is not a contraindication for attaching an AED to a patient?
    a. an unresponsive patient with a radial pulse
    b. CPR was not started prior to attaching the AED
    c. an unresponsive patient with no breathing and a carotid pulse
    d. an AED that has fully charged batteries, but did not discharge on a test at the beginning of the shift

11. You are alone in the back of the ambulance treating and transporting a patient for chest pain when suddenly she becomes unresponsive, pulseless, and stops breathing. Now you should:
    a. attach and turn on the AED.
    b. start CPR and attach the AED.
    c. advise the driver to turn on the siren and lights.
    d. attach the AED, start CPR, and ventilate the patient.

12. The role of the EMT-B in the chain of survival is early:
    a. access and CPR.
    b. advanced life support.
    c. CPR and defibrillation.
    d. defibrillation and advanced care.

13. For the morbidly obese patient, defibrillation:
    a. has a better response to high-energy doses.
    b. is less successful than in patients of normal weight.
    c. is more successful than in patients of normal weight.
    d. is administered in energy doses that are the same as for any other patient.

14. Defibrillation for a child under the age of 8 or weighing less than 25 kg (55 lbs) is:
    a. never recommended.
    b. possible with a biphasic defibrillator only.
    c. possible with a monophasic defibrillator only.
    d. possible with an AED using pediatric pads (electrodes).

15. A patient with crushing chest pain and no difficulty breathing also complains of weakness and dizziness when he tries to walk. The most likely position of comfort for this patient will be _____ position.
    a. semi-Fowler's
    b. high Fowler's
    c. Trendelenburg
    d. left lateral recumbent

16. For the patient with acute breathing difficulty, crackles in the lungs, and a history of congestive heart failure, the most likely position of comfort will be:
    a. lying down.
    b. sitting upright.
    c. lying on the side.
    d. Trendelenburg position.

17. You are treating an 85-year-old female who woke up in the middle of the night with difficulty breathing and severe chest pain. While you are taking her vital signs, her mental status decreases significantly and you lay her down. At this point you:
    a. suction her airway and insert an OPA.
    b. do nothing, as she is still breathing on her own.
    c. attempt to insert an OPA and begin to ventilate with a BVM.
    d. make sure the non-rebreather mask fits properly and then turn up the flow rate.

18. The primary goal of airway management for the patient who is in cardiac arrest is:
    a. to suction for no longer than 15 seconds.
    b. to insert an OPA and maintain cervical stabilization.
    c. to hyperventilate the patient until her color improves.
    d. to maintain a good mask seal and assure chest rise.

19. You are working with a paramedic when a call comes in for a cardiac arrest. The paramedic asks you to provide basic life support while he prepares his equipment. You begin by:
    a. checking vital signs, suctioning, and ventilating with a BVM.
    b. verifying pulselessness and starting CPR.
    c. hyperventilating the patient so that the paramedic can intubate.
    d. directing bystanders to assist with CPR so you can set up the IV bag.

20. You have successfully converted a witnessed cardiac arrest with three shocks from the AED. The patient now has a pulse, is breathing, and is awakening. At this point you should:
    a. cancel ALS and transport.
    b. be prepared for the patient to arrest again.
    c. take the AED off the patient and transport.
    d. be prepared to give the patient nitroglycerin if chest pain returns.

21. Which of the following statements about early defibrillation is most correct?
    a. V-tach with or without a pulse will always result in death without early defibrillation.
    b. In cardiac arrest due to V-fib, the rhythm will deteriorate into a nonshockable rhythm after two minutes.
    c. In cardiac arrest due to asystole, the victim has a better chance of survival with an AED than with CPR.
    d. A sudden death patient has the best chance of survival when an AED is available (and used) before EMS arrives at the victim's side.

22. When the heart is unable to produce effective contractions because of disorganized electrical conduction, the AED will rapidly:
    a. indicate "No shock advised."
    b. reanalyze after 60 seconds.
    c. recognize V-fib as a shockable rhythm.
    d. recognize slow V-tach as a shockable rhythm.

23. A 32-year-old female is complaining of chest pain in the left lower side of her chest. She denies shortness of breath, but states that it hurts to take a deep breath. You find an antibiotic, which she is taking for a respiratory infection. She is also a smoker with a new productive cough. Your treatment should include:
    a. oxygen, attachment of the AED, and nitroglycerin.
    b. oxygen, warmth, position of comfort, and nitroglycerin.
    c. position of comfort, routine transport, and reassessment.
    d. oxygen, warmth, position of comfort, and routine transport.

24. You have assisted a 56-year-old male to take his nitroglycerin. His chest pain came on suddenly as he was shoveling snow, and was totally relieved with oxygen and the nitroglycerin. Now you should:
    a. let the patient sign a refusal and refer him to his cardiologist.
    b. attach the AED, monitor him, and transport the patient to the hospital.
    c. attach the AED and give another nitroglycerin if his blood pressure is adequate.
    d. continue oxygen therapy and perform serial assessments en route to the hospital.

25. When Advanced Cardiac Life Support (ACLS) is available in the prehospital setting to patients with a cardiac emergency,:
    a. the AED will never be needed.
    b. the patient will always have a better outcome.
    c. defibrillation is secondary to the medications the patient can receive.
    d. advanced airway management and emergency medications may improve survival.

26. For the victim of cardiac arrest, the chance of survival is:
    a. highest when ACLS is available in the prehospital setting.
    b. higher when ACLS is available upon arrival at the hospital.
    c. low if ACLS is not available in the prehospital setting.
    d. best when ACLS is available immediately following early defibrillation.

27. Upon completing a focused history and physical exam of a 74-year-old female with severe chest pain, you determine that her blood pressure is quite low, making it a contraindication for assisting with nitroglycerin. You should now:
    a. do not move her, call for ALS, and wait for them to provide IV fluids before transporting.
    b. call medical control and ask for an order for nitroglycerin, because the pain is getting worse.
    c. gently lay her supine on your stretcher, treat her for shock, and rapidly transport her to the hospital.
    d. administer high-flow oxygen, place her in Trendelenburg position, and make a routine transport.

28. The patient you are caring for has chest pain and shortness of breath, and appears to be in severe distress. The ALS unit you called for is 15 minutes away and your patient is in the ambulance ready for transport. Because the hospital is 10 minutes away, you decide to:
    a. begin rapid transport to the hospital.
    b. assist the patient with nitroglycerin and meet the ALS unit en route.
    c. get an order to assist with nitroglycerin while you wait for the ALS unit to arrive.
    d. begin routine transport to the hospital and attempt to meet the ALS unit en route.

29. A/an _____ AED delivers approximately 200 joules for the initial shock to an adult in cardiac arrest.
    a. biphasic
    b. implanted
    c. monophasic
    d. investigational

30. A _____ AED supplies nonescalating defibrillation energy doses for patients 25 kg (55 lbs) and larger.
    a. 12-lead
    b. limb-lead
    c. biphasic
    d. monophasic

31. The difference between a fully automated and a semi-automated defibrillator is that the:
    a. automated defibrillator uses less power.
    b. automated defibrillator requires no training.
    c. semi-automated defibrillator requires someone to interpret the rhythm.
    d. semi-automated defibrillator indicates when it is time to press the shock button.

32. The EMT-B may find a/an _____ AED, prescribed by a physician, in the home of a cardiac patient who is at high risk for V-fib or V-tach.
    a. implanted
    b. experimental
    c. investigational
    d. fully automated

33. While traveling through the airport, you observe a crowd of excited people at the next gate and hear someone yelling "Call 9-1-1." You go over and see an elderly male unresponsive on the floor and an airline employee attaching AED pads to his chest. The employee stops what he is doing when he discovers that the patient's internal defibrillator is firing. What should you do now?

    a. Stand by and watch, as the employee is doing a good job so far.
    b. Offer to do CPR while you wait for the internal defibrillator to stop firing.
    c. Quickly identify yourself as an EMT-B and push the "Analyze" button on the AED.
    d. Identify yourself as an EMT-B, offer to help, and quickly encourage the employee to begin the AED sequence.

34. You have responded to the local high school track for a man who has collapsed on the oval track. It is raining, the patient is soaked, and he is unresponsive, not breathing, and has no pulse. What must be done before utilizing an AED?

    a. Move the patient into the ambulance.
    b. Remove all the wet clothes from the patient.
    c. Check to see if the patient has an implanted defibrillator.
    d. Dry off the patient's chest before applying the electrode.

35. The patient you have been treating for respiratory distress has progressively worsened and now is apneic. Which of the following actions should you take?

    a. Begin CPR, attach the AED pads, turn on the AED, and press "Analyze."
    b. Perform CPR for one minute and then assess breathing and pulse.
    c. Move the patient to a long backboard and assess for pulselessness.
    d. Insert an OPA, begin ventilations with a BVM, and check for a pulse.

36. Many EMS agencies have a policy stating that the AED should not be used when a patient is found to be breathing or has a pulse. The reason for this is:

    a. to prevent accidental or inappropriate defibrillation.
    b. that the AED cannot verify if the patient has a pulse.
    c. AEDs are designed only for use on cardiac arrest victims.
    d. all of the above.

37. Which of the following conditions may result in inappropriate defibrillation of a patient?

    a. The patient is not lying flat on her back.
    b. The patient is in respiratory arrest and is attached to an AED.
    c. The patient is too obese for the AED to monitor adequately.
    d. The patient is too small for the AED to monitor adequately.

38. Which of the following reasons is rarely the cause of inappropriate shocks?

    a. The user has not been trained in the use of AED.
    b. The AED was giving the prompt "Shock advised."
    c. The AED is one month past due for routine maintenance.
    d. The patient was being moved at the time of rhythm analysis.

39. During the transport to the hospital with an adult patient who is in cardiac arrest, how often should CPR be interrupted when using the AED?

    a. every 5 minutes
    b. every 10 minutes
    c. every 15 minutes
    d. CPR should not be interrupted during transport

40. After attaching AED pads to a patient, at which point during two-person CPR is it appropriate to interrupt CPR to analyze the patient?

    a. immediately
    b. after the next ventilation is complete
    c. after the patient has been placed on a long backboard
    d. after completing the current cycle of compressions and ventilations

41. AEDs have the capability of recording each event for review after the call, and are used for quality assurance purposes by the medical director of an agency. This feature is considered to be a/an:

    a. disadvantage for the user.
    b. advantage of the AED device.
    c. disadvantage in the event of a lawsuit.
    d. nuisance for the recordkeeper of an EMS agency.

42. _____ is/are a disadvantage of using AEDs.

    a. Ongoing training and routine maintenance
    b. The minimal steps needed to complete the shock sequence
    c. The time it takes to verify apnea and pulselessness
    d. The amount of time it takes to determine if a rhythm is shockable

43. The amount of time it takes to apply the pads of an AED to a patient, turn on the device, and initiate the analyzing mode:
    a. is a disadvantage of the device.
    b. is easy for most individuals to work within.
    c. impedes the time for delivering the first shock.
    d. takes more than two minutes for a trained rescuer.

44. With training and continued practice, the EMT-B is expected to be able to deliver three successive shocks within _____ seconds after arriving at the side of a victim who is in cardiac arrest.
    a. 30
    b. 60
    c. 90
    d. 120

45. Defibrillating a patient with an AED is considered to be _____ because the energy is delivered to the patient through remote adhesive pads.
    a. hands-on
    b. hands-off
    c. dangerous
    d. spontaneous

46. The possibility of the user being shocked by an AED is very low because:
    a. of the infrequent use of the device.
    b. the amount of electricity is too weak to reach the user.
    c. of the use of remote defibrillation through adhesive pads.
    d. of the amount of training required for proficiency with the device.

47. After administering several shocks over a period of 15 minutes to a patient who is in cardiac arrest, with no successful conversion, the AED should remain attached and turned on during transport because:
    a. the pads are too difficult to remove.
    b. the hospital will need to check if pad placement is correct.
    c. all patients in cardiac arrest must be monitored for no less than 30 minutes.
    d. the AED will continue to monitor the patient and advise if a change in rhythm is detected.

48. Which statement about AED rhythm monitoring is most correct?
    a. An AED will never advise you to shock a conscious patient.
    b. The AED will monitor a patient only when in the analyze mode.
    c. All patients at risk for cardiac arrest should be monitored with an AED.
    d. Some AEDs will advise you to shock a patient who is in a fast V-tach rhythm even if the patient has a pulse.

49. Before the AED is used on a patient who is in cardiac arrest, the EMT-B should:
    a. establish an airway, begin CPR, and call for ALS.
    b. check with the family for a do not resuscitate (DNR) order.
    c. search the patient for a medical identification tag or bracelet.
    d. have checked the batteries and run a test at the start of his shift.

50. Select the correct sequences of steps for use of the semi-automatic AED once the device reaches the patient.
    a. Turn on the device, attach the pads, stop CPR, activate the AED sequence, and shock if advised.
    b. Verify pulselessness, attach the pads, turn on the device, stop CPR, and activate the AED sequence.
    c. Attach the pads, verify pulselessness, stop CPR, turn on the device, and activate the AED sequence.
    d. Stop CPR, verify pulselessness, turn on the device, attach the pads, activate the AED sequence, and shock if advised.

51. After being on the scene of a cardiac arrest for 10 minutes, you have begun transport to the nearest hospital, which will take 20 minutes. When you are 5 minutes away from the hospital, the AED continues to advise you to shock the patient. You should now:
    a. continue CPR only.
    b. change the batteries in the AED.
    c. continue to shock the patient as advised.
    d. run a test to be sure the AED is working properly.

52. You resume CPR after administering three shocks to an apneic and pulseless patient. Now you should:
    a. continue CPR and wait for ALS to arrive.
    b. stop CPR and reanalyze every 10 minutes.
    c. search for a do not resuscitate directive.
    d. continue CPR and place the patient on a long backboard.

53. Shortly after giving three shocks and resuming CPR, the AED does an analysis and reads "No shock advised." You prepare the patient for transport and re-analyze the patient, but this time the AED advises you to deliver a shock. At this point you:
    a. clear the patient and shock as advised.
    b. disregard the "shock advised" message because of the prior reading.
    c. assume that the AED read the patient's movement as V-fib and reanalyze.
    d. disregard the "shock advised" message because the patient has been down too long.

54. Two bystanders in an airport successfully converted a pulseless patient with an AED that was hanging on the wall. The patient awoke after being defibrillated twice. While you are getting the patient on the stretcher, he becomes unresponsive, stops breathing, and loses his pulse. What should you do first?

    a. Start CPR.
    b. Check for a blood pressure.
    c. Reanalyze and shock if indicated.
    d. Immobilize the patient's neck and back.

55. When two EMT-Bs with an AED arrive at the side of a patient who is not breathing and has no pulse, they should first:

    a. perform CPR for 1 minute, call for more help, and attach the AED.
    b. apply the AED as quickly as possible and check for a shockable rhythm.
    c. place the patient on a long backboard, then check for a shockable rhythm.
    d. perform CPR for 3 minutes, then attach the AED and assess for a shockable rhythm.

56. When a single rescuer with an AED arrives at the side of a patient who is not breathing and has no pulse, the steps to take, in order, are:

    a. call for help, turn on and attach the AED, and shock if advised.
    b. attach and turn on the AED, call for help, and shock if advised.
    c. perform CPR for one minute, call for help, attach and turn on the AED.
    d. call for help, perform CPR for one minute, attach and turn on the AED.

57. You are about to deliver the first shock with an AED to a pulseless patient. The next pulse check should be taken after:

    a. the first shock.
    b. 1 minute of CPR.
    c. switching positions with your partner.
    d. the third shock, or when no shock is advised.

58. When delivering the first three shocks with an AED, the EMT-B should:

    a. check for a pulse between each shock, because the AED cannot verify a pulse.
    b. not check for a pulse between each shock, to avoid delay in delivering the shocks.
    c. check for a pulse between each shock, to be sure the patient does not have a pulse.
    d. always check for a pulse before and after each shock, to avoid an unnecessary shock.

59. Shortly after delivering three shocks with an AED, two paramedics arrive on the scene to assist you. What steps should you take now?

    a. Stop CPR and go get the stretcher.
    b. Turn off and remove the AED and let the paramedics attach their monitor.
    c. Continue CPR and report any patient information you have obtained so far.
    d. Deliver another set of three shocks while you give verbal report to the paramedics.

60. For the last link in the chain of survival to be effective, there has to be:

    a. prehospital ACLS available in every community.
    b. rapid transport of the cardiac arrest patient to the emergency department.
    c. an emergency department within a 10-minute transport for each cardiac arrest victim.
    d. practical coordination between ACLS trained providers and the personnel using the AED.

61. After shocking the victim of an electrocution twice with the AED, the patient has a return of pulses and no further shocks are advised. What should be done next?

    a. Immobilize the patient to a long backboard.
    b. Quickly search for entrance and exit wounds.
    c. Assist ventilations and obtain a blood pressure.
    d. Administer high-flow oxygen with a non-rebreather mask.

62. Which of the following should the EMT-B include in the postresuscitation care of a patient resuscitated from V-fib?

    a. Leave the AED attached and turned on.
    b. Leave the AED attached, but turn it off.
    c. Remove the AED pads from the patient.
    d. Allow the patient to assume a position of comfort.

63. For the victim of cardiac arrest with a return of pulses and respirations, _____ is a critical factor in postresuscitation care.

    a. warmth
    b. rapid transport
    c. airway management
    d. C-spine stabilization

64. The victim of a near-drowning, who was initially pulseless, is now breathing and has a pulse after CPR and one shock from the AED. Which of the following complications can you expect with this type of patient?

    a. vomiting
    b. hypoxia
    c. hypothermia
    d. all of the above

65. Which of the following is not an appropriate step in the postresuscitation care of a patient revived from a cardiac arrest?
   a. telling the family that the patient is going to be all right
   b. assisting an ACLS provider with ventilation and intubation
   c. obtaining the patient's past medical history from a family member
   d. explaining to the family what is happening and what they can expect at the hospital

66. Postresuscitation care for every victim of cardiac arrest includes:
   a. obtaining one set of vital signs.
   b. endotracheal intubation.
   c. advanced cardiac life support.
   d. rapid transport to the nearest trauma center.

67. You are working with a partner who has been out of work for several months. He asks you to help him get comfortable using the AED again. How can you best help him?
   a. Give him a testing form and let him practice with a simulator.
   b. Have him practice alone with a mannequin and a training video.
   c. Give him a testing form to review and let him watch a training video.
   d. Using a mannequin, practice with him and provide him with feedback.

68. One of the best ways for an EMT-B to stay proficient at the use of AEDs is to:
   a. rehearse with a simulator monthly.
   b. watch a training videotape monthly.
   c. complete the operator's checklist each shift.
   d. complete a recertification course once every two years.

69. The AED operator's shift checklist should be completed by:
   a. the supervisor.
   b. the most junior crew member.
   c. the most senior crew member.
   d. anyone on the crew trained to use the AED.

70. One of the most common reasons for failure of an AED to work properly when needed is:
   a. dead batteries.
   b. operator error from lack of practice.
   c. aging of the internal components of the AED.
   d. failure to complete a checklist on a regular basis.

71. For citizens in a community to have the best chance of surviving a cardiac event, which of the following elements has to be in place?
   a. high numbers of citizens trained in CPR
   b. an EMS system with ACLS-trained personnel
   c. an active public access defibrillation program
   d. all of the above

72. In the American Heart Association's "Chain of Survival," early _____ is the first link where the possible use of an AED is set in motion.
   a. CPR
   b. access
   c. defibrillation
   d. advanced life support

73. Before the EMT-B who works within an EMS agency may use an AED, she must:
   a. meet the medical director.
   b. directly observe its use on a patient.
   c. be trained and certified in its use for at least 30 days.
   d. meet the training requirements of the medical director.

74. The role of the medical director regarding use of an AED is to:
   a. oversee training and recordkeeping.
   b. provide guidance in the selection and purchase of AEDs.
   c. follow up with the family of every patient on whom an AED was used.
   d. be involved directly or through a designee with each aspect relating to the AED.

75. A case review should be completed following the use of the AED because:
   a. it is a state and federal health care mandate.
   b. if you make a mistake your partner will not be faulted.
   c. it is an effective tool for improving future skills performance.
   d. if your paperwork gets lost, the AED will have a record of the events.

76. When the victim of a cardiac arrest does not survive, how can the EMT-B be assured that his skill performance on the call was appropriate?
   a. Talk to the patient's family.
   b. Obtain a copy of the autopsy report.
   c. Ask the supervisor to evaluate the patient care report.
   d. Obtain feedback on the case review with the medical director.

77. Which of the following is generally not included in a case review of a cardiac arrest for which an AED was used?
    a. the time it took to deliver the first shock
    b. appropriate assessment and interventions
    c. following the EMS agency's AED protocol
    d. the outcomes for patients with anterior infarcts versus lateral infarcts

78. Your medical director is going to do a case review with you for the last cardiac arrest call you had. Which component(s) of the care review might he discuss with you?
    a. run times and documentation
    b. frequency of AED training and practice
    c. ACLS integration with BLS providers
    d. all of the above

79. Which of the following is typically considered a goal of quality improvement regarding AED use?
    a. assessing training and skills needs
    b. making all the links in the "Chain of Survival" stronger
    c. tracking and reporting data relating to respiratory arrests calls
    d. disciplining for incorrect actions or inappropriate defibrillation

80. You have been asked to participate in your EMS agency's quality improvement program. Your role in this program will be to:
    a. act as a liaison between your agency and mutual aid agencies.
    b. help determine appropriate disciplinary action for coworkers who have poor patient skills.
    c. participate in case reviews and help strengthen your link in the "Chain of Survival."
    d. ask each of your patients to complete an evaluation form on your performance after the call.

81. When you assess the pulse of your patient, you find that it is quite irregular. How can you best obtain an accurate count?
    a. Attach the AED and monitor the rhythm.
    b. Count the number of beats for 1 minute.
    c. Listen to the heartbeats with a stethoscope and count for 2 minutes.
    d. Have the most senior crew member assess the pulse.

82. When a patient tells you that he has an implanted defibrillator, this means that:
    a. the patient is at high risk for a cardiac event.
    b. the patient has definitely had a heart attack in the past.
    c. the heart's natural pacemaker does not work anymore.
    d. the patient has had more than one heart attack in the past.

83. Within minutes of assisting a patient with chest pressure to take her nitroglycerin, you reevaluate her blood pressure and find that it has dropped below 100 systolic. The patient still has chest pressure, so what should you do now?
    a. Lay her down and assist her with another nitroglycerin pill.
    b. Do nothing, because a drop in blood pressure is normal after taking nitroglycerin.
    c. Elevate her legs; the blood pressure will come up after a few minutes.
    d. Lay her down, begin transport, and call medical control to advise of the change in blood pressure.

84. After completing a focused history and physical exam of a 58-year-old male with a complaint of chest pain that radiates into the neck and jaw, you discover that before calling EMS, the patient took one dose of nitroglycerin with no relief. Now you are going to:
    a. utilize your local protocol for additional doses of nitroglycerin.
    b. transport the patient with oxygen only, as nitroglycerin did not work.
    c. give the patient a dose of aspirin, provide high-flow oxygen, and transport.
    d. call medical control and request an order for aspirin, as nitroglycerin did not work.

85. Before you assist a patient with nitroglycerin, you must complete each of the following, except:
    a. obtain an OPQRST and SAMPLE history.
    b. verify that the patient has a cardiac history.
    c. assure that the blood pressure is adequate.
    d. obtain an order from the patient's physician.

86. Which one of the following group of patient complaints is an indication for the use of nitroglycerin?
    a. chest tightness, weakness, and labored breathing
    b. slurred speech, shortness of breath, and weakness in the left arm
    c. difficulty breathing, wheezing, and tingling in the hand, arms, and face
    d. a brief fainting episode followed by sweating, nausea, and vomiting

87. Your patient is complaining of shortness of breath and a heavy feeling in his chest. He has a history of angina, but tells you that this pain is different. His vital signs are: respirations 36, shallow; pulse 58, irregular; BP 90/50. Which of these findings is a contraindication for the use of nitroglycerin with this patient?
    a. hypotension
    b. the shortness of breath
    c. pain that is not his typical angina pain
    d. pulse is too slow and respirations are too fast

88. You have been ordered by medical control to assist a patient complaining of chest discomfort to take his nitroglycerin for the first time. However, the physician has asked you to explain the possible side effects of the medication. You tell the patient:

    a. that the taste is unpleasant.
    b. that he will experience a burning sensation.
    c. to lean forward, as he might feel nauseated and vomit.
    d. to lie back on the stretcher, as he might feel dizzy or lightheaded.

89. Which of the following statements is most correct regarding the controls on an AED?

    a. All AEDs have the same functions and controls.
    b. All semi-automated AEDs have voice prompts.
    c. Every AED has different functions and control buttons.
    d. Each brand of AED has standardized functions so that they can be used in the same manner.

90. Which of the following tasks is considered maintenance for an AED?

    a. recharging the batteries every day
    b. changing the defibrillation pads after each use
    c. rotating the defibrillation pads on a monthly basis
    d. following the instructions in the user's manual for recommended service

Chapter 18 Answer Form

	A	B	C	D		A	B	C	D
1.	❏	❏	❏	❏	33.	❏	❏	❏	❏
2.	❏	❏	❏	❏	34.	❏	❏	❏	❏
3.	❏	❏	❏	❏	35.	❏	❏	❏	❏
4.	❏	❏	❏	❏	36.	❏	❏	❏	❏
5.	❏	❏	❏	❏	37.	❏	❏	❏	❏
6.	❏	❏	❏	❏	38.	❏	❏	❏	❏
7.	❏	❏	❏	❏	39.	❏	❏	❏	❏
8.	❏	❏	❏	❏	40.	❏	❏	❏	❏
9.	❏	❏	❏	❏	41.	❏	❏	❏	❏
10.	❏	❏	❏	❏	42.	❏	❏	❏	❏
11.	❏	❏	❏	❏	43.	❏	❏	❏	❏
12.	❏	❏	❏	❏	44.	❏	❏	❏	❏
13.	❏	❏	❏	❏	45.	❏	❏	❏	❏
14.	❏	❏	❏	❏	46.	❏	❏	❏	❏
15.	❏	❏	❏	❏	47.	❏	❏	❏	❏
16.	❏	❏	❏	❏	48.	❏	❏	❏	❏
17.	❏	❏	❏	❏	49.	❏	❏	❏	❏
18.	❏	❏	❏	❏	50.	❏	❏	❏	❏
19.	❏	❏	❏	❏	51.	❏	❏	❏	❏
20.	❏	❏	❏	❏	52.	❏	❏	❏	❏
21.	❏	❏	❏	❏	53.	❏	❏	❏	❏
22.	❏	❏	❏	❏	54.	❏	❏	❏	❏
23.	❏	❏	❏	❏	55.	❏	❏	❏	❏
24.	❏	❏	❏	❏	56.	❏	❏	❏	❏
25.	❏	❏	❏	❏	57.	❏	❏	❏	❏
26.	❏	❏	❏	❏	58.	❏	❏	❏	❏
27.	❏	❏	❏	❏	59.	❏	❏	❏	❏
28.	❏	❏	❏	❏	60.	❏	❏	❏	❏
29.	❏	❏	❏	❏	61.	❏	❏	❏	❏
30.	❏	❏	❏	❏	62.	❏	❏	❏	❏
31.	❏	❏	❏	❏	63.	❏	❏	❏	❏
32.	❏	❏	❏	❏	64.	❏	❏	❏	❏

	A	B	C	D		A	B	C	D
65.	❏	❏	❏	❏	78.	❏	❏	❏	❏
66.	❏	❏	❏	❏	79.	❏	❏	❏	❏
67.	❏	❏	❏	❏	80.	❏	❏	❏	❏
68.	❏	❏	❏	❏	81.	❏	❏	❏	❏
69.	❏	❏	❏	❏	82.	❏	❏	❏	❏
70.	❏	❏	❏	❏	83.	❏	❏	❏	❏
71.	❏	❏	❏	❏	84.	❏	❏	❏	❏
72.	❏	❏	❏	❏	85.	❏	❏	❏	❏
73.	❏	❏	❏	❏	86.	❏	❏	❏	❏
74.	❏	❏	❏	❏	87.	❏	❏	❏	❏
75.	❏	❏	❏	❏	88.	❏	❏	❏	❏
76.	❏	❏	❏	❏	89.	❏	❏	❏	❏
77.	❏	❏	❏	❏	90.	❏	❏	❏	❏

CHAPTER 19

Diabetes, Altered Mental Status, and Seizures

1. A 30-year-old female with a history of diabetes was found unresponsive. The patient's husband tells you that she does not take insulin because she controls her blood sugar with her diet. What type of diabetes does the patient most likely have?

   a. type 1
   b. type 2
   c. type 3
   d. type 4

2. The adult female patient you are assessing appears dazed. She responds to her name but is confused about the day of the week and other questions you ask her. A neighbor who is on the scene tells you he thinks she is an insulin-dependent diabetic. In an effort to confirm this, you ask your partner to:

   a. perform a prehospital stroke exam.
   b. look in the refrigerator for her insulin.
   c. search the apartment for needles and syringes.
   d. check her blood pressure to see if she is hypotensive.

3. You are dispatched on a call for a sick person who is vomiting. Upon arrival, you form a general impression of a conscious elderly male who is sitting up at his desk complaining of a tingling sensation in his face. In slow speech, he keeps repeating the phrase "I am low." Your next action would be to:

   a. administer oral glucose.
   b. complete an initial assessment.
   c. consider that the patient is having a stroke.
   d. consider that the patient is hyperventilating.

4. You have responded to a call for a fall and find that the patient is in bed. He appears awake, yet stunned. Family members tell you that the patient is an insulin-dependent diabetic who was fine before tripping and falling. What step(s) should you take first?

   a. Perform a rapid trauma exam.
   b. Take C-spine precautions, then assess and manage the ABCs.
   c. Ask a family member to use the patient's glucometer to check his blood sugar.
   d. Apply high-flow oxygen and assist the patient with high-concentration oral glucose.

5. A patient with an altered mental status is taking diabetic medicine and has a history of diabetes. If you are unable to measure the blood sugar or are uncertain, you should:

   a. call for ALS.
   b. assume that the blood sugar is low.
   c. assume that the blood sugar is high.
   d. look for another cause of altered mental status.

6. The mother of an 11-year-old patient who is unresponsive and has a history of diabetes tells you that they checked the blood sugar reading an hour ago and it was 130 mg/dl. No trauma was involved, so you suspect that:

   a. there may have been a medication dosing error.
   b. the patient's glucometer is not properly calibrated.
   c. the cause of the altered mental status is low blood sugar until proven otherwise.
   d. all of the above.

7. You have been called to transport a male teenager who was witnessed drinking alcohol. He appears to be very intoxicated but is cooperative getting into the ambulance. This patient is at high risk for _____, making airway management a high priority.

   a. vomiting
   b. seizures
   c. hypoglycemia
   d. hyperglycemia

8. Select the adjunct most appropriate for an adult male who is unresponsive and seizing.
    a. oropharyngeal airway
    b. nasopharyngeal airway
    c. soft-tip suction catheter
    d. rigid-tip suction catheter

9. An unresponsive 19-year-old female is suspected of having taken an overdose of sleeping pills. She is breathing shallowly in a regular pattern at a rate of 12 bpm. You begin airway management by:
    a. ventilating with a BVM at 20 to 24 bpm.
    b. administering oxygen by nasal cannula and suctioning with a rigid-tip catheter.
    c. administering oxygen by nasal cannula and suctioning with a soft-tip catheter.
    d. attempting to insert an airway adjunct and administering high-flow oxygen by NRB.

10. You are to assist a patient with a slightly altered mental status to take some oral high-concentration glucose gel. Before you do so, you need to:
    a. taste the gel to see if it is fresh.
    b. get suction ready in case of vomiting.
    c. call for ALS in case the oral glucose does not work.
    d. confirm a diabetic history and/or check for diabetic medications.

11. Orange juice, non-diet sodas, and oral gel-type high-glucose in toothpaste-like tubes are all:
    a. dangerous for the patient who has type 1 diabetes.
    b. contraindicated for use in the patient with no history of diabetes.
    c. commercial oral high-concentration glucose products for diabetic emergencies.
    d. high-concentration glucose products that may be ingested to raise the blood sugar.

12. One method of assisting a conscious diabetic patient with an altered mental status is to place oral high-concentration glucose gel between the cheek and gum. This method works to improve mental status by:
    a. reducing the risk of hypoxia.
    b. stimulating the release of insulin.
    c. increasing a person's sensitivity to insulin.
    d. the rapid absorption of glucose through a highly vascular area.

13. A diabetic patient who had an altered mental status was assisted to eat a tube of high-concentration glucose gel. Approximately 15 minutes later, the patient has become more alert. Management of this patient will now include:
    a. continuing to reassess and beginning transportation.
    b. doing nothing until a blood sugar reading is obtained.
    c. calling for ALS, as the patient is going to need IV glucose.
    d. calling medical control and asking to assist with two additional tubes of glucose.

14. When caring for a patient with a possible diabetic problem, the EMT-B should call medical direction:
    a. only if ALS is not available.
    b. according to local protocols.
    c. only if the patient appears to be going into respiratory arrest.
    d. after completing a focused history and physical exam and before beginning treatment.

15. The wife of an unresponsive patient who has a history of diabetes tells you that she tried to give her husband orange juice prior to your arrival but was unsuccessful. The patient has an open airway, is breathing adequately, and has a strong pulse. The management steps for this patient include:
    a. rapid transport, serial vital signs, and a detailed physical exam while en route.
    b. high-flow oxygen, monitor vital signs, contact medical control, and transport.
    c. assist with oral glucose gel under the tongue, obtain vital signs, and transport.
    d. assist with oral glucose gel between the cheek and gum, obtain vital signs, and perform a focused history and physical exam.

16. When a diabetic gets too much insulin, the effects on the body include:
    a. a decrease in mental status.
    b. cells becoming starved for glucose.
    c. a significant drop in blood sugar levels.
    d. all of the above.

17. For a diabetic patient who meets the criteria, the quick administration of oral glucose by the EMT-B means that:
    a. a diabetic emergency is being managed appropriately.
    b. blood sugar levels will return to normal within 30 minutes.
    c. the patient may complain of abdominal pain after awakening.
    d. transport to the hospital will not be necessary once the patient awakens.

18. When the blood sugar falls to a hypoglycemic state, the longer a patient remains hypoglycemic the more likely there will be:
    a. urinary incontinence.
    b. a drop in blood pressure.
    c. a fruity smell on the breath.
    d. permanent damage to brain cells.

19. The function of insulin is to:
    a. carry sugar from the blood into the cells.
    b. carry sugar from the cells into the blood.
    c. break down glucagon and create energy.
    d. prevent too much sugar from being released into the bloodstream.

20. The most common cause of seizures in toddlers is:
    a. trauma.
    b. poison ingestion.
    c. drug or alcohol related.
    d. a rapid increase in body temperature.

21. You are assessing a patient with an altered mental status. She is very confused, but is becoming more awake as you obtain vital signs and complete a rapid trauma exam. The patient is wearing a medic alert device which tells you she has seizures. Your primary concern for this patient now is:
    a. to be prepared for another seizure.
    b. to be alert for incontinence and take precautions.
    c. to call medical control and request to assist the patient with oral glucose.
    d. to wait for the patient to become more alert, then assist with oral glucose.

22. When a patient has two or more seizures without a period of consciousness in between, the condition is known as status epilepticus. The danger that makes this a true emergency is that:
    a. the patient can swallow his tongue.
    b. the patient is at risk for traumatic injury.
    c. prolonged seizures can cause brain damage.
    d. prolonged seizures cause extreme states of hypoglycemia.

23. A family has called EMS because Grandpa had fallen several times in the last 2 days. They described him having had a couple of periods of "fogginess and forgetfulness." This patient has an extensive history of heart disease and high blood pressure, and recently he had surgery on his leg for vascular problems. Which of the following do you suspect is the cause of the change over the last 2 days?
    a. infection
    b. mini-strokes
    c. dehydration
    d. new onset of diabetes

24. This morning the wife of an elderly patient had trouble waking her husband, so she called EMS. She tells you he is not a diabetic, but takes medication for high blood pressure, and that this has never happened before. The patient does not respond to you verbally and you find a complete weakness on the left side of the body during your physical exam. Management of this patient will include:
    a. being prepared for a seizure, administering high-flow oxygen, and observing for vomiting.
    b. obtaining a temperature if possible, administering high-flow oxygen, and treating for shock.
    c. high-flow oxygen, supportive care, and early notice to the hospital for a possible stroke.
    d. high-flow oxygen, contacting medical control to assist with oral glucose, and rapid transport.

25. The family of an elderly woman has called EMS because they noticed that during lunch she had a brief period of looking stunned, followed by a change in speech. She now seems better. The patient has no past medical history and takes only vitamins. You suspect that the:
    a. patient had a mini-stroke.
    b. patient is developing dementia.
    c. patient had low blood sugar, which improved after she finished her lunch.
    d. family may not be fully forthcoming because they are trying to get the woman admitted to the hospital for a while.

26. Which of the following conditions in a diabetic patient, left untreated, can cause altered mental status due to hypoglycemia?
    a. infection
    b. wheezing
    c. asthma attack
    d. traumatic injury

27. The roommate of a 23-year-old female returned home from the drug store to find that her friend was difficult to awaken. She was sweaty and hot to the touch as well. Except for the patient becoming suddenly sick during the night, there is no significant past medical history, no medications, and no allergies. Which of the following is most likely the cause of the altered mental status in this patient?
    a. seizure
    b. infection
    c. hypoglycemia
    d. hyperglycemia

28. The EMT-B should consider altered mental status in an elderly patient to be associated with _____ until proven otherwise.
    a. stroke or TIA
    b. tachycardia
    c. abuse or neglect
    d. hypoxia or hypoglycemia

29. You have responded to a call for abdominal pain. When you meet the patient, it is obvious that her eyes and skin are yellow. After obtaining a focused history, you have learned that she has unknowingly taken an excessive amount of acetaminophen over the past two days for a toothache. After managing the ABCs, you call medical control and discuss:
    a. the use of activated charcoal.
    b. the reporting of a possible suicide attempt.
    c. the reporting of an accidental overdose.
    d. withholding oxygen due to abnormal hemoglobin binding.

30. The parents of a teenager called EMS because they found their daughter in her bed in a sluggish state and two empty pill bottles in her room. The parents tell you that she has been depressed and is taking medication. Your first action(s) is/are to:
    a. manage the ABCs.
    b. estimate how many pills are missing.
    c. call medical control or poison control for directions.
    d. consider hypoxia and low blood sugar as a cause of the altered mental status.

31. A woman called EMS because her mother had fainted and fallen at home. Your general impression is that of a 64-year-old female who is sitting up with no apparent signs of distress or injury. The daughter reports that the patient has a history of hypertension and arthritis, and that she had been well prior to the brief loss of consciousness. Your initial assessment findings are that the patient is unable to talk; she has an open airway with adequate respiratory effort, clear lung sounds, strong and regular distal pulse, and skin is pink, warm, and dry. What action would be appropriate next?
    a. Administer oral glucose.
    b. Assess the patient further for signs of stroke.
    c. Search the residence for alcohol or drugs that are commonly abused.
    d. Perform a rapid trauma assessment, while remaining alert for signs of physical abuse.

32. (Continuing with the preceding question) You now administer oxygen, and finish obtaining a SAMPLE history and OPQRST information from the daughter as your partner obtains vital signs. The patient is compliant with her medications, has no allergies, and has never had a similar episode. The patient is able to answer questions by moving her head, and she denies any difficulty breathing, pain, or injury. Vital signs are: respiratory rate 16; pulse 66, strong and regular; BP 148/90; SpO2 is 100%. The patient has weakness, which requires that you lift her onto the stretcher. As you settle the patient into the ambulance, she begins to speak, but has slurring. What do you suspect is happening to the patient, and what can you do to confirm your suspicions?
    a. The patient has signs and symptoms of a transient ischemic attack. Perform serial assessments using a stroke scale.
    b. The patient may have an alcohol or substance abuse problem and now the effects of the alcohol or substance are probably wearing off. Take any medications found at the residence to the hospital.
    c. The patient has signs and symptoms of a head injury. Perform an ongoing assessment focusing on mental status and vital signs.
    d. The patient may have a new onset of diabetes and be hypoglycemic. Continue to administer additional oral glucose and watch for signs of improvement.

33. EMS was dispatched for an unresponsive male in his fifties. When you enter the residence, you find the patient on the floor with his eyes closed. He appears disoriented, as he repeatedly waves his right arm in small circles. His airway is clear and he is breathing adequately; his skin is pale, moist, and very cold. He will not respond to you. Family members state that they found him on the floor when they got up this morning and that he is a diabetic. They have a glucagon kit for emergencies, but are not sure how to use it. You confirm that ALS is en route and will arrive within 5 minutes. During that time, what actions should you take?
    a. Administer one tube of oral glucose.
    b. Administer glucagon from the patient's emergency kit.
    c. Administer oxygen, move the patient off the cold floor, and provide warmth.
    d. Administer oxygen and immobilize the patient to keep him from harming himself.

34. You have been dispatched to a call for severe headache. At the residence you find the patient to be a 24-year-old female who is alert and sitting up, complaining of pain from the worst headache she has ever experienced. The pain started suddenly after she came home from jogging. The patient also has extreme weakness and numbness in the right arm and leg and is unable to stand up. The vital signs are: respiratory rate 22; pulse rate 90, strong and regular; BP 180/110; skin CTC is pink, warm, and moist. Management of this patient will include:

   a. administration of oxygen, protection of the weak and numb extremities, and rapid transport to a stroke center.
   b. observation only of the patient, as she has most likely hyperventilated to cause the presenting symptoms.
   c. fully immobilizing the patient on a long backboard, as her symptoms are consistent with a traumatic head injury.
   d. administering oxygen, determining if the patient is pregnant, providing supportive care, and transporting to the hospital of her choice.

35. The wife of a 71-year-old male calls EMS because she thinks her husband is having a stroke. When you arrive, she tells you that the patient was watching television when the symptoms began. She says that her mother had a stroke and that she recognized her husband as having very similar symptoms. As part of the stroke assessment, which of the following will you examine the patient for?

   a. facial droop, arm drift, and abnormal speech
   b. evidence of hypertension and inability to move all extremities
   c. abnormal speech, equal grip strength, and ability to walk a straight line
   d. arm drift or weakness, evidence of headache, or new onset of hearing loss

Chapter 19 Answer Form

	A	B	C	D			A	B	C	D
1.	❑	❑	❑	❑		19.	❑	❑	❑	❑
2.	❑	❑	❑	❑		20.	❑	❑	❑	❑
3.	❑	❑	❑	❑		21.	❑	❑	❑	❑
4.	❑	❑	❑	❑		22.	❑	❑	❑	❑
5.	❑	❑	❑	❑		23.	❑	❑	❑	❑
6.	❑	❑	❑	❑		24.	❑	❑	❑	❑
7.	❑	❑	❑	❑		25.	❑	❑	❑	❑
8.	❑	❑	❑	❑		26.	❑	❑	❑	❑
9.	❑	❑	❑	❑		27.	❑	❑	❑	❑
10.	❑	❑	❑	❑		28.	❑	❑	❑	❑
11.	❑	❑	❑	❑		29.	❑	❑	❑	❑
12.	❑	❑	❑	❑		30.	❑	❑	❑	❑
13.	❑	❑	❑	❑		31.	❑	❑	❑	❑
14.	❑	❑	❑	❑		32.	❑	❑	❑	❑
15.	❑	❑	❑	❑		33.	❑	❑	❑	❑
16.	❑	❑	❑	❑		34.	❑	❑	❑	❑
17.	❑	❑	❑	❑		35.	❑	❑	❑	❑
18.	❑	❑	❑	❑						

CHAPTER

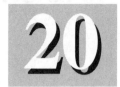

Allergies

1. A patient who is experiencing an allergic reaction might have which of the following findings associated with the upper airway?
   a. stridor
   b. wheezing
   c. bronchospasm
   d. pulmonary edema

2. Which group of symptoms suggests an allergic reaction that has not progressed to anaphylaxis?
   a. wheezing, abdominal cramps, and nausea
   b. hives on the upper arms, sweating, and confusion
   c. blotches and itching on the arms, back, chest, and thighs
   d. pale skin color, dizziness, and rash on the chest and arms

3. In the patient who is experiencing an allergic reaction, which of the following findings associated with the skin is typically not present?
   a. redness or rash
   b. hives and swelling
   c. pallor and sweating
   d. jaundice and blisters

4. You are working with a new partner today. You are returning to service from the last call when you notice that your partner's hands are red and slightly swollen. He tells you that his hands are itchy, but otherwise he feels fine. What should you do next?
   a. Call your supervisor and ask to be placed with another partner.
   b. Suspect a possible latex allergy and go back to the emergency department.
   c. Have your partner wash his hands thoroughly and report the incident to the supervisor.
   d. Go back to the emergency department and try to determine if your last patient has an infectious disease.

5. At a standby for a soccer game, a parent approaches you with her 8-year-old son who has two bee stings on his lower leg. The mother tells you that she removed the stingers but she would like you to look at the child. Which of the following findings would you consider significant, requiring treatment by EMS?
   a. swelling of the lips
   b. the child is crying
   c. local swelling at the site of the sting
   d. all of the above

6. Responding to a call for a possible allergic reaction, you find a 36-year-old female who took a new antibiotic prescription two hours ago and now feels very sleepy. Her vital signs are: respirations 20, adequate; pulse 78, regular; BP 114/68; skin CTC is pink, warm, and dry. She denies difficulty breathing, but feels there is something wrong. Management of this patient includes:
   a. treatment for shock and rapid transport.
   b. administration of oxygen, position of comfort, reassessment, and transport.
   c. administration of high-flow oxygen, assistance with an epi auto-injector, and rapid transport.
   d. calling medical control for permission to let the patient sign off and follow up with her own physician.

7. While playing football, a 16-year-old male disturbed a wasp nest and was stung approximately 10 times. He has redness at the sites and is developing a rash on his chest. He is also complaining of chest tightness. You begin airway management with:
   a. high-flow oxygen by non-rebreather mask.
   b. inspecting the mouth for stings and swelling.
   c. assisting the patient to use his epinephrine auto-injector.
   d. removal of any remaining stingers, to prevent further exposure to antigens.

8. While at school, a 14-year-old girl ate a cookie not knowing that it contained a nut to which she has a known allergy. She is complaining of chest tightness and swelling of the tongue, and her respiratory rate is 30. How should you manage the airway?

    a. Lay the patient down with legs elevated and assist ventilations with a BVM.

    b. Keep the patient calm and administer oxygen with a nasal cannula at 6 lpm.

    c. Keep the patient calm, place an NPA in the right nostril, and administer high-flow oxygen with a non-rebreather mask.

    d. Allow the patient to stay in a position of comfort, administer high-flow oxygen with a non-rebreather mask, and be prepared to assist ventilations with a BVM.

9. Your unit is dispatched for an unresponsive 28-year-old male. His wife tells you that the patient complained of being bitten or stung by an insect in the lower left leg before collapsing. You quickly determine that he has inadequate breathing and is cyanotic. You begin to manage the airway by:

    a. inserting an OPA and assisting ventilations with a BVM.

    b. suctioning as needed and assisting ventilations with a BVM.

    c. suctioning the airway, inserting an OPA, and administering high-flow oxygen with a non-rebreather mask.

    d. inserting an NPA, suctioning, and then assisting ventilations with a pocket mask connected to oxygen.

10. _____ is the trade name for the medication in an auto-injector prescribed for severe allergic reactions.

    a. Adrenalin

    b. Benadryl

    c. Epinephrine

    d. Epi Pen Jr.

11. _____ is the generic name for the medication in an auto-injector prescribed for severe allergic reactions.

    a. Epi Pen

    b. Adrenalin

    c. Epinephrine

    d. Bronchodilator

12. For a severe allergic reaction with respiratory distress, the administration of epinephrine is a high priority because:

    a. the effects reduce toxicity from antigens.

    b. it is an antidote for many types of allergens.

    c. it relaxes the smooth muscles of the airways.

    d. the effects are similar to that of an anesthetic.

13. Select the proper order of steps in the procedure for the use of an epinephrine auto-injector.

    a. Remove the cap, place the injector tip against the patient's thigh, push the injector, and hold in place for 10 seconds.

    b. Remove the cap and discard it in a sharps container, shake the injector gently, aim the tip into the patient's upper arm, and inject for 15 seconds.

    c. Shake the injector gently, hold the injector with the tip down, place against the patient's thigh, avoiding any area of hives, and inject.

    d. Shake the injector vigorously, record the time, place the injector tip against the patient's upper arm, and dispose of the injector in a sharps container.

14. The form of epinephrine that comes in an auto-injector is a:

    a. gel.

    b. liquid.

    c. spray.

    d. crystal.

15. When assessing a patient who is experiencing an allergic reaction, which of the following findings would prompt you to call medical control immediately?

    a. skin flushing

    b. swelling of the hands

    c. the presence of shock

    d. hives on the arms and legs

16. Which of the following is not an indication for the use of an epinephrine auto-injector?

    a. The patient has a history of multiple allergies.

    b. The patient has signs and symptoms of severe allergic reaction.

    c. Medical direction has authorized the use of the auto-injector online.

    d. Medical direction has authorized the use of the auto-injector offline.

17. For the patient with signs and symptoms of progressive allergic reaction, the EMT-B should contact medical control:

    a. as soon as possible.

    b. only when signs and symptoms become severe.

    c. only when signs of respiratory distress are present.

    d. only if administration of the first epinephrine auto-injector does not begin to work within 10 minutes.

18. You are treating and transporting the victim of a low-speed MVC. You have the patient fully immobilized because of a suspected spinal injury. On the way to the hospital, you notice that the patient's skin is red where you have placed adhesive tape. How would you manage this patient now?

    a. Ask the patient if she has ever had to use an epinephrine auto-injector.
    b. Leave the patient secured as is and continue to monitor and reassess her.
    c. Call medical control right away and discuss the use of an epinephrine auto-injector.
    d. Remove the adhesive tape and perform a focused physical exam for a possible allergic reaction.

19. Which of the following factors is a good indicator that a mild allergic reaction may progress to a severe allergic reaction?

    a. multiple prior exposures to the antigen
    b. no known prior exposures to the antigen
    c. the amount of body surface area covered with hives
    d. the speed of onset of symptoms from time of exposure

20. An office manager calls EMS because one of the employees has suddenly developed blotchy redness on her face, neck, and arms over the past 2 hours. The employee says that she has had a runny nose and nasal congestion for three days, but the redness is new. She has no other complaints. What do you suspect is wrong with this patient and how will you manage her?

    a. She has signs of a severe reaction and needs epinephrine and rapid transport.
    b. She has signs of a mild allergic reaction, so provide supportive care and transport for evaluation.
    c. There are no significant findings and the patient has no serious complaints, so help her contact her own physician to follow up.
    d. She is progressing to a severe reaction, so be prepared to assist with an epinephrine auto-injector and begin rapid transport.

21. Which of the following statements is most correct about the use of an epinephrine auto-injector for anaphylaxis?

    a. Epinephrine does not work with allergens that have been inhaled.
    b. The use of epinephrine for anaphylaxis will always save the patient's life.
    c. Any patient with signs and symptoms of anaphylaxis needs to be treated with epinephrine.
    d. For best results, epinephrine should be administered within the first 30 minutes after exposure to the allergen.

22. For the patient experiencing anaphylactic shock with hypotension and no respiratory distress, the use of an epinephrine auto-injector is:

    a. contraindicated.
    b. not a BLS treatment.
    c. for medical direction to decide.
    d. a priority and will increase the blood pressure.

23. Select the proper steps in the management of a patient who is experiencing anaphylaxis.

    a. Treat for shock, assist with an epinephrine auto-injector if available, and transport.
    b. Assist with an epinephrine auto-injector if available, administer high-flow oxygen, and transport.
    c. Begin rapid transport to the nearest hospital, administer high-flow oxygen, and assist with an epinephrine auto-injector if available.
    d. Maintain airway support, assist with an epinephrine auto-injector if available, treat for shock, and transport to the nearest hospital.

24. The main goal in the treatment of anaphylaxis is to:

    a. alleviate hives and rash.
    b. relieve abdominal cramping.
    c. relieve itching and swelling.
    d. restore respiratory and cardiac efficiency.

25. Which of the following side effects is typical with the use of epinephrine in anaphylaxis?

    a. seizure
    b. tachycardia
    c. nausea or vomiting
    d. headache or dizziness

26. After assisting a patient who is experiencing anaphylactic shock to administer his own epinephrine auto-injector, you should expect:

    a. breathing effort to improve.
    b. tachycardia and palpitations.
    c. the blood pressure to improve.
    d. all of the above.

27. The use of epinephrine in the elderly comes with a precaution because:

    a. it can cause hypertension.
    b. the side effects are long-lasting.
    c. it increases the workload on the heart.
    d. of its incompatibility with other prescribed medications.

28. The dose of epinephrine in an auto-injector is _____ mg for adults and _____ mg for pediatrics.

    a. 0.3, 0.15
    b. 3.0, 1.5
    c. 1.5, 0.3
    d. 0.03, 0.015

29. Epinephrine has several side effects, of which _____ is/are the most serious.
    a. nausea
    b. anxiety
    c. cardiac dysrhythmias
    d. respiratory depression

30. The effects of epinephrine are:
    a. slow onset and short-lasting.
    b. slow onset and long-lasting.
    c. rapid onset and short-lasting.
    d. rapid onset and long-lasting.

Chapter 20 Answer Form

	A	B	C	D			A	B	C	D
1.	❏	❏	❏	❏		16.	❏	❏	❏	❏
2.	❏	❏	❏	❏		17.	❏	❏	❏	❏
3.	❏	❏	❏	❏		18.	❏	❏	❏	❏
4.	❏	❏	❏	❏		19.	❏	❏	❏	❏
5.	❏	❏	❏	❏		20.	❏	❏	❏	❏
6.	❏	❏	❏	❏		21.	❏	❏	❏	❏
7.	❏	❏	❏	❏		22.	❏	❏	❏	❏
8.	❏	❏	❏	❏		23.	❏	❏	❏	❏
9.	❏	❏	❏	❏		24.	❏	❏	❏	❏
10.	❏	❏	❏	❏		25.	❏	❏	❏	❏
11.	❏	❏	❏	❏		26.	❏	❏	❏	❏
12.	❏	❏	❏	❏		27.	❏	❏	❏	❏
13.	❏	❏	❏	❏		28.	❏	❏	❏	❏
14.	❏	❏	❏	❏		29.	❏	❏	❏	❏
15.	❏	❏	❏	❏		30.	❏	❏	❏	❏

CHAPTER

21

Poisoning/Overdose

1. Children are at highest risk for exposure to toxic substances by:
   a. injection.
   b. ingestion.
   c. inhalation.
   d. absorption.

2. Carbon monoxide poisoning is an example of an _____ exposure to a toxic substance.
   a. injection
   b. ingestion
   c. inhalation
   d. absorption

3. _____ is a toxic substance that is typically introduced into the body by absorption.
   a. Lead paint
   b. A pesticide
   c. Carbon monoxide
   d. A poisonous mushroom

4. Of the following statements, which is most correct regarding the signs and symptoms of poisoning?
   a. The effects of toxic substances will not be immediately apparent.
   b. Signs and symptoms vary widely and depend on the substance and amount taken into the body.
   c. Any time a toxic substance is taken into the body, the patient will have signs of an altered mental status.
   d. Any patient with a decreased pulse and respiratory rate should be considered for exposure to a toxic substance.

5. The most dangerous toxic substances affect the _____ system(s).
   a. respiratory
   b. nervous
   c. endocrine and gastrointestinal
   d. respiratory, nervous, and endocrine

6. The most significant findings associated with signs and symptoms of poisoning are:
   a. age-related.
   b. headache and seizures.
   c. changes in the size of the pupils.
   d. those that affect the ABCs.

7. The police have called you to transport an intoxicated patient. You assess a 52-year-old male who is conscious, but has slurred speech, smells of alcohol, has filthy clothing, and does not answer your questions appropriately. Management of this patient will include:
   a. performing a detailed physical exam and being alert for vomiting or seizures.
   b. getting him on the stretcher and letting him sleep during the transport to the hospital.
   c. obtaining vital signs, assessing for incontinence, and removing his clothing prior to arrival at the hospital.
   d. obtaining vital signs and performing a physical exam while being alert for any other causes of altered mental status.

8. An elderly patient's home health aide has called EMS because she found three empty medication bottles that should be nearly full according to the dates on the bottles. Initial assessment of the patient reveals that she is conscious but confused; she does not recall taking any medications. Her vital signs are: respirations 18, adequate; pulse 60, regular; BP 148/90. What should you do next?
   a. Administer activated charcoal.
   b. Verify the home health aide's credentials.
   c. Obtain a focused history and perform a physical exam.
   d. Attempt to get the patient to vomit and take the vomitus to the hospital.

9. The father of a toddler calls EMS because he thinks his child has eaten an entire box of throat lozenges. The father is quite upset and the child is crying. What should you do next?

   a. Notify dispatch to send a crisis counselor to the scene.
   b. Call the child's pediatrician and notify her about the incident.
   c. Talk to the father and obtain a focused history, while your partner assesses the child.
   d. Tell the father there is nothing to worry about, as there is no potential danger from ingesting throat lozenges.

10. Two women custodians who used cleaning products in a confined space for approximately one hour are now complaining of dizziness and nausea. They deny difficulty breathing, chest pain, or vomiting. Lung sounds are clear and neither of them has red eyes or tearing. The emergency medical care for these patients begins with:

    a. decontaminating the patients.
    b. calling the poison control center for instructions.
    c. locating the material safety data sheet (MSDS).
    d. removing them from the confined area and providing high-flow oxygen.

11. You are obtaining a focused history from a patient with suspected poisoning. Which of the following questions is of least significance for the EMT-B?

    a. How much was ingested?
    b. When did the poisoning occur?
    c. Has this substance been ingested before?
    d. What, if anything, has been done for treatment so far?

12. Your next-door neighbor calls you and says that her 20-month-old son has eaten an unknown amount of toothpaste; she wants to know what to do. What steps should you take now?

    a. Tell her to flush out the child's mouth and give him milk to drink.
    b. Call poison control and get instructions before going next door to help.
    c. Call 9-1-1 for the neighbor, then go over and begin assessing the child.
    d. Tell her to call 9-1-1, because you really cannot give any advice while off-duty.

13. A 16-year-old female is suspected of taking multiple prescriptions in a suicide attempt. She is unresponsive to pain with the following vital signs: respirations 8, shallow and inadequate; pulse 58, regular; BP 100/40. Your first steps in managing this patient include:

    a. hyperventilating the patient with a BVM.
    b. suctioning and administering high-flow oxygen by non-rebreather mask.
    c. attempting oropharyngeal airway insertion and assisting ventilations with a BVM.
    d. inserting a nasopharyngeal airway and administering high-flow oxygen by non-rebreather mask.

14. EMS was called to a residence where a party is going on. Friends of the unresponsive patient describe him as having had way too much to drink, and they are unable to wake him. The patient has snoring respirations at a rate of 12 per minute; distal pulse of 60, strong and regular; skin is normal color, warm, and dry. Initial airway management should include:

    a. placing the patient in the recovery position.
    b. suctioning, and assisting ventilations with a BVM.
    c. inserting an OPA and administering high-flow oxygen by non-rebreather mask.
    d. inserting an NPA and administering high-flow oxygen by non-rebreather mask.

15. A contractor accidentally splashed liquid chlorine into his face. He is alert and breathing adequately, but complains of severe burning pain in both eyes. The initial management for this patient includes:

    a. calling medical control for advice prior to touching him.
    b. not touching the patient until the fire department arrives to decontaminate him.
    c. removing the patient's clothing and continuously irrigating the eyes and face.
    d. irrigating the eyes and face for five minutes, administering high-flow oxygen, and rapid transport.

16. Due to the unpleasant appearance of activated charcoal, it should be administered by:

    a. putting a blindfold on the patient.
    b. pinching the nose shut and closing the eyes.
    c. having the patient close her eyes and chug.
    d. sipping through a straw out of a foam cup.

17. The generic name for the antidote used for ingested poisons is:

    a. Super char.
    b. charcola.
    c. Charco aide.
    d. activated charcoal.

18. You are about to assist your partner with administering activated charcoal to a patient who has ingested a poison. What form of medication will you be using?
    a. liquid
    b. oral spray
    c. slow-acting tablets
    d. fast-dissolving capsules

19. A family of five is complaining of symptoms of carbon monoxide poisoning. Before you arrived, the fire department took the family outside into the fresh air. All five patients have severe headache, three are vomiting violently, and two have nausea. Select the correct steps in the management of these patients.
    a. Triage, contact medical control, then treat and transport.
    b. Manage the ABCs, declare a multiple casualty incident, and triage.
    c. Declare a multiple casualty incident, then triage, treat, and transport.
    d. Call dispatch and ask for four more ambulances, then triage and contact medical control.

20. You are treating a patient who ingested a chemical product thinking it was his coffee. He is alert and complaining of burning in his mouth and throat. His vital signs are stable. Your protocols allow you to administer activated charcoal on standing orders, but you think the chemical may be corrosive. What should you do?
    a. Call medical control for instructions.
    b. Have the patient gargle with an antiseptic.
    c. Have the patient flush out his mouth with milk.
    d. Administer the activated charcoal on standing orders.

21. The fire department carried a victim out of a confined space that had noxious fumes in it. The patient is conscious but confused. While you are listening to his breath sounds, he begins to seize. You protect the patient from injury and ask your partner to:
    a. suction and insert an oropharyngeal airway.
    b. call medical control for decontamination instructions.
    c. administer high-flow oxygen and be prepared to assist with ventilations.
    d. call medical control and request an order to administer activated charcoal.

22. A frantic young mother calls EMS because one of her preschool-aged children ingested an entire bottle of baby aspirin, thinking it was candy. The use of activated charcoal in this patient is:
    a. not indicated, because of the child's age.
    b. contraindicated for aspirin ingestion.
    c. indicated and will work for aspirin overdose.
    d. indicated, but probably will not work for aspirin overdose.

23. One hour after ingesting a full bottle of prescription sleeping pills, the patient vomited the pills. Now that the patient has vomited, the use of activated charcoal is:
    a. indicated, as it will help decrease the effects of depression.
    b. indicated, as it will absorb toxins still present in the GI tract.
    c. not indicated, because the patient has eliminated the toxins.
    d. not indicated, because there was not enough time for the toxins to become dangerous.

24. In a case of severe poisoning, the primary precaution associated with the administration of activated charcoal is:
    a. vomiting.
    b. hypotension.
    c. abdominal bloating.
    d. a decreased mental status.

25. In the prehospital management of a poisoned or overdosed patient, the EMT-B should contact medical direction early, because:
    a. it takes a while to prepare the activated charcoal.
    b. if you wait too long to give activated charcoal, it will not be effective.
    c. medical control clarifies treatment options recommended by poison control.
    d. all of the above.

26. A 48-year-old female attempted suicide by taking 20 pills of her mother's prescription pain medication. The mother discovered the attempt moments after the ingestion. After obtaining vital signs, a focused history, and physical exam, you quickly call medical control to get an order for activated charcoal, because:
    a. activated charcoal is indicated for many ingested poisons.
    b. the sooner the activated charcoal is administered, the quicker it can bond to the toxin.
    c. many pain medications cause an altered mental status, which would prevent you from giving the activated charcoal.
    d. all of the above.

27. After assessing and providing high-flow oxygen to a patient who accidentally ingested too much of a prescription antibiotic, you call medical control to obtain an order to administer activated charcoal. You explain to the patient that the actions of activated charcoal are:
    a. slow.
    b. delayed.
    c. immediate.
    d. long-lasting and require only one dose.

28. Common side effects of the use of activated charcoal for management of a poisoning include all of the following, except:

    a. constipation.
    b. nausea and vomiting.
    c. abdominal cramping.
    d. decreased mental status.

29. The standard adult dose of activated charcoal for the management of poisoning is:

    a. 50 grams.
    b. 50 milligrams.
    c. 50 ounces.
    d. 50 micrograms.

30. You respond to a call for a sick person and upon arrival find a 65-year-old male and his wife who promptly tell you they think they have food poisoning. They are complaining of abdominal cramping, vomiting, and diarrhea. The symptoms began early this morning and the husband's symptoms have gotten worse. They both ate hamburgers last night at a local restaurant. What should you do you next?

    a. Call the fire department to check out a possible high CO exposure.
    b. Obtain vital signs, get a focused history, and perform a physical exam.
    c. Manage the ABCs and call medical control to request an order to assist with activated charcoal.
    d. Find out which restaurant the patients ate at and report it to dispatch for notification to the health department.

Chapter 21 Answer Form

	A	B	C	D			A	B	C	D
1.	❏	❏	❏	❏		16.	❏	❏	❏	❏
2.	❏	❏	❏	❏		17.	❏	❏	❏	❏
3.	❏	❏	❏	❏		18.	❏	❏	❏	❏
4.	❏	❏	❏	❏		19.	❏	❏	❏	❏
5.	❏	❏	❏	❏		20.	❏	❏	❏	❏
6.	❏	❏	❏	❏		21.	❏	❏	❏	❏
7.	❏	❏	❏	❏		22.	❏	❏	❏	❏
8.	❏	❏	❏	❏		23.	❏	❏	❏	❏
9.	❏	❏	❏	❏		24.	❏	❏	❏	❏
10.	❏	❏	❏	❏		25.	❏	❏	❏	❏
11.	❏	❏	❏	❏		26.	❏	❏	❏	❏
12.	❏	❏	❏	❏		27.	❏	❏	❏	❏
13.	❏	❏	❏	❏		28.	❏	❏	❏	❏
14.	❏	❏	❏	❏		29.	❏	❏	❏	❏
15.	❏	❏	❏	❏		30.	❏	❏	❏	❏

CHAPTER

22

Environmental Emergencies

1. It is a hot day and you see a sun worshipper tanning in the park. She is spraying a water mister to keep cool. What method of cooling is she enjoying?
   a. radiation
   b. convection
   c. conduction
   d. evaporation

2. You are trying to cool a patient who is suffering from heat exposure. By allowing a fan to blow over the patient, you are cooling him by which method?
   a. radiation
   b. convection
   c. conduction
   d. evaporation

3. You have been called to care for a person found lying outside in the snow. You find the patient, who is cold and shivering. This patient has lost a significant amount of body heat in a short time, primarily by means of:
   a. radiation.
   b. conduction.
   c. convection.
   d. evaporation.

4. You have just discovered a person who has been exposed to the cold for a prolonged period of time and has frostbite on a distal extremity. Which signs and symptoms can you expect to find?
   a. The extremity will appear white and feel numb.
   b. The extremity will look shriveled, but have normal color.
   c. The extremity will feel cold, look red, and the patient will have severe pain.
   d. The extremity will appear black and blue and the patient will have severe pain.

5. For the victim of sudden exposure to extremely cold temperatures, such as falling through the ice into freezing water, decreased coordination and motor function are _____ findings.
   a. early
   b. very late
   c. unreliable
   d. nonassociated

6. For a victim of prolonged cold exposure, which of the following signs indicates that the condition is critical?
   a. frost nip
   b. urinary incontinence
   c. decreased mental status
   d. decreased fine motor function

7. A 60-year-old male went to get the newspaper and fell in his driveway between high snow banks. He lay there for nearly an hour before being discovered. He is alert, cold, wet, and appears to have a severely deformed open fracture of his ankle. The steps in management of this patient include:
   a. move him out of the cold, splint the ankle, administer high-flow oxygen, and transport rapidly.
   b. check ABCs, splint the ankle, move the patient into the ambulance, remove his wet clothing, and provide warmth.
   c. check ABCs, remove the wet clothing, splint the ankle and control any bleeding, and move the patient out of the cold and provide warmth.
   d. control any bleeding, splint the ankle and elevate the leg, administer high-flow oxygen, move the patient into the ambulance, and transport.

8. You are dispatched for an elderly patient who has fallen. Upon arrival you find a conscious and confused woman who may have been on the floor for more than 18 hours. She is incontinent of urine and is complaining of being really cold. The first priority after managing the ABCs is to:
   a. stop ongoing heat loss.
   b. provide warm, humidified oxygen.
   c. cover the patient with a blanket and begin transport in a warm ambulance.
   d. call medical control for an order to assist with oral high-concentration glucose.

9. Two men who were out snowshoeing became lost for a few hours, then found their way out of the woods. EMS was called because one had developed frostbite on the toes of his left foot. Management of the extremity includes:

 a. beginning to warm the extremity while keeping it elevated.

 b. splinting the extremity and keeping it from further cold exposure.

 c. keeping the extremity from warming until the patient reaches the hospital.

 d. placing the foot in tepid water for 5 minutes, and then splinting the extremity.

10. The EMT-B can recognize dehydration associated with prolonged exposure to heat by the patient's:

 a. sweaty skin.

 b. inability to sweat.

 c. past medical history.

 d. signs and symptoms.

11. A healthy person with a mild to moderate heat exposure might be expected to have which of the following signs and symptoms?

 a. shock.

 b. weak pulse.

 c. altered mental status.

 d. nausea and vomiting.

12. Which of the following signs and symptoms of heat exposure are most severe?

 a. confusion or dizziness

 b. any compromise to the ABCs

 c. muscle twitching and sweating

 d. increased body temperature and intense thirst

13. You have been dispatched to a vehicle that is stopped in a parking lot, for a 2-year-old child who is having seizures. When you arrive, the parents tell you that the child's eyes rolled back into his head, he began to seize, and appeared to have stopped breathing. They also state that this has never happened before. The child appears to be sleeping and is slowly waking. He is bundled up in a snowsuit, which is appropriate for the weather. What are your next management steps?

 a. Remove some of the clothing, provide oxygen, and transport the child in his car seat.

 b. Let the mother hold the child with an oxygen mask on the child's face and transport them together.

 c. Pour cool water over the child's head, provide oxygen, and transport him immobilized on a short board.

 d. Let the mother hold the child outside of the vehicle in the cold to lower his temperature, and then transport the child on a stretcher.

14. Your crew is standing by at a soccer tournament on a very warm afternoon. The humidity is high and the players have been participating in multiple games. A player has collapsed, apparently from the heat. He is conscious but not alert. You begin to treat him by giving him high-flow oxygen by non-rebreather mask, followed by:

 a. removing his clothing.

 b. blowing a fan on him and misting him with water.

 c. putting him into your air-conditioned ambulance as soon as possible.

 d. all of the above.

15. If rapid cooling is not begun for the victim of a severe heat disorder, _____ may result.

 a. hypertension

 b. hypoglycemia

 c. congestive heart failure

 d. permanent brain damage

16. A group of water skiers were on the lake practicing when one went down in the water. He was unconscious when pulled from the water and brought to shore. When you arrive, he is awake but does not recall what happened. What should you do next?

 a. Consider that the patient may be hyperthermic.

 b. Attempt to obtain a SpO2 and blood glucose reading.

 c. Consider that the patient may have a heart condition.

 d. Take spinal precautions and prepare to fully immobilize the patient.

17. Two boaters were tossed into the water when their canoe overturned. Both had life preservers (PFDs) on, but one could not swim, and it took them nearly 2 hours to get to shore. The nonswimmer was acting confused, so EMS was called. The patient appears cyanotic and is cold to the touch. Vital signs are: respirations 16, adequate; pulse 68, regular; BP 100/50. What do you suspect is the primary problem at this point?

 a. shock

 b. hypoxia

 c. hypothermia

 d. near-drowning

18. You are dispatched to the local marina for a sick person. Upon arrival, you find the patient complaining of motion sickness, headache, and aches in the neck and shoulders. She denies difficulty breathing or chest pain. The patient is a new employee of a dive shop and she did not dive today, but she did two dives yesterday. How should you manage this patient?

    a. Be prepared for this patient to go into respiratory arrest.
    b. Consider that this patient needs decompression therapy.
    c. She has no life-threatening injuries, so refer her to her own physician.
    d. Consider this to be a decompression emergency only if she dove below 33 feet.

19. Which of the following statements regarding near-drowning is most accurate?

    a. Kidney failure is common following a near-drowning episode.
    b. Aspiration of either salt water or fresh water results in hypoxia.
    c. The EMT-B must treat every victim of near-drowning for hypothermia.
    d. All victims of near-drowning should be placed in Trendelenburg position, to allow drainage of the lungs.

20. In the initial assessment of the victim of a near-drowning, the patient may appear normal. In the on-going assessment, however, the EMT-B should expect signs and symptoms of problems related to:

    a. infection.
    b. breathing.
    c. decompression sickness.
    d. all of the above.

21. Which of the following factors is typically not associated with victims of near-drowning?

    a. alcohol
    b. frostbite
    c. spinal injury
    d. hypothermia

22. During a domestic dispute, one patient sustained human bites on the back and upper left arm. There are no other injuries and the patient denies any other symptoms. This patient should be transported for evaluation:

    a. only if she is over 60 years of age.
    b. only if she is less than 16 years of age.
    c. only if the biter has not been vaccinated for tetanus.
    d. if the bites have broken through the skin and are bleeding.

23. A victim of snakebite is alert and shows you two fang marks on his left calf. The bite occurred 20 minutes ago. He is not sure what type of snake it was, but remembers that it was brown. Emergency medical care for this type of injury includes supporting the ABCs and:

    a. elevating and icing the extremity.
    b. cleaning the wound using suction.
    c. applying a tourniquet above the injury site.
    d. splinting the extremity and keeping the patient still.

24. The patient you are assessing was bitten multiple times on the lower arms and hands in an attack by a strange dog. She complains of severe pain at the injury site and is bleeding from the wounds. Emergency medical care for this patient begins with:

    a. supporting the ABCs.
    b. wrapping and splinting the arms and hands.
    c. determining if the dog has had its immunizations.
    d. determining when the patient's last tetanus shot was.

25. SCUBA is an acronym associated with diving and represents:

    a. selective compression under baro-atmosphere.
    b. self-contained underwater breathing apparatus.
    c. sea cylinder used below atmospheric pressure.
    d. sealed canister used beneath atmospheric pressure.

26. The formation of nitrogen bubbles in the blood or tissues, associated with diving, is known as:

    a. the bends.
    b. nitrogen narcosis.
    c. hyperbaric sickness.
    d. recompression sickness.

27. Which of the following would not cause decompression sickness?

    a. scuba diving in a dry suit
    b. snorkeling down to a depth of 20 feet
    c. scuba diving at a depth of no more than 33 feet
    d. diving using an air hose running from the surface for breathing

28. _____ is the formation of ice crystals within the tissues as a result of prolonged exposure to cold temperatures.
    a. Frostnip
    b. Frostbite
    c. Air embolism
    d. Decompression illness

29. Which of the following conditions is not a predisposing factor for hypothermia?
    a. child less than 1 year old
    b. an elderly person who is living alone
    c. a female in the third trimester of pregnancy
    d. a person who is intoxicated with alcohol

30. For the victim of a sting from a marine life form, the general approach to emergency care includes:
    a. rapid transport for evaluation.
    b. splinting and/or elevating the affected area.
    c. assisting with an epinephrine auto-injector.
    d. applying ice to reduce the pain and swelling.

31. EMS was called for a 12-year-old female who was having a seizure in the pool. Another child described the patient as having lost consciousness. A parent was nearby when the seizure began and quickly pulled the patient from the pool. Your general impression is that of a conscious patient with an open airway who is coughing. Underneath the blanket she is wrapped in, you can see that her skin is pink, warm, and still wet. She is alert and appropriately responsive to you, and her lung sounds are clear. You administer oxygen and obtain vital signs. She has no history of seizures, takes no medicine, and has no allergies. What action is appropriate next?
    a. Perform a rapid trauma assessment and ongoing assessments.
    b. Perform a rapid medical assessment followed by a detailed physical exam.
    c. Perform a focused assessment based on the seizure activity and the submersion.
    d. Finish obtaining vital signs and continue to observe the patient for a few more minutes before making a transportation decision.

32. (Continuing with the preceding question) There was no apparent traumatic MOI. After talking to the patient and the other child, you discover that the seizure activity began when they were swimming underwater and competing to see who could hold their breath the longest. The patient appears well and is moving all extremities. Vital signs are: respiratory rate 20, with good effort; pulse 84, strong and regular; BP 118/74; SpO2 100%. The patient's father is convinced that she did not swallow any water, and says he will follow up with the child's own pediatrician for the possible seizure activity. He is willing to sign your patient refusal paperwork, but you try to convince him to have the patient seen in the ED because:
    a. the seizure activity could be a new onset of epilepsy.
    b. the patient may attempt to go back into the water and could have another seizure.
    c. serious complications, including death, can occur many hours after a submersion.
    d. you believe the father is making an irrational decision that could be considered child neglect.

33. Your ambulance is dispatched for a 54-year-old male who has abdominal pain. When you arrive at his residence, he is alert and in distress from severe muscle spasms in the abdomen. He says that he has never experienced anything like this before and denies difficulty breathing, chest pain, or loss of consciousness. His wife asks you to look at his hand and says that he was in the attic earlier and was bitten by an insect, perhaps a spider. She wants to know if the muscle spasms are related to the bite. The area of the bite is red and swollen and the patient states that there is a dull ache. Which of the following insect bites or stings could produce these symptoms?
    a. tick
    b. fire ant
    c. black widow spider
    d. brown recluse spider

34. (Continuing with the preceding question) You quickly obtain a SAMPLE history and focused physical exam. The cramping did begin after the bite. The patient is taking medications for hypertension and high cholesterol, he has no known allergies, and his last meal was lunch (soup and ham sandwich). His vital signs are: respiratory rate 22, nonlabored; pulse 90, weak and irregular; BP 100/50. The patient's abdomen is rigid and now he is feeling weak. Select the appropriate management steps for the patient.

    a. Treat for shock and provide wound care for the hand.

    b. Apply ice to the area of the bite and perform a detailed physical exam.

    c. Pour vinegar over the area of the bite to denature the toxin or sprinkle meat tenderizer over the area.

    d. Place a tourniquet above the area of the bite, splint the extremity, and transport the patient to the nearest trauma center.

35. Dispatch has sent your crew to the city park for a possible alcohol overdose. The police are on the scene with a male in his 50s who smells of alcohol and urine. His pants are wet and he is shivering uncontrollably, even though the ambient temperature is nearly 70°F. The police tell you that they got reports that the patient has been lying in the bushes for hours. The patient is able to answer your questions and understands where he is and what is happening. He denies any injury, but is hungry. This patient's mental status and body shivering indicate that:

    a. his body is trying to generate heat.

    b. his core body temperature is below 90°F.

    c. his core body temperature is critically low.

    d. he has suffered chronic exposure to mild temperatures.

Chapter 22 Answer Form

	A	B	C	D			A	B	C	D
1.	❏	❏	❏	❏		19.	❏	❏	❏	❏
2.	❏	❏	❏	❏		20.	❏	❏	❏	❏
3.	❏	❏	❏	❏		21.	❏	❏	❏	❏
4.	❏	❏	❏	❏		22.	❏	❏	❏	❏
5.	❏	❏	❏	❏		23.	❏	❏	❏	❏
6.	❏	❏	❏	❏		24.	❏	❏	❏	❏
7.	❏	❏	❏	❏		25.	❏	❏	❏	❏
8.	❏	❏	❏	❏		26.	❏	❏	❏	❏
9.	❏	❏	❏	❏		27.	❏	❏	❏	❏
10.	❏	❏	❏	❏		28.	❏	❏	❏	❏
11.	❏	❏	❏	❏		29.	❏	❏	❏	❏
12.	❏	❏	❏	❏		30.	❏	❏	❏	❏
13.	❏	❏	❏	❏		31.	❏	❏	❏	❏
14.	❏	❏	❏	❏		32.	❏	❏	❏	❏
15.	❏	❏	❏	❏		33.	❏	❏	❏	❏
16.	❏	❏	❏	❏		34.	❏	❏	❏	❏
17.	❏	❏	❏	❏		35.	❏	❏	❏	❏
18.	❏	❏	❏	❏						

CHAPTER 23

Behavioral Emergencies

1. Which of the following is not considered a behavioral emergency?
   a. fasting
   b. anxiety attack
   c. suicide gesture
   d. suicide attempt

2. Abnormal behavior that results from a crisis in a person's life is interpreted as a/an:
   a. emotion.
   b. adaptive behavior.
   c. emotional disorders.
   d. behavioral emergency.

3. A strong feeling that is typically accompanied by physical findings such as increased heart rate is a/an:
   a. emotion.
   b. mental disorder.
   c. behavioral disorder.
   d. psychiatric disorder.

4. You are assessing a patient who may have experienced a fainting episode. He is now awake but is acting very strangely. Which of the following conditions should you consider first as being the cause?
   a. pain
   b. hypoxia
   c. abnormal blood sugar
   d. history of personality disorder

5. Factors that may cause unusual changes in a patient's behavior include:
   a. genetics and a history of emotional illness.
   b. severity of injury and perceived degree of pain.
   c. past experiences and the severity of the current illness.
   d. all of the above.

6. Which of the following statements reported by a patient would indicate that she is currently experiencing a behavioral emergency?
   a. I am feeling overwhelmed.
   b. I am a recovering alcoholic.
   c. I am taking medication for depression.
   d. There is a history of schizophrenia in my family.

7. The sudden death of a parent, a sudden change in the course of an acute disease, or the inability to accept a new role in life, such as becoming a grandparent, are all examples of:
   a. phobias.
   b. personality disorders.
   c. the need for crisis intervention.
   d. reasons for psychological crisis.

8. _____ is any acute, severe disruption in the balance of an individual or group.
   a. Crisis
   b. Anxiety
   c. Distress
   d. Emotion

9. Which of the following statements is most correct regarding the potential for a crisis situation?
   a. The reaction to a crisis will be the same for each individual.
   b. Every illness or injury is associated with some type of psychological stress.
   c. The patient in crisis usually has a history of drug or alcohol dependency.
   d. A person with a previous emotional illness is most likely to lapse into a crisis situation.

10. Which of the following characteristics is typically an unassociated risk factor for suicide?
    a. paranoia
    b. serious illness
    c. lack of self-esteem
    d. the loss of a significant loved one

11. A patient who makes a suicide gesture:
    a. is not really serious about suicide.
    b. typically uses a violent method of self-destruction.
    c. is most likely to be noncompliant with medications.
    d. must be treated and transported for evaluation by a psychiatrist.

12. One of the most common behavioral disorders, which can lead to suicide and other psychological and medical disorders, is:
    a. anxiety.
    b. dementia.
    c. depression.
    d. bipolar disorder.

13. _____ involves great medical and legal considerations for the EMT-B.
    a. Treating a victim of assault
    b. Caring for the victim of a rape
    c. Physically restraining a patient
    d. Attempted resuscitation of a victim of suicide

14. When the EMT-B is assessing and treating a patient who is impaired due to alcohol intoxication, the EMT-B is responsible for:
    a. arranging transportation to a detoxification facility.
    b. classifying the impairment as behavioral or psychiatric in nature.
    c. transporting the patient to a facility capable of providing a psychiatric evaluation.
    d. following both local protocols and state laws regarding persons with an altered mental status.

15. When entering a crime scene to care for a patient who is experiencing a behavioral emergency, the first priority is to:
    a. protect yourself.
    b. preserve the crime scene.
    c. preserve any evidence found on the patient.
    d. get the patient into the ambulance quickly.

16. A behavioral emergency can be caused by organic or emotional problems and should be treated:
    a. as nonurgent.
    b. as a physical problem.
    c. promptly, but without rushing the patient.
    d. as though the patient will require restraints.

17. Each of the following is a common misconception about behavioral illnesses, except:
    a. all mental patients are unstable.
    b. all mental patients are dangerous.
    c. abnormal behavior is always weird.
    d. behavioral illnesses often have an organic cause.

18. When managing a patient who is experiencing a behavioral emergency, it is necessary to:
    a. begin crisis intervention after the initial assessment.
    b. allow the police to be included in all phases of the call.
    c. begin crisis intervention after the focused physical exam.
    d. assess for physical causes that may mimic a behavioral emergency.

19. A factor that may cause an individual to become violent on the scene of an EMS call include the:
    a. age of the patient.
    b. gender of the patient.
    c. history of depression.
    d. patient's perception of the EMT-B.

20. A sign indicating that a patient may become violent is:
    a. memory loss.
    b. the patient raising his tone of voice.
    c. unusual odors on the breath.
    d. the appearance of being withdrawn.

21. A patient who is acting out in a hostile and violent manner is most likely:
    a. at high risk for suicide.
    b. experiencing depression.
    c. to be a disturbed teenager looking for attention.
    d. making an attempt to gain control of the situation.

22. The use of physical restraints on a patient who is displaying violent behavior is:
    a. dangerous for the patient and the rescuers.
    b. no longer a legal or moral treatment option.
    c. an acceptable method of calming the patient.
    d. necessary with all patients who are at risk for violence.

23. The police have called your crew to transport a teenager who punched his mother in the face. The patient is talking continuously in a loud tone and frequent use of vulgar language. He is in handcuffs and an officer is accompanying you. Your approach to calming this patient should include:
    a. helping the patient to maintain his dignity.
    b. asking for the patient's permission to take vital signs.
    c. not attempting to touch the patient if that is his desire.
    d. all of the above.

24. In managing a patient with an acute attack of anxiety, the EMT-B can help calm the patient by:
    a. keeping eye contact whenever possible.
    b. keeping a distance of a minimum of six feet.
    c. explaining to the patient that she is overreacting.
    d. telling the patient that you are here to help and that she can expect help from you.

25. You are faced with the problem of having to transport a patent against his will, because he poses a possible danger to himself or others. It is necessary to:
    a. display authoritative and threatening actions.
    b. impose a physical assessment on the patient.
    c. follow local protocols together with medical control.
    d. assure the patient that he will not be able to harm anyone while in your care.

26. The patient who is experiencing a behavioral emergency may become violent as a result of an action that would not normally lead to violence. Therefore, the EMT-B who responds to care for such a patient should:

    a. remain calm and professional at all times.
    b. not let the patient verbally express any anger or frustration.
    c. restrain every patient who is experiencing a behavioral emergency.
    d. request a police escort for every transport that involves behavioral emergency.

27. While performing a physical exam on a patient, which of the following findings would cause you to suspect that the patient has a history of a behavioral or psychiatric disorder?

    a. The patient has urinated on himself.
    b. The patient has a strong odor of alcohol.
    c. The patient has a strong odor of cigarettes.
    d. The patient shows an abnormal lack of regard for personal hygiene.

28. Generally, the time you spend with a patient who is experiencing a behavioral emergency will be:

    a. the same as with any other patient.
    b. longer, because of the time it takes to restrain the patient.
    c. longer, because of the special needs of this type of patient.
    d. shorter, because the patient will usually refuse to be touched.

29. In the management of a patient who intentionally took an overdose of medication, with the intent to harm himself, the EMT-B should:

    a. listen carefully to what the patient wants to say.
    b. avoid asking the patient if this is the first attempt at suicide.
    c. be indirect and nonspecific with communications and actions.
    d. not allow the patient to discuss his problems until the police are present.

30. Statistics show that _____ make more many more suicide attempts and that _____ are more successful at suicide.

    a. females, males
    b. males, females
    c. teenagers, females
    d. the elderly, males

Chapter 23 Answer Form

	A	B	C	D			A	B	C	D
1.	❏	❏	❏	❏		16.	❏	❏	❏	❏
2.	❏	❏	❏	❏		17.	❏	❏	❏	❏
3.	❏	❏	❏	❏		18.	❏	❏	❏	❏
4.	❏	❏	❏	❏		19.	❏	❏	❏	❏
5.	❏	❏	❏	❏		20.	❏	❏	❏	❏
6.	❏	❏	❏	❏		21.	❏	❏	❏	❏
7.	❏	❏	❏	❏		22.	❏	❏	❏	❏
8.	❏	❏	❏	❏		23.	❏	❏	❏	❏
9.	❏	❏	❏	❏		24.	❏	❏	❏	❏
10.	❏	❏	❏	❏		25.	❏	❏	❏	❏
11.	❏	❏	❏	❏		26.	❏	❏	❏	❏
12.	❏	❏	❏	❏		27.	❏	❏	❏	❏
13.	❏	❏	❏	❏		28.	❏	❏	❏	❏
14.	❏	❏	❏	❏		29.	❏	❏	❏	❏
15.	❏	❏	❏	❏		30.	❏	❏	❏	❏

CHAPTER

24

Obstetrics/Gynecology

1. The umbilical cord consists of:
   a. a muscular tube.
   b. one artery and two veins.
   c. one vein and two arteries.
   d. a self-contained feeding system.

2. *Afterbirth* is a lay term for which of the following organs or components of childbirth?
   a. uterus
   b. placenta
   c. amniotic fluid
   d. umbilical cord

3. Physical assessment of a contraction is best palpated:
   a. over the umbilicus.
   b. over the symphysis pubis.
   c. on the fundus (top) of the uterus.
   d. on the cervix (bottom) of the uterus.

4. The contents of an obstetric kit are:
   a. sterile.
   b. clean, but not sterilized.
   c. enough to care for two babies.
   d. only for use by a trained and certified EMT-B.

5. An obstetric kit usually includes one or two large plastic bags, which are used for:
   a. transporting the placenta.
   b. wrapping the baby's head for warmth.
   c. catching any vomitus from the mother.
   d. catching amniotic fluid lost from childbirth.

6. A commercially prepared obstetric kit includes which of the following items?
   a. items to manage the umbilical cord
   b. items to measure and weigh a baby
   c. items to control heavy vaginal bleeding after delivery
   d. all the necessary PPE for the delivery and management of a baby

7. You have just finished immobilizing the driver of a vehicle that was involved in a MVC. She is complaining of neck and low back pain and she is pregnant, in her 38th week. When you put her into the ambulance, she becomes unconscious. What step do you take next?
   a. Elevate her legs.
   b. Administer high-flow oxygen.
   c. Check for breathing and a pulse.
   d. Tilt the backboard slightly up to the left side.

8. A pregnant 32-year-old patient, in the third trimester, is complaining of severe abdominal pain, which began suddenly. She denies any vaginal bleeding or discharge. When you palpate her abdomen, you find that the uterus is rigid. What life-threatening condition do you suspect?
   a. preeclampsia
   b. placenta previa
   c. abruptio placenta
   d. ectopic pregnancy

9. You respond to a call for pregnancy with vaginal bleeding and discover a 24-year-old female in her third trimester of pregnancy. She is frightened and tells you that suddenly she began having heavy vaginal bleeding. She denies any pain or traumatic injury and reports that the bleeding has not stopped. What life-threatening condition do you suspect?
   a. placenta previa
   b. premature labor
   c. abruptio placenta
   d. ectopic pregnancy

10. During the transport of a woman in active labor, the patient tells you that the baby is coming. You examine her and find the baby crowning. The hospital is 5 minutes away, so now you:
    a. stop the ambulance and assist with the delivery.
    b. continue transport and assist with the delivery en route.
    c. continue transport and tell the mother to close her legs until you arrive.
    d. continue transport and instruct the mother not to push with contractions.

11. Prior to transporting a woman in active labor, you assessed her for crowning and saw none. During transport, the contractions become stronger and closer together. Which of the following signs is an indication of an imminent delivery?

    a. severe back pain
    b. abdominal cramping
    c. the patient feels an urge to move her bowels
    d. the patient has been leaking clear fluid for several hours

12. You have responded to a residence for a young woman in labor. She called EMS because she has no other way of getting to the hospital. Her contractions are strong, regular, occur every 5 minutes, and last for 30 seconds. You should:

    a. transport the patient.
    b. request a second ambulance.
    c. prepare the mother for delivery.
    d. instruct the mother to close her thighs together.

13. Your unit has been called to transfer a high-risk pregnant patient woman to the hospital for admission. The staff reports that the patient is 25 weeks pregnant and is experiencing Braxton Hicks contractions. Her vital signs are stable. Management of this patient includes:

    a. declining transport and calling an ALS ambulance.
    b. position of comfort, high-flow oxygen, and rapid transport.
    c. supportive care, position of comfort, and routine transport.
    d. having a staff member ride along on the transport.

14. EMS has been called for a woman who is having seizures. Upon arrival, you confirm that there was a brief seizure and find a pregnant female who is conscious, confused, and complaining of severe headache. She is 36 weeks along in gestation and is being treated for hypertension. Your initial assessment findings, together with the patient's history, indicate that the patient is experiencing:

    a. eclampsia, a life-threatening condition.
    b. preeclampsia, a life-threatening condition.
    c. eclampsia, a non-life-threatening condition.
    d. preeclampsia, a non-life-threatening condition.

15. (Continuing with the preceding question) After completing a focused physical exam, you find swelling in the patient's face, hands, lower legs, and feet. Her vital signs are: pulse 110, regular; respiration 20, regular; BP 186/100; skin CTC is flushed, warm, and dry. Management of this patient should include:

    a. high-flow oxygen, calling for ALS, and rapid transport.
    b. high-flow oxygen, position of comfort, and rapid transport.
    c. notifying her physician's office and offering to transport her there.
    d. low-flow oxygen, position of comfort, and routine transport.

16. During emergency childbirth, which of the following factors should the EMT-B be alert for as a possible cause of an airway problem?

    a. nausea and vomiting
    b. the patient biting her tongue during a contraction
    c. the patient holding her breath during a contraction
    d. the patient putting her face into a pillow to scream

17. When preparing the mother for delivery in emergency childbirth, the EMT-B should:

    a. use only absolutely sterile equipment.
    b. allow the mother to go to the toilet before she delivers.
    c. allow the husband or friend to be present during delivery.
    d. allow only one other person to be present during delivery.

18. Once you have determined that birth is imminent, you will need to prepare the mother for delivery by:

    a. asking her to empty her bladder.
    b. letting her take a position of comfort.
    c. administering high-concentration oxygen.
    d. positioning her on her back on the stretcher.

19. To which of the following body fluids is the EMT-B at low risk of exposure during an emergency childbirth?

    a. amniotic fluid
    b. urine and blood
    c. cerebral spinal fluid
    d. vomitus and breast milk

20. In addition to gloves and a face mask, which item found in an obstetrical kit will help reduce the risk of exposure for the EMT-B?

    a. gown
    b. plastic bag
    c. disposable sheets
    d. umbilical cord clamps

21. During an emergency childbirth, the need for body substance isolation is _____ because the potential for exposure is _____.

    a. great, high
    b. negligible, low
    c. average, moderate
    d. often excessive, minimal

22. Management of the third stage of delivery includes:

    a. watching for the baby's head to push through the vaginal opening.
    b. frequently assessing the patient for signs of hypertension and eclampsia.
    c. waiting to begin transport, but calling the ED to advise of the current status.
    d. coaching the patient to deliver the placenta and assessing for signs of shock.

23. Immediately after the baby's head is delivered, the next step in assisting with a delivery is to:
    a. prepare to deliver the upper shoulder.
    b. prepare to deliver the lower shoulder.
    c. check for the cord around the baby's neck.
    d. wipe the head off so that it is not so slippery.

24. A woman in active labor is crowning and pushing with contractions. She tells you the baby is coming. She is in the delivery position and you see the baby's head emerging. The next step is to:
    a. wipe the baby's head and assess for meconium.
    b. use a sterile dressing to prepare to catch the baby.
    c. take a suction bulb in one hand and get ready to suction.
    d. place your hand on the baby's head to prevent an explosive delivery.

25. The priority in care of the baby as the head delivers is:
    a. suctioning the airway.
    b. assessing the skin CTC.
    c. wiping the eyes clear of fluid with a sterile pad.
    d. not to stimulate the infant to breathe until it is delivered.

26. The steps in suctioning the baby during delivery begin with:
    a. suctioning the nose, then the mouth after the baby is delivered.
    b. using a bulb syringe to rapidly evacuate the mouth, nose, and ears.
    c. keeping the baby's head in a slightly downward position for drainage.
    d. suctioning the mouth, then the nose once the baby's head is delivered.

27. The most common presentation of the baby's head from the vaginal opening is:
    a. face up.
    b. face down.
    c. turned to the left side.
    d. turned to the right side.

28. The umbilical cord may be safely cut by:
    a. using a sterile, sharp knife.
    b. snipping with sterile scissors.
    c. slicing with a sterile surgical blade.
    d. each of the above.

29. When assisting with an emergency childbirth, the EMT-B should clamp and cut the cord:
    a. when a prolapsed cord is present.
    b. only after the baby has been delivered.
    c. only after the placenta has been delivered.
    d. when it cannot be unwrapped from around the neck.

30. After clamping and cutting the umbilical cord, you observe that the end of the cord attached to the baby is leaking blood. You should manage this by:
    a. pinching the stump of the cord until it stops bleeding.
    b. carefully placing a second clamp proximal to the first.
    c. elevating the cord and placing an ice pack on the stump.
    d. keeping the cord warm and letting the natural clotting process stop the bleeding.

31. When the placenta is delivered and a portion is visibly missing, the EMT-B can expect:
    a. significant vaginal bleeding to follow.
    b. the remaining portion to deliver within minutes.
    c. the remaining portion to deliver within the hour.
    d. no problems during the time it takes to finish transport.

32. When assisting the mother to deliver the placenta, the EMT-B should expect:
    a. that the cord can easily become entangled in the placenta.
    b. no bleeding following expulsion of the placenta.
    c. significant bleeding following expulsion of the placenta.
    d. contractions that are painful and similar to those occurring with delivery of the baby.

33. When delivery of the placenta occurs in the prehospital setting, the EMT-B is required to bring the placenta to the hospital for which of the following reasons?
    a. proper disposal
    b. blood typing
    c. stem cell research
    d. inspection of completeness

34. A home delivery for the third child of a woman in her late twenties was assisted by a midwife. The delivery of the baby and placenta was reported as uncomplicated, but the mother has heavy vaginal bleeding and transport to the hospital is requested. Care for this patient includes:
    a. considering the possibility of delivery of a second baby.
    b. treating for shock, calling for ALS, and rapid transport.
    c. calling for ALS and treating for shock until the paramedics arrive.
    d. treating the patient and notifying child protective services about the home delivery.

35. Following delivery, the EMT-B may have to manage a rip in the skin and bleeding from the mother in the area known as the:
    a. anus.
    b. pubis.
    c. placenta.
    d. perineum.

36. After assisting the mother with an uncomplicated emergency delivery, management of the mother should be focused on:
   a. rapid transport and treatment for shock.
   b. letting the mother hold the baby if she is capable.
   c. performing uterine massage to reduce pain and bleeding.
   d. supportive care, comfort, and reassessment for signs of shock.

37. After 30 seconds of drying, warming, suctioning, and stimulation, a newborn baby is not responding well. The heart rate is slow and breathing is inadequate. The next step in resuscitation is to:
   a. start chest compressions.
   b. retilt the head and suction again.
   c. check the umbilical cord for bleeding.
   d. administer oxygen and prepare to assist ventilations.

38. Stimulating a newborn baby to breathe can be accomplished by any of the following methods, except:
   a. rubbing the baby's back.
   b. clicking the bottom of the feet.
   c. drying the baby with clean, dry towels.
   d. holding the baby upside down to allow fluids to drain.

39. Within 1 minute of delivery of a newborn, if the heart rate is less than _____ beats per minute and is not increasing with stimulation and oxygenation, the EMT-B should begin chest compressions.
   a. 90
   b. 80
   c. 70
   d. 60

40. For the baby that presents with the buttocks first in the mother's vaginal opening, the EMT-B should first:
   a. place the mother on her back with legs elevated and transport quickly.
   b. place the mother on her side with both legs closed and transport quickly.
   c. place her gloved fingers into the vagina to keep the baby's airway open.
   d. support the buttocks and legs as the baby delivers, to prevent injury to the baby's neck.

41. A frightened young mother-to-be has called EMS because her water broke and she is having contractions. When you assess her for crowning, you see about six inches of the umbilical cord hanging out of the vaginal opening and no baby. At this point you should:
   a. do nothing, as this is not an uncommon finding.
   b. quickly prepare for delivery, as birth is imminent.
   c. keep the mother still while you wait for ALS to arrive.
   d. consider this a true emergency and begin rapid transport.

42. Which of the following abnormal deliveries should not be attempted in the prehospital setting?
   a. twins or triplets
   b. premature baby
   c. limb presentation
   d. breech presentation

43. Twins that are born from the same placenta will always be:
   a. premature.
   b. the same size.
   c. the same gender.
   d. one of each gender.

44. The size of each twin baby will be different at birth, yet the EMT-B can expect both twins to be _____ single babies.
   a. larger than
   b. smaller than
   c. the same size as
   d. always premature compared to

45. The procedure for assisting with delivery of twins is _____ that for single babies, and the EMT-B can typically expect the first baby to appear _____.
   a. different from, feet first
   b. different from, head first
   c. the same as for, feet first
   d. the same as for, head first

46. The danger associated with the presence of meconium in amniotic fluid is:
   a. that the baby will be difficult to stimulate or resuscitate.
   b. that the baby has likely suffered irreversible brain damage.
   c. that the immature lungs cannot tolerate aggressive suctioning.
   d. aspiration of meconium, leading to respiratory distress syndrome.

47. When meconium is present during the delivery, the EMT-B should suction the baby:
   a. as soon as the head appears.
   b. immediately after the baby is delivered.
   c. only after the umbilical cord is clamped.
   d. after the umbilical cord is clamped and cut.

48. Meconium staining in the amniotic fluid is a sign of:
   a. a traumatic labor.
   b. a premature infant.
   c. imminent cardiac arrest.
   d. fetal distress during the pregnancy.

49. Premature babies are prone to lose body heat very easily because:

    a. they have a very small amount of body fat.
    b. the temperature regulating system is immature.
    c. they have a larger body surface area in relation to their weight.
    d. all of the above.

50. A baby that is born prematurely is at increased risk for:

    a. hypercarbia.
    b. hypothermia.
    c. hyperglycemia.
    d. hyperventilation syndrome.

51. The EMT-B can recognize a premature infant because the baby:

    a. weighs less than 5.5 pounds.
    b. is born before 39 weeks gestation.
    c. has a darker skin color than a full-tern baby.
    d. has a lighter skin color than a full-term baby.

52. You are assessing a 56-year-old female who has severe abdominal pain. She tells you she has a history of hypertension and had a hysterectomy 4 years ago. She looks pale, is tachycardic, and her blood pressure is 110/50. Management of this patient should begin with:

    a. calling ALS for pain management.
    b. an examination for vaginal bleeding.
    c. high-flow oxygen and treatment for shock.
    d. attention to the ABCs and suspicion of an ectopic pregnancy.

53. Abdominal pain, low back pain, fever, nausea, and abnormal vaginal discharge are signs and symptoms associated with:

    a. kidney stones.
    b. ectopic pregnancy.
    c. urinary tract infection.
    d. sexually transmitted disease.

54. A 21-year-old female is complaining of abdominal pain with cramping in the left lower quadrant. She denies being pregnant and has no vaginal discharge. Which condition should be suspected first?

    a. appendicitis
    b. kidney stone
    c. sexual trauma
    d. ectopic pregnancy

55. Which of the following can cause irregular fetal development when the mother is taking it or is exposed to it?

    a. calcium
    b. folic acid
    c. vitamin A
    d. vitamin C

56. If a pregnant woman sustains an injury that results in shock, her body will engage a self-protective mechanism that:

    a. masks signs of shock in the baby.
    b. delays the normal signs of shock in the baby.
    c. directs blood from the baby to keep the mother alive.
    d. directs blood from the mother to keep the baby alive.

57. A serious motor vehicle collision has resulted in the cardiac arrest of a woman in her thirties who appears to be in the third trimester of pregnancy. CPR has been started and she will be ready for transport quickly. The fetus's chance of survival in this case:

    a. is near-zero.
    b. depends on the quality of prenatal care.
    c. is better if the bag of waters has not ruptured.
    d. depends on aggressive resuscitation of the mother.

58. The normal term of gestation (pregnancy) is _____ weeks.

    a. 36 to 40
    b. 38 to 42
    c. 40 to 44
    d. 42 to 46

59. The _____ is actually fetal membranes which are commonly called the "bag of waters."

    a. embryo
    b. placenta
    c. amniotic sac
    d. amniotic fluid

60. The _____ is the area around the external opening in the bottom of the pelvis.

    a. vagina
    b. rectum
    c. perineum
    d. symphysis pubis

Chapter 24 Answer Form

	A	B	C	D		A	B	C	D
1.	❏	❏	❏	❏	31.	❏	❏	❏	❏
2.	❏	❏	❏	❏	32.	❏	❏	❏	❏
3.	❏	❏	❏	❏	33.	❏	❏	❏	❏
4.	❏	❏	❏	❏	34.	❏	❏	❏	❏
5.	❏	❏	❏	❏	35.	❏	❏	❏	❏
6.	❏	❏	❏	❏	36.	❏	❏	❏	❏
7.	❏	❏	❏	❏	37.	❏	❏	❏	❏
8.	❏	❏	❏	❏	38.	❏	❏	❏	❏
9.	❏	❏	❏	❏	39.	❏	❏	❏	❏
10.	❏	❏	❏	❏	40.	❏	❏	❏	❏
11.	❏	❏	❏	❏	41.	❏	❏	❏	❏
12.	❏	❏	❏	❏	42.	❏	❏	❏	❏
13.	❏	❏	❏	❏	43.	❏	❏	❏	❏
14.	❏	❏	❏	❏	44.	❏	❏	❏	❏
15.	❏	❏	❏	❏	45.	❏	❏	❏	❏
16.	❏	❏	❏	❏	46.	❏	❏	❏	❏
17.	❏	❏	❏	❏	47.	❏	❏	❏	❏
18.	❏	❏	❏	❏	48.	❏	❏	❏	❏
19.	❏	❏	❏	❏	49.	❏	❏	❏	❏
20.	❏	❏	❏	❏	50.	❏	❏	❏	❏
21.	❏	❏	❏	❏	51.	❏	❏	❏	❏
22.	❏	❏	❏	❏	52.	❏	❏	❏	❏
23.	❏	❏	❏	❏	53.	❏	❏	❏	❏
24.	❏	❏	❏	❏	54.	❏	❏	❏	❏
25.	❏	❏	❏	❏	55.	❏	❏	❏	❏
26.	❏	❏	❏	❏	56.	❏	❏	❏	❏
27.	❏	❏	❏	❏	57.	❏	❏	❏	❏
28.	❏	❏	❏	❏	58.	❏	❏	❏	❏
29.	❏	❏	❏	❏	59.	❏	❏	❏	❏
30.	❏	❏	❏	❏	60.	❏	❏	❏	❏

Trauma

CHAPTER

25

Bleeding and Shock

1. The primary function of the circulatory system is to:
   a. prevent obstruction in circulation to the heart.
   b. provide a continuous source of nutrients to tissues.
   c. prevent the formation of diseased states of the body.
   d. maintain pressure within the inner walls of the blood vessels.

2. The fluid that transports cells and nutrients to all body tissues is:
   a. lymph.
   b. plasma.
   c. platelet.
   d. marrow.

3. Blood is involved in all of the following functions, except:
   a. nutrition.
   b. fluid balance.
   c. temperature regulation.
   d. nerve impulse regulation.

4. A woman called 9-1-1 after she accidentally cut her arm with a utility knife. She has wrapped a cloth around the arm and it is soaked through with dark red blood. You suspect that the bleeding is:
   a. venous.
   b. arterial.
   c. capillary.
   d. life-threatening.

5. A 23-year-old male put his hand through a glass door; the injury resulted in bleeding that is pulsating and difficult to control. You recognize this as _____ bleeding.
   a. arterial
   b. venous
   c. internal
   d. capillary

6. A 12-year-old boy injured his wrist while skateboarding. While splinting his arm, you notice bloodstains on the knees of his jeans. Your partner exposes the patient's knees and finds abrasions on both legs. This type of bleeding is typically:
   a. arterial.
   b. venous.
   c. capillary.
   d. difficult to control.

7. The method of using elevation to control external bleeding works best when:
   a. the wound is below the waist.
   b. ice has been applied to the wound.
   c. the wound is raised above the level of the heart.
   d. the wound is more than 2 inches in length or diameter.

8. The first step in controlling a bleed from a deep gash on the forearm is to:
   a. apply an ice pack.
   b. elevate the extremity.
   c. pack the wound with gauze.
   d. apply direct pressure using a dressing.

9. A tourniquet applied on an extremity to control a life-threatening bleed is:
   a. used on lower extremities only.
   b. used on upper extremities only.
   c. no longer used in the prehospital setting.
   d. a method of last resort to control bleeding in the prehospital setting.

10. Body substance isolation is a method of personal protection that is based on the belief that:
    a. immunizations should be kept current.
    b. all blood and body fluids are potentially infectious.
    c. health care providers should wash their hands after every patient contact.
    d. the incidence of disease would resolve if everyone washed their hands before and after every patient contact.

11. _____ is the most common serious infectious disease that is transmitted by exposure to external bleeding.
   a. HIV
   b. Hepatitis
   c. Meningitis
   d. Tuberculosis

12. Which of the following is not considered a significant exposure as a result of managing a hemorrhage?
   a. spray into the mouth
   b. splatter into the eye(s)
   c. contact with broken skin
   d. soaking the uniform pant leg

13. While standing by at a soccer tournament, you witness a player run face-first into the goal. He appears to have broken his nose and is bleeding steadily. After several minutes of pinching the nostrils, you are unsuccessful in controlling the bleeding, and now the patient is complaining of nausea. How would you manage the airway now?
   a. Suction the nose and mouth.
   b. Pack the nostrils and apply an ice pack.
   c. Tilt the head back and apply an ice pack to the nose.
   d. Tilt the head forward and have the patient spit out the blood.

14. You are transporting a large female who is immobilized to a long backboard. She complained of neck pain after her vehicle was struck from behind. During the ride in, she develops nausea and states that she is going to vomit. The next action to take should be to:
   a. turn on the suction and begin suctioning.
   b. take off her collar and loosen the straps on the board.
   c. tell the driver to use the lights and siren and hurry to the ED.
   d. loosen the stretcher straps enough to be able to tilt the board.

15. A worker fell from a height of approximately 40 feet. You have determined that he is apneic and pulseless and direct your partner to perform manual spinal immobilization. You insert an OPA and attempt to ventilate him with a BVM while another rescuer starts compressions. The ventilations are poor and air is escaping, so you attempt to correct the problem by:
   a. suctioning the airway.
   b. improving the mask seal.
   c. tilting the head and lifting the jaw.
   d. all of the above.

16. In a motor vehicle collision, internal injuries may occur from which of the following MOIs?
   a. rapid deceleration
   b. rapid acceleration
   c. compression forces
   d. all of the above

17. The fire department has extricated the driver of a vehicle that struck a pole. The airbag deployed, but he was not wearing a seat belt. He has a large bruise on his forehead and a deformed ankle. The patient has an altered mental status and his vital signs are: respirations 18, adequate; pulse 120, weak and regular; blood pressure 80/40. Which injury do you suspect is the cause of shock?
   a. head injury
   b. ankle injury
   c. spinal injury
   d. internal bleeding

18. A 19-year-old male was stabbed in the upper right quadrant of his abdomen by another teenage male, who used a 3-inch knife. Which organs are most likely to be injured?
   a. liver, large intestine, and lung
   b. heart, aorta, diaphragm, and spleen
   c. stomach, appendix, and small intestine
   d. diaphragm, liver, large intestine, and lung

19. Early signs indicating that a patient has intraabdominal bleeding include:
   a. hypertension, headache, and nausea.
   b. hyperventilation, hypoxia, and constipation.
   c. bradycardia, hypotension, and irregular pulse.
   d. sustained tachycardia, and normal or low blood pressure.

20. Which of the following signs is not a reliable finding associated with internal bleeding?
   a. tarry stool
   b. bowel sounds
   c. rigid abdomen
   d. blood in the urine

21. The mother of a 12-year-old male has called you because her son fainted. Your initial assessment finds a patient who is conscious, pale, and moist with a weak, rapid pulse. The patient denies any recent injury or illness and his mother agrees; also, he has no significant past medical history and takes no medications. Your initial treatment plan is to:
   a. prepare for vomiting.
   b. consider the use of MAST/PASG.
   c. administer high-flow oxygen and treat for shock.
   d. perform a focused physical exam of the abdomen.

22. A 52-year-old male patient with symptoms of nausea, dizziness, and vomiting blood has a history of gastric reflux. His vital signs are: respirations 24, adequate; pulse 120, regular; BP 96/50; skin CTC cool, moist, and pasty-looking. Management of this patient should include:

a. oxygen by cannula, observation for vomiting, and routine transport.

b. high-flow oxygen, position of comfort, warmth, and routine transport.

c. supine with legs flexed for comfort, high-flow oxygen, and rapid transport.

d. supine position, high-flow oxygen, warmth, rapid transport, and call for ALS.

23. After falling approximately 25 feet from a roof, a construction worker was unconscious for approximately 30 seconds. He is now alert and complaining of severe low back pain. There is blood trickling out of his left ear. The bleeding from this injury should be managed by:

a. packing the ear with sterile gauze.

b. direct pressure and elevation of the head.

c. a sterile dressing taped over the outside of the ear.

d. turning the patient on his left side to allow drainage.

24. A driver who was involved in a moderate-speed MVC appears to have struck his face on the steering wheel during the incident. There is blood draining from his nose. Bleeding should be controlled by which method?

a. direct pressure

b. pressure dressing

c. use of a pressure point

d. packing the nose with a sterile dressing

25. The skin signs of a patient experiencing hypoperfusion include:

a. cold, white, and dry.

b. cool, pale, and moist.

c. hot, cyanotic, and dry.

d. hot, flushed, and moist.

26. Severe hemorrhage results in the loss of _____, causing a decrease in oxygenation of the body tissues.

a. plasma

b. platelets

c. red blood cells

d. white blood cells

27. When the adult body senses a loss of blood volume, one of the body's first responses is:

a. fainting.

b. respiratory distress.

c. an increased pumping rate of the heart.

d. to initiate a process that leads to kidney failure.

28. A woman has called EMS because her husband fainted this morning. He is lying in bed and appears very weak and pale. There is a strong odor of stool, and the wife confirms that the patient has had diarrhea and vomiting during the night and all morning. The vital signs are: respirations 24, labored; pulse 110, regular but weak; BP 70/40. After you administer high-flow oxygen, the next steps in the emergency medical care of this patient include:

a. providing rapid transport only.

b. attaching the AED, requesting an ALS intercept, and beginning rapid transport.

c. requesting ALS and preparing the patient for transport while waiting for ALS to arrive.

d. elevating the legs, providing warmth, beginning rapid transport, and requesting ALS intercept.

29. Dispatched for a traumatic injury, you arrive on the scene to find a 50-year-old male who has nearly cut off one of his fingers with a chainsaw. He is pale and has beads of sweat on his forehead. A family member has a cold wet bandage on the finger and has controlled the bleeding. Your initial assessment of this patient prompts you to treat this patient for _____ shock.

a. cardiogenic

b. psychogenic

c. compensating

d. decompensating

30. The rider of a motorcycle was traveling at a moderate speed when she was cut off by a car and knocked to the ground. The patient is conscious now, but bystanders report that she was unconscious for about a minute. Her helmet is cracked and both of her thighs appear to have closed fractures. Her airway is clear; skin CTC is pale, moist, and cool; and her vital signs are: respirations 18, adequate; pulse 126, regular; BP 80/40. Your management of this patent will be to treat for:

a. compensating shock due to the head injury.

b. decompensating shock due the head injury.

c. compensating shock due to the internal bleeding.

d. decompensating shock due to the internal bleeding.

31. Each additional minute spent on the scene for a patient with life-threatening traumatic injuries:

a. increases the trauma score.

b. increases the criteria for rapid transport.

c. reduces the patient's chance for survival.

d. reduces the time it takes for ALS to reach the patient.

32. The decision to provide rapid transport for a trauma patient is typically based on:
    a. the MOI.
    b. signs of shock.
    c. external bleeding.
    d. signs of shock and /or the MOI.

33. When you suspect that a patient is bleeding internally, the interventions you provide will be rapid because definitive care is:
    a. often surgical.
    b. accomplished on scene.
    c. available at any hospital.
    d. performed en route to the hospital.

34. Abdominal trauma is the second leading cause of trauma death, because:
    a. most abdominal trauma occurs in children.
    b. blunt trauma to the abdomen is always overlooked.
    c. significant blood loss occurs before signs of distention are apparent.
    d. injury to solid organs can produce severe bleeding that progresses rapidly.

35. The severity of a hemorrhage can best be determined by which of the following factors?
    a. arterial versus venous bleeding
    b. internal versus external bleeding
    c. how much blood has been lost
    d. the age and height of the patient

Chapter 25 Answer Form

	A	B	C	D		A	B	C	D
1.	❏	❏	❏	❏	19.	❏	❏	❏	❏
2.	❏	❏	❏	❏	20.	❏	❏	❏	❏
3.	❏	❏	❏	❏	21.	❏	❏	❏	❏
4.	❏	❏	❏	❏	22.	❏	❏	❏	❏
5.	❏	❏	❏	❏	23.	❏	❏	❏	❏
6.	❏	❏	❏	❏	24.	❏	❏	❏	❏
7.	❏	❏	❏	❏	25.	❏	❏	❏	❏
8.	❏	❏	❏	❏	26.	❏	❏	❏	❏
9.	❏	❏	❏	❏	27.	❏	❏	❏	❏
10.	❏	❏	❏	❏	28.	❏	❏	❏	❏
11.	❏	❏	❏	❏	29.	❏	❏	❏	❏
12.	❏	❏	❏	❏	30.	❏	❏	❏	❏
13.	❏	❏	❏	❏	31.	❏	❏	❏	❏
14.	❏	❏	❏	❏	32.	❏	❏	❏	❏
15.	❏	❏	❏	❏	33.	❏	❏	❏	❏
16.	❏	❏	❏	❏	34.	❏	❏	❏	❏
17.	❏	❏	❏	❏	35.	❏	❏	❏	❏
18.	❏	❏	❏	❏					

CHAPTER 26

Soft-Tissue Injuries

1. One of the major functions of the skin is:
   a. production of fat tissue.
   b. temperature regulation.
   c. the formation of white blood cells.
   d. the release of glucose into the blood.

2. The skin is part of the largest organ system of the body and is the:
   a. first line of defense against infection.
   b. juncture for the formation of red blood cells.
   c. structure that provides nourishment for the cells.
   d. structure that helps stimulates hormone production.

3. When a significant portion of a person's skin is involved in a burn injury, that person is at high risk for _____ shock.
   a. spinal
   b. cardiogenic
   c. anaphylactic
   d. hypovolemic

4. In order from the surface to the underlying muscle or tissue, the layers of the skin are:
   a. hypodermis, epidermis, and dermis.
   b. epidermis, hypodermis, and dermis.
   c. epidermis, dermis, and subcutaneous tissues.
   d. dermis, epidermis, and subcutaneous tissues.

5. The subcutaneous tissue:
   a. supports the production of calcium.
   b. aids in the production of male hormones.
   c. helps to maintain the growth of hair and nails.
   d. attaches the skin to the underlying bone or muscle.

6. You are evaluating a 16-year-old male who ripped open an area of skin on the inside of his upper arm. The injury is approximately 4 inches long. You see fat or adipose tissue and recognize this as part of the:
   a. dermis.
   b. epidermis.
   c. sebaceous glands.
   d. subcutaneous tissue.

7. First responders have immobilized a 23-year-old male who was knocked off an ATV after striking a tree. They report that he is complaining of neck and back pain, and he has a large contusion on his forehead and a very large hematoma on his left flank. Before you begin your examination, you put on your minimum level of PPE, which includes:
   a. gloves.
   b. gloves and a mask.
   c. gloves and eye protection.
   d. gloves, eye protection, and a mask.

8. An 8-year-old child who fell while skateboarding has sustained abrasions on both knees and his left elbow, but has no other injuries. Before treating his injuries, at a minimum you put on:
   a. gloves.
   b. gloves and a mask.
   c. gloves and eye protection.
   d. gloves, eye protection, and a mask.

9. The victim of an assault has contusions and lacerations on her face and scalp. Her nose is bleeding and she is spitting blood. You take body substance isolation precautions that include:
   a. gloves and a gown.
   b. placing an oxygen mask on the patient.
   c. gloves, eye protection, and a mask.
   d. gloves and a face mask for the patient.

10. You are dispatched to the parking lot of the local supermarket for a traumatic injury. Upon arriving, you find a toddler crying. His mother says his fingers were accidentally slammed in the car door. Two fingers are purple under the nails, but the skin is not broken and the fingers do not appear to be broken. This injury can be described as:
    a. closed.
    b. splintering.
    c. compound.
    d. complicated.

11. When a soft-tissue injury results in leakage of fluid from capillaries or larger vessels, the condition is called:
    a. painful.
    b. edema.
    c. life-threatening.
    d. simple compression.

12. Shortly after the accident occurred, EMS was called for a 30-year-old male who walked into a door and struck his forehead. The patient has no altered mental status, but developed swelling, pain, and tenderness at the site. The skin is intact and there is no bleeding, so you determine that this type of injury is a/an:
    a. contusion.
    b. hematoma.
    c. ecchymosis.
    d. possible fracture.

13. An elderly patient tripped on a curb and fell on her face. She has a hematoma and swelling under the left eye. There is no external bleeding, and she denies neck or back pain or losing consciousness. In addition to the closed soft-tissue injury, you must suspect:
    a. facial fractures.
    b. that she is confused about why she fell.
    c. that she is lying about the loss of consciousness.
    d. that this type of blood loss can progress to shock.

14. A babysitter calls EMS for an eye injury. While having a pillow fight, one of the children in her care was struck in the eye. The 8-year old boy has blood present in the sclera (white part) of the left eye. He denies any pain or vision disturbance. The parents are on their way home. Which actions do you take next?
    a. Apply cold over the closed eye and lay the patient down.
    b. Cover both eyes with a dressing and transport the patient.
    c. Apply heat over the closed eye and keep the patient sitting up.
    d. Do not touch the eye, but offer to transport the patient for evaluation.

15. A neighbor knocks on your station door and shows you her thumb. She was cleaning a window when it came down hard on her hand, and now her thumb is swollen and throbbing with pain. She can move and bend it and wants some advice on how to care for it right now; she does not want to go to the hospital. In addition to recommending that she see her physician, you advise her to:
    a. apply cold and elevation.
    b. keep it dry until it has been X-rayed.
    c. let you splint it and transport her to the ED.
    d. apply heat first, then alternate cold and heat.

16. When managing a penetrating injury to the chest, the EMT-B will use an occlusive dressing, which:
    a. provides an airtight seal.
    b. decreases cardiac preload.
    c. controls severe hemorrhage.
    d. prevents subcutaneous emphysema.

17. On a transport to the emergency department, you learn that a patient you treated last week for a GSW to the chest died from a pericardial tamponade. You recall that this injury can result in death because:
    a. of the loss of pulse pressure.
    b. it impairs the filling of the heart.
    c. it causes the vena cava to kink.
    d. of the increase in tracheal deviation.

18. The victim of a stabbing has a wound to the chest and is having difficulty breathing. While you remove her shirt, you hear a sucking sound each time she:
    a. inhales.
    b. coughs.
    c. exhales.
    d. tries to speak.

19. While at a construction site, a worker dropped his nail gun, which accidentally discharged. A coworker was struck with a nail that entered his chest near the right border of the sternum. There is no exit wound, and the patient is complaining of difficulty breathing. The first treatment step for this patient is to:
    a. apply an occlusive dressing.
    b. assist ventilations with a BVM.
    c. determine if the nail was galvanized.
    d. apply a bulky bandage and direct pressure.

20. The victim of an assault is a 20-year-old female who was stabbed with a 12-inch knitting needle. The penetration is 4 inches into the upper left quadrant of her abdomen. Care for this wound includes:
    a. stabilizing the object in place with bulky dressings.
    b. applying an occlusive dressing and direct pressure.
    c. immobilizing the object, but allowing the wound to drain.
    d. removing the object in the opposite direction of entry and applying direct pressure.

21. The police secured the scene at a residence where there was a domestic violence incident. The patient is a 30-year-old male who was reported as being stabbed in the upper back, over the scapula, with a fork. The bleeding is minor, but it continues to trickle. The patient denies difficulty breathing or any other injuries. Care for this wound includes:
    a. occlusive dressing.
    b. direct pressure and bandage.
    c. direct pressure and sitting the patient upright.
    d. pressure bandage with patient lying on his back.

22. Your crew is dispatched to assist a nonambulatory patient with getting back to bed. While assisting the patient, you note one of the following conditions that warrants a trip to the hospital for evaluation. Which is it?

    a. an abdominal hernia
    b. abnormal spinal curvature
    c. peripheral edema in both legs
    d. a lower extremity that is red and hot

23. A motorcycle rider lost control of his bike on a curve, hit a guard rail, and tore open his lower abdomen. The lower right quadrant has an evisceration with a portion of the small bowel exposed. This wound should be managed by:

    a. applying a pressure dressing.
    b. covering with a dry dressing and applying direct pressure.
    c. covering the bowel with a moist sterile dressing and keeping the area warm.
    d. rinsing the bowel, then scooping it back into the abdomen and covering it with a bulky dressing.

24. The police have called EMS for a GSW from a drive-by shooting. The patient is a 25-year-old woman who was shot in the stomach. There is an entrance wound in the upper left quadrant, but no exit wound. In addition to wounds involving abdominal organs, what is another primary associated injury that must be considered?

    a. fracture
    b. chest trauma
    c. spinal cord injury
    d. all of the above

25. An example of a severe burn that should be treated at a burn specialty center is a/an:

    a. electrical burn.
    b. 20 percent BSA partial-thickness burn.
    c. 9 percent BSA superficial burn to a child.
    d. 15 percent BSA superficial burn to an adult.

26. While cooking on a stove, a woman accidentally dumped a pot of boiling water on her right leg. She has redness and blisters on the front of the entire upper leg. The severity of this burn is:

    a. mild.
    b. severe.
    c. moderate.
    d. complicated.

27. Superficial, partial thickness, and full thickness, are all classifications of burns by the:

    a. depth.
    b. source.
    c. location.
    d. severity.

28. While attempting to light a gas grill, a woman lit a match and experienced a sudden burst of flame. She singed her eyebrows, bangs, and arm hairs. She was left with painful reddened skin on the front of both arms and her face. This burn can be classified as a:

    a. superficial burn involving 18 percent BSA.
    b. superficial burn involving 13½ percent BSA.
    c. partial-thickness burn involving 18 percent BSA.
    d. partial-thickness burn involving 27 percent BSA.

29. You have been called to care for the victim of a flash burn. The scene is safe and the patient is sitting down with coworkers who are helping him cool his face with a wet cloth. His entire face and neck is red and he states that he cannot see and that his eyes and face hurt. This burn can be classified as:

    a. superficial.
    b. fourth degree.
    c. full thickness.
    d. partial thickness.

30. A superficial or first-degree burn:

    a. is the most painful type of burn.
    b. involves the outer surface of the skin only.
    c. is characterized as having unbroken blisters.
    d. typically causes painful muscle contractions.

31. When a toddler was lowered into the bathtub, he began screaming. The parents did not test the bath water. The parents call EMS, and when you arrive the child has stocking burns on the legs just below the knees and red spots (splashing) on the thighs. There is severe redness and blisters are beginning to form. This type of burn can be classified as:

    a. child abuse.
    b. partial thickness only.
    c. second and third degree.
    d. superficial and partial thickness.

32. A thermal burn that damages the epidermis and a portion of the dermis, excluding the muscle tissue, is classified as _____ degree.

    a. first
    b. second
    c. third
    d. fourth

33. Persons who suffer a burn injury are at risk for infection:

    a. with any burn.
    b. only with third-degree burns.
    c. when the severity is full thickness or greater.
    d. when the severity is partial thickness or greater.

34. While lighting firecrackers, a 10-year-old male burned his hands, face, and neck. His airway and breathing are clear and adequate, but his face and neck are red and peppered with black powder. Fortunately, his eyes and vision were not affected. His hands are red and blistered and two fingers appear fused together with blisters. Which of his burns is considered the most serious?

    a. first-degree burns on the face
    b. first-degree burns on the neck
    c. partial-thickness burns on the hands
    d. each of these burns is equally serious because of the location

35. A second-degree burn is typically very painful and requires pain management. This is because of the affected:

    a. nerves.
    b. sweat glands.
    c. blood vessels.
    d. sebaceous glands.

36. Which of the following structures is not typically affected by a partial-thickness burn?

    a. nerves
    b. hair follicles
    c. blood vessels
    d. subcutaneous fat

37. A full-thickness burn affects:

    a. every layer of the skin.
    b. only the dermis and epidermis.
    c. more than 30 percent BSA in adults.
    d. more than 15 percent BSA in children.

38. A furnace blast has injured a 32-year-old male. His hands and one arm are critically burned into the soft tissue and muscle. He is conscious but confused, and has hearing loss and audible wheezing. Which of his injuries is an immediate life-threatening condition?

    a. inhalation injuries
    b. acute hearing loss
    c. full-thickness burns
    d. altered mental status

39. A firefighter came to the emergency department a couple of hours after working at a fire. On the back of his right calf he has a burn that apparently resulted from an ember that settled into his boot while he was working. He did not realize he had an injury until he showered, when he noticed that the area involved was dark and felt rough and dry. What type of burn does he have?

    a. first degree
    b. second degree
    c. third degree
    d. first, second, and third degree

40. A worker at a construction site was working with cement and did not realize that the gloves he was wearing were too porous for the job. EMS was called when he removed his gloves and saw that his fingers were graying-white with the skin peeling. His palms were red and had no skin. What type of burn is this?

    a. third degree
    b. a thermal burn
    c. second degree
    d. second and third degree

41. Which of the following characteristics describes a full-thickness burn?

    a. burned or singed hair
    b. an associated fracture
    c. a complication with the airway
    d. damaged blood vessels, fat, or muscle

42. You arrive at one of the local nursing homes for a burn injury call. The victim is an elderly resident who has a burn on the left arm. An electric heating pad was being used for a preexisting injury to the elbow and was accidentally left on overnight. Approximately two-thirds of the arm is blistered with oozing. The center area of the burn is dry and leathery. This burn can be classified as critical because of the:

    a. age of the patient.
    b. location of the burn.
    c. amount of BSA involved.
    d. type or source of the burn.

43. The mother of a toddler called EMS because her daughter was splashed on the arms with very hot water. The mother tried to calm the child's crying by rubbing butter on the superficial splatter areas on the arms, with no success. With the help of the mother, you:

    a. wrap and immobilize both arms in splints.
    b. use ice cubes to cool and wipe off the butter.
    c. rinse the burned areas with cool water for several minutes.
    d. apply a second coat of butter and wrap the arms in sterile dressings.

44. Before providing the correct emergency care for a burn, the EMT-B needs to determine the:

    a. age of the patient.
    b. source of the burn.
    c. weight of the patient.
    d. medications the patient is taking.

45. Emergency care for sunburn that involves the entire posterior surface of the body includes:

    a. applying ice.
    b. cooling the burn.
    c. applying a commercial soothing ointment.
    d. not touching the burn and transporting rapidly.

46. A customer at the town garden center had lime powder spill onto his skin and clothing while lifting a bag into his cart. He is now complaining of a burning sensation. To stop the burning process prior to flushing him with water, you carefully brush off as much of the powder as you can and then instruct the patient to:

    a. remove his clothing, socks, and shoes.
    b. lie face down while you hose him off.
    c. lie on his back while you hose him off.
    d. close his eyes and hold his breath while you hose him off.

47. An adult who was exposed to a flash burn received partial-thickness burns over her entire chest, abdomen, anterior legs, and arms. You do not have enough sterile burn dressing to cover the entire area. What do you do next?

    a. Leave the area uncovered.
    b. Wrap the injured area with plastic cling wrap.
    c. Cover the area with a clean dry sheet.
    d. Cover the area with a clean wet sheet.

48. A woman sustained partial-thickness burns on both hands and arms while putting out a stovetop grease fire. The firefighters are bringing her out of the apartment as you arrive. As you begin your assessment, your partner helps you cut away the patient's sleeves and remove her rings and watch. You do this because:

    a. it helps to prevent blisters.
    b. it helps to prevent swelling.
    c. this will help the healing process.
    d. those items can retain heat and continue to burn the patient.

49. The care of a patient with full-thickness burns over 15 percent BSA or more includes:

    a. administering oxygen.
    b. preventing further heat loss.
    c. covering the burn with sterile dressings.
    d. all of the above.

50. A full-thickness extremity burn that is circumferential should be treated as:

    a. a life-threatening emergency.
    b. a limb-threatening emergency.
    c. the same as any other burn.
    d. like a fracture and be fully immobilized.

51. While working in a lab, a janitor spilled a chemical container and a coworker received severe burns to both lower legs. After cutting away his clothing, you see that the affected skin is white, dry, and leathery, with skin peeling away. The first step in the care of this burn is to:

    a. prevent shock.
    b. administer oxygen.
    c. decontaminate with flushing.
    d. determine the severity of the burn.

52. For a laceration that is deep and bleeding continuously, the use of a dressing will help to:

    a. keep the wound sterile.
    b. prevent further contamination.
    c. cool the injury and stop the bleeding.
    d. prevent heat loss associated with shock.

53. One advantage of quickly applying a dressing to an open wound on a child is:

    a. that the child will always stop crying.
    b. the child will gain trust in the EMT-B.
    c. it will help hide the severity of the injury from the child.
    d. that the parents or caregiver will be more compassionate.

54. The function of a bandage is to:

    a. hold a dressing in place.
    b. reduce arterial blood flow.
    c. occlude venous blood flow.
    d. reduce the risk of a hematoma.

55. Large blisters resulting from steam burns are best managed by:

    a. covering with dressings to keep them from rupturing.
    b. rupturing the blisters first, then wrapping them with bandages.
    c. splinting whenever possible, with dressings over the splint.
    d. wrapping first with dressings, then rupturing the blisters with pressure.

56. The use of a bandage will substantially aid in:

    a. stopping arterial blood flow.
    b. preventing movement at the injury site.
    c. reducing the risk of contamination and infection.
    d. all of the above.

57. A traumatic injury at a work site has left a 45-year-old male with a large laceration across the lower abdomen. When you cut away the clothing, you see abdominal contents protruding and you quickly apply a bandage over the evisceration. The goal of application of this type of dressing is to:

    a. retain moisture and warmth.
    b. prevent nausea and vomiting.
    c. absorb any blood lost from abdominal organs.
    d. absorb any contents spilled from abdominal organs.

58. You are making a pressure bandage for bleeding from an open wound on an extremity. Which of the following pieces of equipment may be used when manual pressure is not enough?

    a. BP cuff
    b. pillow splint
    c. traction splint
    d. padded-board splint

59. To stop the bleeding of an open wound, a pressure bandage may be applied _____ the wound site.
    a. on
    b. below
    c. under
    d. above

60. Before a pressure bandage is applied to control bleeding, the EMT-B should:
    a. apply oxygen.
    b. apply an ice pack.
    c. locate the pressure point.
    d. use direct pressure and elevation.

61. Police called EMS for the victim of a stabbing. When you arrive, the police officers take you to a young woman who is unresponsive with labored breathing. She is lying on a couch with a 6-inch knife protruding from her abdomen. The knife appears to be pointed up toward the chest and you suspect serious internal injuries. Each of the following is a potential injury associated with this type of MOI, except:
    a. torn diaphragm.
    b. punctured lung.
    c. perforated heart.
    d. lacerated trachea.

62. You are called to a local baseball field for a traumatic injury with difficulty breathing. A player was struck in the chest by a full swing of a bat. He is alert, anxious, spitting up blood, and working to breathe. Lung sounds are present in the apices, but decreased in both bases. He has an unstable rib segment and you suspect a hemothorax. Emergency care for this injury begins with:
    a. calling ALS for help with chest decompression.
    b. immobilizing the C-spine and beginning rapid transport.
    c. splinting the ribs, assisting ventilations, and watching for vomiting.
    d. stabilizing the flail section, administering high-flow oxygen, and assisting ventilations if necessary.

63. In which of the following situations would you suspect a potentially serious airway injury from a burn?
    a. a mechanic who is in severe pain after splashing fuel in his eyes
    b. an electrician who received a high-voltage shock and is stunned
    c. a customer who burnt her lips and tongue on extremely hot coffee
    d. a firefighter who is wheezing after working in an overhaul after a fire

64. A major complication commonly associated with an improperly applied dressing includes:
    a. death.
    b. loss of limb.
    c. patient discomfort.
    d. increased tissue damage.

65. After unsuccessfully attempting to control an arterial bleed from the lower leg with every method you have been trained to use, you now decide to apply a tourniquet. Which of the following items should be used to control the bleeding?
    a. a strand of string
    b. a wide band of cloth
    c. a piece of rope or wire
    d. 2-inch or 3-inch tape wrapped around the upper leg

66. You and your partner are attempting to control an arterial bleed of the upper arm. Direct pressure, elevation, and pressure on a pressure point appear to have stopped the bleeding. In an effort to prevent the bleeding from starting again, you:
    a. apply a tourniquet.
    b. maintain elevation and apply a pressure bandage.
    c. remove the soaked dressing and apply a dry sterile dressing.
    d. remove the soaked dressing and apply an ice pack over a pressure dressing.

67. The victim of an assault has been sliced on the face from the ear to the tip of her nose, and stabbed in the leg with a 3-inch pocketknife, which is still in the wound. She is alert and spitting blood. Which action do you take first?
    a. Manage the ABCs.
    b. Stabilize the knife wound.
    c. Put on your eye protection and gloves.
    d. Apply direct pressure to the facial wound.

68. Teenagers at a backyard pool party were playing with a Frisbee when an 18-year-old girl slipped and fell backward into a glass door. She did not lose consciousness, but she has multiple lacerations on her back, arms, and legs. Upon closer examination, you find a large piece of glass remaining in a wound in her right flank area. Management of her wounds includes:
    a. controlling bleeding, bandaging, and stabilizing the glass in place.
    b. removing all the glass, controlling the bleeding, and immobilizing her on a long backboard.
    c. removing only the largest pieces of glass and immobilizing her on a long backboard.
    d. each of the actions listed here is inappropriate.

69. Moving or removing an object that has impaled the foot can result in:
    a. nausea and vomiting.
    b. acute hypovolemic shock.
    c. an increased risk of infection, and bleeding.
    d. damage to blood vessels, nerves, and muscles.

70. The objective of managing an amputated body part is to:
    a. prevent damage to the exposed nerves.
    b. control bleeding of the stump and the amputated part.
    c. prevent blood vessels from closing and becoming damaged.
    d. control bleeding of the stump and save the part for possible reattachment or reimplantation.

71. The use of dry ice in the emergency care of an amputated body part is not recommended because:
    a. it can actually burn the tissue.
    b. there is no way to control the bleeding of the part.
    c. it is difficult to wrap or seal the part with the dry ice.
    d. dry ice is not an effective method of cooling or freezing.

72. While working with a chainsaw to trim tree limbs, an elderly male lost control of the saw and cut off the first two fingers of his left hand. He looks pale, is trembling, and is bleeding through the rag he used to wrap his hand. You begin to manage this patient by:
    a. wrapping the amputated fingers in sterile moist gauze pads.
    b. laying him down and controlling the bleeding of the stump with direct pressure.
    c. sitting him down and using direct pressure and ice packs to control the bleeding.
    d. dressing the stump with a compression bandage and placing the amputated fingers in a bag of ice.

73. While working in a machine shop, an employee took off his hard hat to wipe his brow and face. Just then, a forklift came by and knocked over a metal sheet that struck the worker in the back of the leg, completely tearing off a large piece of skin. When you arrive, coworkers have controlled the bleeding with bandages and have the skin in a plastic bag with ice cubes. You begin to assess the patient and ask your partner to:
    a. try to thaw any parts of the amputated part that may have frozen.
    b. take the amputated part out of the ice and place it in a dry sterile dressing.
    c. place the bag with the amputated part in the ambulance so it is not left behind.
    d. wrap the amputated part in a sterile, moist gauze pad and place it in another plastic bag, and then place the bag on ice.

74. A worker in an industrial setting has splashed a chemical into his eyes. Before you arrived, coworkers got him to an eyewash station and began flushing. The patient tells you that he cannot see and that he has a great deal of pain. When you examine his eyes you see that he is wearing contact lenses. Management for this injury includes:
    a. calling for ALS, as the patient is going to need analgesia.
    b. removing the lenses or assisting the patient to do so.
    c. not touching the eyes or lenses and continuing to flush the eyes.
    d. not touching the eyes or lenses and beginning transport to the hospital.

75. The police have called you to care for one of their officers. During the arrest of a person who was combative, they used pepper spray and one officer was sprayed in the face. Treatment for this exposure begins with:
    a. wiping off any wet spray that is left on the skin and flushing with milk.
    b. instructing the officer to spit, blow his nose, and not rub the eyes or face.
    c. sponging off the exposed area without rubbing and flushing the eyes with water.
    d. moving the officer to a sink and flushing the entire head, face, and neck with cold water.

76. EMS is dispatched to a hazmat scene where a worker was reported to have spilled concentrated sodium hydroxide on his arm. You look up the chemical in your hazmat reference and see that it is a strong alkali that will require flushing with water. You prepare to flush the patient and recall that:
    a. alkalis are weaker than acids and require less flushing.
    b. cold water is better than warm water for this type of care.
    c. inhalation injuries are common with this type of exposure.
    d. alkalis are stronger than acids and require a lot of flushing.

77. A golfer who was struck by lighting is lying in the wet grass on the fairway. As you approach, he appears to be unresponsive and a witness tells you he was struck and thrown backward. The first step in emergency care for this patient is to:
    a. start CPR if he has no pulse.
    b. immobilize him to a long backboard.
    c. assess for entrance and exit wounds.
    d. get the patient out of the rain and into the ambulance.

78. A homeowner who was last seen by his wife digging in the front yard was found collapsed on the ground. Dispatch is unable to determine if the patient is breathing because the caller is hysterical. As you approach the patient, it becomes clear that he struck an underground wire with his shovel. They next step in the care of this patient is to:
    a. start CPR if he has no pulse.
    b. back off and call the power company.
    c. move the patient onto a long backboard.
    d. let the fire department extricate the patient from his present location.

79. The weekend handyman was attempting to do his own wiring in the basement fuse box when the power went out. His wife called EMS because he was knocked out. When you get to him, he is responsive to pain, breathing adequately, and has a strong distal pulse. There are obvious black burns on his hands and you look for an exit wound first on his:
    a. feet.
    b. head.
    c. back.
    d. face.

80. Which type of burn can cause the most injury to the lower airways?
    a. arc
    b. flash
    c. steam
    d. chemical

81. An ATV rollover crash involving a 20-year-old male has left him conscious, but not alert. He has an open wound across the nose and the left eyeball has been knocked out of the socket. Care for this injury includes:
    a. continuous flushing of the eye to keep it moist.
    b. replacing the eyeball in the socket and covering it with a dressing.
    c. covering the eye with a moist dressing without replacing it in the socket.
    d. replacing the eyeball in the socket and covering both eyes with a dressing.

82. A circumferential partial- or full-thickness burn to the upper torso is considered a serious injury to the respiratory system because:
    a. of the BSA involved.
    b. of the increased risk of heart attack.
    c. it impedes the ability of the chest wall to expand.
    d. of the rapid onset of shock associated with this area of the body.

83. The three sources of electrical burns are:
    a. first, second, and third degree.
    b. arcing, contact, and flash burns.
    c. open, closed, and partial penetration.
    d. superficial, partial thickness, and full thickness.

84. A couple was painting their apartment when the husband stood up under a ladder and cut open his head. You see evidence of a lot of bleeding, and when you assess the wound you see a 6-inch flap of skin folded down over the right ear. You manage this wound by:
    a. replacing the flap and applying a dry sterile bandage.
    b. palpating the skull for a fracture and evidence of brain tissue.
    c. leaving the flap down and applying compression with a dry sterile bandage.
    d. taping the flap down with an occlusive dressing and covering it with a trauma bandage.

85. (Continuing with the preceding question) After you have finished applying a dressing and bandage, you see that the bleeding has not stopped and has soaked the dressing. What steps can you take next?
    a. Apply pressure to the nearest pressure point.
    b. Sit the patient down and apply direct pressure over the wound.
    c. Remove the first dressing and rewrap with a pressure dressing.
    d. Lay the patient down and elevate his legs while holding pressure on the wound.

Chapter 26 Answer Form

	A	B	C	D
1.	❏	❏	❏	❏
2.	❏	❏	❏	❏
3.	❏	❏	❏	❏
4.	❏	❏	❏	❏
5.	❏	❏	❏	❏
6.	❏	❏	❏	❏
7.	❏	❏	❏	❏
8.	❏	❏	❏	❏
9.	❏	❏	❏	❏
10.	❏	❏	❏	❏
11.	❏	❏	❏	❏
12.	❏	❏	❏	❏
13.	❏	❏	❏	❏
14.	❏	❏	❏	❏
15.	❏	❏	❏	❏
16.	❏	❏	❏	❏
17.	❏	❏	❏	❏
18.	❏	❏	❏	❏
19.	❏	❏	❏	❏
20.	❏	❏	❏	❏
21.	❏	❏	❏	❏
22.	❏	❏	❏	❏
23.	❏	❏	❏	❏
24.	❏	❏	❏	❏
25.	❏	❏	❏	❏
26.	❏	❏	❏	❏
27.	❏	❏	❏	❏
28.	❏	❏	❏	❏
29.	❏	❏	❏	❏
30.	❏	❏	❏	❏
31.	❏	❏	❏	❏
32.	❏	❏	❏	❏

	A	B	C	D
33.	❏	❏	❏	❏
34.	❏	❏	❏	❏
35.	❏	❏	❏	❏
36.	❏	❏	❏	❏
37.	❏	❏	❏	❏
38.	❏	❏	❏	❏
39.	❏	❏	❏	❏
40.	❏	❏	❏	❏
41.	❏	❏	❏	❏
42.	❏	❏	❏	❏
43.	❏	❏	❏	❏
44.	❏	❏	❏	❏
45.	❏	❏	❏	❏
46.	❏	❏	❏	❏
47.	❏	❏	❏	❏
48.	❏	❏	❏	❏
49.	❏	❏	❏	❏
50.	❏	❏	❏	❏
51.	❏	❏	❏	❏
52.	❏	❏	❏	❏
53.	❏	❏	❏	❏
54.	❏	❏	❏	❏
55.	❏	❏	❏	❏
56.	❏	❏	❏	❏
57.	❏	❏	❏	❏
58.	❏	❏	❏	❏
59.	❏	❏	❏	❏
60.	❏	❏	❏	❏
61.	❏	❏	❏	❏
62.	❏	❏	❏	❏
63.	❏	❏	❏	❏
64.	❏	❏	❏	❏

	A	B	C	D			A	B	C	D
65.	❏	❏	❏	❏		76.	❏	❏	❏	❏
66.	❏	❏	❏	❏		77.	❏	❏	❏	❏
67.	❏	❏	❏	❏		78.	❏	❏	❏	❏
68.	❏	❏	❏	❏		79.	❏	❏	❏	❏
69.	❏	❏	❏	❏		80.	❏	❏	❏	❏
70.	❏	❏	❏	❏		81.	❏	❏	❏	❏
71.	❏	❏	❏	❏		82.	❏	❏	❏	❏
72.	❏	❏	❏	❏		83.	❏	❏	❏	❏
73.	❏	❏	❏	❏		84.	❏	❏	❏	❏
74.	❏	❏	❏	❏		85.	❏	❏	❏	❏
75.	❏	❏	❏	❏						

CHAPTER 27

Musculoskeletal Care

1. The intercostal muscles of the chest are classified as _____ muscle.
   a. skeletal
   b. smooth
   c. cardiac
   d. tensile-strength

2. When muscles contract, the normal result is:
   a. pain.
   b. strain.
   c. pressure.
   d. body movement.

3. Muscles are named according to their:
   a. size.
   b. shape.
   c. location.
   d. all of the above.

4. Cartilage, tendons, and ligaments are connective tissues associated with:
   a. the production of blood cells.
   b. beating of the heart muscle.
   c. movement of the skeletal system.
   d. movement of food through the digestive system.

5. A metabolic function of support provided by the skeletal system is the:
   a. production of blood cells.
   b. destruction of blood cells.
   c. regulation of blood glucose.
   d. stimulation of hair and nail growth.

6. The thorax (rib cage), spinal column, and skull are bones that:
   a. stimulate muscle growth.
   b. protect organs of the body.
   c. aid in movement of the body.
   d. contain storage sites for hormones.

7. While splinting a patient who has a possible ankle fracture/dislocation, you consider the bones that make up the ankle; you know that the _____ is not a bone in that grouping.
   a. talus
   b. tibia
   c. fibula
   d. metatarsal

8. The bones of the hands that make up the fingertips are the:
   a. tarsals.
   b. carpals.
   c. phalanges.
   d. metacarpals.

9. Which of the following is not a bone of the thorax?
   a. sternum
   b. costal arch
   c. floating ribs
   d. manubrium

10. The shoulder girdle is comprised of the:
    a. clavicle, humerus, and scapula.
    b. manubrium, clavicle, and scapula.
    c. acromion process, scapula, and manubrium.
    d. acromioclavicular (A/C) joint, clavicle, and cervical spine.

11. When the EMT-B describes a musculoskeletal injury in a verbal or written report, the information that should be included is the anatomical area involved, the level of discomfort, a description of the painful or swollen deformity, and:
    a. whether it was an open or closed injury.
    b. the name of each bone involved.
    c. a diagnosis of a fracture or sprain.
    d. the name of each muscle involved.

12. On a Saturday morning, you are dispatched to the local elementary school for a traumatic injury. While playing basketball, a 32-year-old male injured his ankle. He states that he landed hard and felt it crack and is now having severe pain. The ankle is grossly deformed and there is blood under the skin in the area of the injury. This injury can be described as:

    a. closed.
    b. open.
    c. sprained.
    d. strained.

13. As the standby ambulance crew at a high school football game, you are signaled to come over to an injured player. The player is writhing in pain as the trainer shows you his kneecap, which appears to be displaced. The area is swollen and deformed and a hematoma is developing. This injury is:

    a. closed.
    b. open.
    c. the type that requires ALS.
    d. the type that cannot be splinted.

14. Splinting a long-bone fracture in _____ will prevent further damage to blood vessels, bones, and muscles.

    a. a straight position
    b. an elevated position
    c. a position of comfort
    d. the position it is found

15. When splinting a dislocation, the EMT-B should immobilize the injury in the _____ while maintaining a good blood supply distal to the injury.

    a. straight position
    b. elevated position
    c. lowered position
    d. position of comfort for the patient

16. When splinting a long-bone fracture, the key objective is to carefully splint the extremity:

    a. within 30 minutes of the time of the injury.
    b. within 15 minutes of the time of the injury.
    c. to minimize the opportunity for the patient to self-splint.
    d. without allowing the bone to protrude through the skin.

17. You have just finished applying a sling and swathe on a teenager who flipped over the handlebars of his bike and appears to have dislocated or fractured his right shoulder. The goal in splinting this type of injury is to:

    a. immobilize the elbow and wrist joint.
    b. eliminate the patient's pain completely.
    c. immobilize the shoulder and elbow joint.
    d. return the shoulder to a position of function.

18. The ongoing assessment of an extremity that was splinted because of a possible fracture includes:

    a. reassessing vital signs every 5 minutes.
    b. applying ice to reduce the pain and swelling.
    c. noting and managing any diminishment in PMS.
    d. reassessing the blood pressure every 15 minutes.

19. An elderly patient who uses a walker fell in her apartment and now has pain in her thigh and is unable to get up. Your partner is holding stabilization on her femur, which appears deformed and swollen. Before applying a traction splint, you:

    a. assess proximal PMS.
    b. assess distal PMS.
    c. move the patient to a long backboard.
    d. determine if the injury is a sprain or strain rather than a fracture.

20. You are en route to the hospital with a patient who has a painful, swollen deformity of the wrist that you splinted on the scene. You perform the ongoing assessment and discover that the patient's fingers are tingling and becoming numb. The cause of this complication is most likely:

    a. that the splint has been applied too loosely.
    b. that the splint has been applied too tightly.
    c. an early sign of permanent nerve damage.
    d. an early indicator of permanent motor function injury.

21. When a splint is incorrectly applied, which of the following conditions may occur?

    a. increased bleeding
    b. increased swelling and pain
    c. increased circulation distal to the injury
    d. increased circulation proximal to the injury

22. The EMT-B is trained to fully immobilize a patient with a serious MOI who complains of neck or back pain to a long backboard. Upon arrival at the ED and after examination by the physician, the most common complication associated with this type of splinting is:

    a. that the chest straps were too loose.
    b. that the cervical collar was incorrectly applied.
    c. a decrease in motor function of the lower extremities.
    d. increased back pain due to lying on a long backboard for a long time.

23. After a prolonged extrication, a driver who was involved in a MVC is freed. He is alert and his vital signs are good; his only injury is to the left upper arm, which is painfully swollen and deformed. The distal pulse is absent and his fingers feel numb. The transport to the hospital will take 40 minutes. What steps do you take next?
    a. Splint the injury on the scene.
    b. Splint the injury during the transport.
    c. Apply an ice pack and do not splint.
    d. Let the patient put the arm in a position of comfort.

24. Friends have asked you out for a day hike. Shortly after you begin the hike, one of them severely twists an ankle. You begin to look for something to make a splint, but the injured friend insists on walking out, so you explain that the longer you wait to splint the injury, the more likely it is that she will suffer an:
    a. increased blood loss.
    b. increased swelling and pain.
    c. increased risk of loss of function.
    d. all of the above.

25. You have responded to a call for a traumatic injury. Upon arrival, a man waves you in and tells you that his neighbor injured her hand while cleaning the lawn mower. The patient is holding a cloth around her hand, which is deformed and bleeding, as she runs toward the ambulance. She is pleading for you to quickly take her to the hospital, which is only 5 minutes away. You explain to the patient that you need to assess and manage the injury before transporting because:
    a. you can stop the bleeding.
    b. she will bleed to death if you don't.
    c. this will prevent the patient from going into shock.
    d. doing so will minimize the opportunity for further injury.

26. Which of the following type of splint is commonly used for musculoskeletal injuries involving the shoulder, humerus, elbow, and forearm?
    a. air splint
    b. rigid splint
    c. traction splint
    d. sling and swathe

27. After falling on an outstretched hand, a 14-year-old male appears to have a dislocation of the right elbow. This type of injury is serious and requires cautious management during immobilization due to the:
    a. age of the patient.
    b. potential for excessive blood loss.
    c. proximity of the radial artery to the injury site.
    d. proximity of the brachial artery to the injury site.

28. Each of the following is an advantage of splinting a painful, swollen, or deformed extremity, except:
    a. splints help to reduce muscle damage.
    b. splints can easily be made from many different materials.
    c. splinting helps to prevent excessive bleeding at the injury site.
    d. splinting can keep a closed fracture from becoming an open fracture.

29. A skier has fallen and has an open fracture of the lower leg. There is bleeding and a bone end is visible. After assessing distal PMS, the next steps in the management of this injury are to:
    a. splint the leg and then control the bleeding.
    b. control bleeding with a compression bandage, then splint.
    c. rinse off the bone end, splint the leg, and then apply a pressure bandage.
    d. place a temporary tourniquet on the upper leg, then splint and release the tourniquet.

30. In the management of a painful, swollen, and deformed extremity, the EMT-B can minimize swelling of the injury site by:
    a. applying an ice pack.
    b. applying a heat pack.
    c. elevating the patient's head when the patient is lying on the stretcher.
    d. frequently raising and lowering the extremity to promote improved circulation.

31. After tripping and falling, an elderly patient tells you that her chest hurts in the area under her left arm. She is sitting still and leaning toward the left side. She has pain with each respiration and is taking shallow breaths. You suspect:
    a. a pneumothorax and call for ALS.
    b. rib fractures and splint her with a sling and swathe.
    c. rib fractures and immobilize her to a long backboard.
    d. cardiac chest pain and respiratory distress and assist her with nitroglycerin.

32. While cleaning a handgun, the owner accidentally discharged the weapon, causing the bullet to go through his right palm. Which bones do you suspect are involved?
    a. carpals and tarsals
    b. tarsals and metatarsals
    c. carpals and metacarpals
    d. metacarpals and metatarsals

33. You are obtaining a history from a patient who was involved in a MVC. She tells you that she has a preexisting sacral spinal injury. You recall that this area is:

    a. the tailbone.
    b. part of the pelvis.
    c. the lower part of the back.
    d. the upper part of the back.

34. A fracture that occurs through a process of weakening from disease is called a/an _____ fracture.

    a. epiphyseal
    b. pathological
    c. osteoporotic
    d. nondisplaced

35. The finding of crepitus in an extremity injury is an indication that the injury is:

    a. open.
    b. a strain.
    c. a sprain.
    d. a fracture.

Chapter 27 Answer Form

	A	B	C	D			A	B	C	D
1.	❏	❏	❏	❏		19.	❏	❏	❏	❏
2.	❏	❏	❏	❏		20.	❏	❏	❏	❏
3.	❏	❏	❏	❏		21.	❏	❏	❏	❏
4.	❏	❏	❏	❏		22.	❏	❏	❏	❏
5.	❏	❏	❏	❏		23.	❏	❏	❏	❏
6.	❏	❏	❏	❏		24.	❏	❏	❏	❏
7.	❏	❏	❏	❏		25.	❏	❏	❏	❏
8.	❏	❏	❏	❏		26.	❏	❏	❏	❏
9.	❏	❏	❏	❏		27.	❏	❏	❏	❏
10.	❏	❏	❏	❏		28.	❏	❏	❏	❏
11.	❏	❏	❏	❏		29.	❏	❏	❏	❏
12.	❏	❏	❏	❏		30.	❏	❏	❏	❏
13.	❏	❏	❏	❏		31.	❏	❏	❏	❏
14.	❏	❏	❏	❏		32.	❏	❏	❏	❏
15.	❏	❏	❏	❏		33.	❏	❏	❏	❏
16.	❏	❏	❏	❏		34.	❏	❏	❏	❏
17.	❏	❏	❏	❏		35.	❏	❏	❏	❏
18.	❏	❏	❏	❏						

CHAPTER

Injuries to the Head and Spine

1. The peripheral nervous system includes which of the following structures?
   a. brain stem
   b. cerebrospinal fluid
   c. brain and spinal cord
   d. 31 pairs of spinal nerves

2. The division of the nervous system that is composed of the brain and spinal cord is the _____ nervous system.
   a. central
   b. peripheral
   c. automatic
   d. autonomic

3. The regulation of activities such as maintaining heart rate and blood pressure are under the control of the _____ nervous system.
   a. central
   b. peripheral
   c. automatic
   d. autonomic

4. _____ cushion(s) and protects the brain and spinal cord from outside impact.
   a. Receptors
   b. Motor nerves
   c. Sensory nerves
   d. Cerebrospinal fluid

5. While playing softball, an outfielder was struck in the head with a ball. In addition to complaining of a headache, the player is having vision disturbances. Which part of the brain has been affected?
   a. frontal
   b. parietal
   c. occipital
   d. temporal

6. The brain is connected to the spinal cord by which of the following structures?
   a. meninges
   b. brain stem
   c. cerebellum
   d. hypothalamus

7. The _____ originate(s) in the spinal cord and lead to the arms, legs, and the trunk of the body.
   a. dura mater
   b. spinal nerves
   c. cranial nerves
   d. accessory nerves

8. The spinal canal is located in an opening in the:
   a. vertebrae.
   b. fontanelle.
   c. mastoid process.
   d. foramen magnum.

9. The main nerve trunk connecting the body to the brain is/are the:
   a. meninges.
   b. spinal cord.
   c. spinal nerves.
   d. cranial nerves.

10. A person who has sustained a significant electrical shock is typically immobilized by EMS personnel because of the potential for head injury caused by:
    a. the exit wound.
    b. trauma from falling.
    c. the entrance wound.
    d. loss of reflex control.

11. You are assessing a patient with a questionable MOI for a potential spinal injury. He wants to be "checked out," but does not want to be strapped to a long backboard. When making the determination that this patient is reliable, which of the following findings would exclude his wishes and make immobilization necessary due to the MOI?
    a. He is sober.
    b. He has a broken ankle.
    c. He is alert and oriented.
    d. He is calm and cooperative.

12. The MOI is one of the most important factors in the assessment and treatment of an injured patient, because:
    a. even patients who have experienced minor MOIs will develop deficits later.
    b. a significant MOI will always cause some form of neurological problem for the patient.
    c. the potential for significant injury is recognized from the MOI, rather than presence or absence of symptoms.
    d. the MOI is the absolute deciding factor in determining the need for spinal immobilization.

13. Filling the voids when splinting the spine will:
    a. minimize the pain from any new injury.
    b. prevent increased pain from preexisting back injuries.
    c. make the patient more comfortable on a long backboard.
    d. prevent the development of pain associated with lying on a backboard for a long time.

14. The patient with a suspected spinal injury is immobilized in a neutral position because:
    a. this position reduces stability.
    b. it is the most perpetual position for the spinal column.
    c. this position allows maximum comfort for the patient.
    d. this position allows the most space for the spinal cord.

15. The primary goal in caring for a potential spinal injury is to:
    a. apply a rigid collar.
    b. prevent further injury.
    c. increase lung expansion.
    d. maintain a neutral position.

16. The victim of a GSW was shot in the abdomen. He is alert, weak, and losing a lot of blood. When you roll him to inspect his back, you find an exit wound. You find no pain or deformity upon palpation of his neck and spine. You quickly place a trauma dressing on the exit wound and fully immobilize him to a long backboard because:
    a. he has the MOI for a spinal injury.
    b. this is the fastest way to move him.
    c. a backboard will be needed if CPR becomes necessary.
    d. all of the above.

17. Which of the following signs or symptoms is an indication of a potential spinal injury?
    a. poorly localized cervical pain
    b. stable cervical spinous processes
    c. no deficit or loss of PMS in one or more extremities
    d. lateral neck and shoulder pain with active movement

18. At the scene of a MVC, you are assessing a backseat passenger with a complaint of low back pain. She is 80 years old, has a history of hypertension, and has arthritis for which she takes medications. When you assess distal PMS in her upper extremities, she has a very weak grip, especially with the right hand. You suspect that this:
    a. is a symptom of stroke and now you will up-triage her.
    b. may be due to the arthritis and ask her if this is normal.
    c. weakness is a result of spinal injury, so you immobilize her to a long backboard.
    d. requires splinting the right extremity, as it may be a possible fracture or dislocation.

19. The patient you are assessing has a questionable MOI and denies neck or back pain. Before making a decision about immobilization, you:
    a. call medical control for direction.
    b. ask her if she has ever been immobilized in the past.
    c. assess for spinal tenderness by palpating each spinous process.
    d. ask her if she has a fear of being restricted with limited movement.

20. The husband of a 38-year-old woman called EMS because his wife slipped going downstairs in their home. She is alert, lying at the bottom of the stairs, and tells you that she slipped near the top and slid down on her back. She has pain on her tailbone, and when you palpate her back there is tenderness next to but not on the lumbar spine. Treatment considerations for this patient are:
    a. do not immobilize if no deficits are noted in the distal PMS.
    b. to immobilize her to a long backboard for a potential spinal injury.
    c. do not immobilize, because there is only tenderness and no local pain.
    d. do not immobilize, because the spinal cord does not reach as far as the tailbone.

21. Neighbors of an elderly man called EMS because they saw him fall approximately five feet off a ladder in his yard. They tell you that he did not lose consciousness and that they kept him lying down while waiting for you to arrive. The patient appears confused, but denies any injuries or pain in the neck, back, or extremities. When you decide if immobilization is appropriate, which of the following factors is not an indication of a spinal injury?
    a. pain with movement of the back
    b. tenderness when the spine is palpated
    c. the MOI, age of the patient, and confused mental status
    d. denial of any injuries or pain in the neck, back, or extremities

22. While returning from the hospital, you and your partner witness a serious MVC at a busy intersection. The driver of one vehicle is slumped on the wheel so that the horn is continuously blowing. You park the ambulance as your partner notifies dispatch. The other two drivers are out of their vehicles and deny having any injuries, but as you approach the last driver it is quickly apparent that he is unconscious, and his breathing is inadequate with snoring respirations. The next step you take is to:
    a. begin a rapid extrication.
    b. suction his airway and apply a cervical collar.
    c. apply a cervical collar and begin ventilations with a BVM.
    d. lift his head into a neutral position and perform a jaw thrust.

23. Dispatch has sent you to a MVC with a motorcycle. When you arrive, the first ambulance on scene directs you to go to a rider who is lying in the road with an EMT-B holding manual stabilization of his C-spine. The rider is conscious, alert, and appears to have an open fracture of the left femur. His airway is clear and he denies difficulty breathing or chest pain. After you complete a rapid trauma exam, you begin to apply a traction splint and then the patient loses consciousness. What steps do you take next?
    a. Remove his helmet and assess his airway and breathing.
    b. Assess his airway and breathing and then remove the helmet.
    c. Assess his ABCs and remove the helmet if you need to manage the airway.
    d. Remove his helmet, apply a cervical collar, and roll him onto a long backboard.

24. The victim of an assault was beaten with a bat on the head, face, and back. She is alert and has bleeding from the nose and facial injuries. As you begin to immobilize her, you consider how to keep her airway clear from all the blood that is draining from her injuries. You will manage her airway by:
    a. holding a jaw thrust and suctioning continuously.
    b. holding a jaw thrust and suctioning her as needed.
    c. tilting the backboard to assist with drainage and suctioning frequently.
    d. tilting the backboard to assist with drainage and suctioning continuously.

25. Dispatch has sent you to a local department store for a fall. When you arrive, you find a crowd at the bottom of an escalator and an elderly woman lying on the ground. She has multiple skin tears and is complaining of neck and back pain. When you attempt to move her head into a neutral position, she cries out in pain. In the next attempt to stabilize her, you:
    a. do nothing and call for ALS to assist.
    b. splint her neck in the position it was found.
    c. ask her to relax and attempt a neutral position again.
    d. ask a couple of bystanders to help you move her into a neutral position using traction.

26. You are helping to teach a new EMT-B course, and the skill you are teaching is C-spine stabilization. You demonstrate to the students how to place the head in a neutral position and maintain stabilization until:
    a. PMS is assessed after immobilization.
    b. the cervical collar is securely fastened.
    c. the MOI is determined to be insignificant.
    d. the patient is properly secured to an immobilization device.

27. A motorcycle rider with a passenger had a crash. The passenger is sitting on the ground holding her helmet in her lap as you approach her. She is crying and says that she cannot feel her legs. The next step you take is to:
    a. give her a hug.
    b. ask the patient to lie down.
    c. place a cervical collar on her neck.
    d. ask the patient not to move her head.

28. Which of the following is not an indication for the use of a cervical spine immobilization device?
    a. patient who is unconscious for no apparent reason
    b. normal vital signs with an isolated extremity injury
    c. patient appears intoxicated and the MOI is questionable
    d. underage patient with a questionable MOI who will not fit securely on a long backboard

29. A 17-year-old female was a driver in the second car of a five-car chain collision. When you arrive, she is standing next to her vehicle talking on her cell phone and crying to someone that her neck hurts. She sits in her vehicle as you approach and perform an initial assessment. You find that she is stable, but needs transport for evaluation of the potential spinal injury. You decide to:
    a. apply a short-board device.
    b. perform a rapid extrication onto a long backboard.
    c. wait for her mother to arrive because she is not an adult.
    d. have the patient stand and perform a standing takedown immobilization.

30. The decision to size and apply a cervical collar is based on the:
    a. MOI only.
    b. chief complaint.
    c. signs and symptoms.
    d. MOI, signs, and symptoms.

31. A victim of an assault was strangled, and has finger and thumb bruises on his neck. He is alert and complaining of neck pain in a strained voice. His lung sounds are clear and his vital signs are stable. As you begin to immobilize him, he tells you that he is having difficulty breathing. You suspect:
    a. injury to C-4 and C-5.
    b. swelling of his tongue.
    c. swelling of his airway tissues.
    d. bleeding of his airway tissues.

32. A child was knocked unconscious at a Little League game by a ball that struck him in the temporal skull area. When you first arrived he was awake, but now he is becoming unconscious again. The patient is at risk for:
    a. dental trauma.
    b. vision disturbances.
    c. vomiting and aspiration.
    d. hemorrhage from an avulsion.

33. After securing an unconscious patient with a head injury to a spinal immobilization device, primary management for the patient includes ensuring:
    a. that hypoxia is prevented.
    b. that the patient is hyperventilated.
    c. adequate distal motor function.
    d. that the blood pressure stays over 110 systolic.

34. The crew chief has asked you to immobilize a stable infant who is still in her car seat. The collision was a significant MOI. The child begins to cry when your partner takes manual stabilization of her head. You now begin to immobilize her by:
    a. fitting a pillow around her head and taping it down.
    b. using a rolled towel and securing it around her neck.
    c. tape the head in place with nothing around the neck.
    d. doing nothing until the child stops crying, to prevent further agitation.

35. The driver of a vehicle that was involved in a low-speed collision is complaining of neck and low back pain. After your initial assessment, you find him stable and call for help to immobilize him, because he weighs more than 400 pounds. You check to see if he will fit into your short spinal immobilization device by:
    a. asking him his height.
    b. sizing the device to the patient.
    c. wrapping a 9-foot strap around him to see if it will close.
    d. asking him to take a deep breath and hold it while you measure his waist.

36. As the second ambulance to arrive at the scene of an MVC, you are directed to immobilize a 6-year-old child with a complaint of neck pain. A first responder is holding spinal stabilization on the patient in the second-row seat of a minivan. You size up a cervical spine immobilization device for the child patient by:
    a. considering the patient's age.
    b. considering the patient's level of distress.
    c. considering the patient's weight and height.
    d. making the adult-size device fit by securing it tighter.

37. You are working with an ALS crew to immobilize a patient who was injured in an industrial accident. The patient is unstable with a head injury, and the crew is ready to roll the patient onto the long backboard. Which responder makes the count to begin the roll?
    a. the most senior responder
    b. the responder stabilizing the head
    c. the responder with the highest level of training
    d. the responder who has established a rapport with the patient

38. The rider of an ATV is lying on the ground with his helmet on; he fell off the vehicle while traveling up a hill. His chief complaint is neck pain and his vital signs are stable. You have decided to leave the helmet in place and are ready to roll him onto a long backboard. The proper sequence of steps to take next is:
    a. roll on the count of three, secure to the long backboard, and assess distal PMS.
    b. roll on the count of three, assess distal PMS, and secure to the long backboard.
    c. assess distal PMS, roll on the count of three, and secure to the long backboard.
    d. assess distal PMS, roll on the count of three, secure to the long backboard, and reassess PMS.

39. A crew of three is going to logroll a patient onto a long backboard because of a suspected spine injury. One member stabilizes the head and the other two members take a position on the patient's side and prepare to roll by taking hold of the patient's:
    a. hip and legs.
    b. shoulder and hip.
    c. stomach and legs.
    d. shoulder and legs.

40. "Bone to board" is a phrase used to describe:
    a. the proper method of securing a patient to a long backboard.
    b. the extrication of a vehicle occupant onto a short-board device.
    c. immobilizing a nontraumatic back pain patient with no cervical tenderness.
    d. those areas of the body that become tender after lying on a long backboard.

41. Your crew is immobilizing an adult patient to a long backboard because of a possible cervical injury following a fall. Now you need to strap him in tightly because you are going to carry him down stairs. The body part(s) you secure last is/are the:
    a. hips.
    b. head.
    c. chest.
    d. lower legs.

42. The proper method of securing a patient to a long backboard is to strap the patient firmly to the board with the straps over the:
    a. upper chest, hips, and legs.
    b. head, abdomen, and ankles.
    c. lower chest, hips, and ankles.
    d. shoulders, abdomen, and thighs.

43. Which of the following hazards would preclude the EMT-B from using a short spine board on a stable patient with a potential spine injury?
    a. broken glass from the driver's door
    b. powder residue from a deployed airbag
    c. exposed metal produced by extrication tools
    d. smoke coming from the engine compartment

44. Dispatch has sent you to a MVC for one patient with back pain. When you arrive, you determine that there was no collision; however, the driver was taking his wife to the hospital for spasms in her back. He pulled over when she nearly passed out from severe pain. Now she is awake and cannot move. Which of the following immobilization devices or techniques is most appropriate for removing this patient from the vehicle?
    a. long backboard
    b. rapid extrication
    c. short spine board
    d. standing takedown

45. The front-seat passenger in a Jeep was injured when the vehicle was rear-ended. She has pain in the right shoulder that radiates into her neck. Both of her knees have abrasions. You complete an initial assessment, find her to be in stable condition, and place a cervical collar on her. Which of the following immobilization devices or techniques is appropriate for removing this patient from the vehicle?
    a. long backboard
    b. rapid extrication
    c. short spine board
    d. standing takedown

46. Which of the following statements is most accurate about the use of a short spine board to immobilize a patient with a potential spine injury?
    a. Only stable patients should be secured to a short spine board.
    b. The short spine board must be secured to a long backboard before the patient is transported.
    c. A properly secured short spine board is more painful for a patient than a long backboard.
    d. A patient who is secured properly to a short spine board not need be secured to a long backboard.

47. You are assisting your partner to immobilize a young adult to a short spine board within a motor vehicle. With a cervical collar in place, you keep the patient in a neutral position and prepare to move him forward. Next, your partner:
    a. assesses distal PMS.
    b. secures the torso straps and then the head.
    c. secures the head and then the torso straps.
    d. places the short spine board between the patient and the seat.

48. When you are using a short spine board device to immobilize a patient who has a potential cervical injury, the patient's head is manually stabilized until the:
    a. torso straps are secure.
    b. patient's torso and head are secured to the device.
    c. short spine board is secured to the long backboard.
    d. short spine board is set in place between the patient and the seat.

49. A vehicle is off the road and appears to have rolled before coming to a stop. The driver is belted in but unconscious when you gain access to the vehicle. When you touch him, he responds by moaning. His breathing is shallow and his pulse is fast and weak. Which of the following immobilization devices or techniques will you use for this patient?
    a. rapid extrication
    b. short spine board
    c. standing takedown
    d. Kendrick Extrication Device (K.E.D.)

50. Which of the following is not an indication for the use of rapid extrication?
    a. hypotensive patient
    b. trauma arrest patient
    c. heavy rainstorm in the dark
    d. spilled gas under the car

51. It is just past midnight when a call comes in for a MVC with multiple patients. When you arrive, the fire department is on scene assessing three patients from a vehicle that struck a tree. One person is out of the vehicle and appears to have minor injuries. The driver is confused but denies injury, and the back-seat passenger is in respiratory arrest. The tree on one side of the vehicle and the driver are blocking access to the back-seat passenger. Rapid extrication is needed for:
    a. both patients still in the vehicle.
    b. just the back-seat occupant.
    c. none of the occupants of this vehicle.
    d. just the driver, to gain access to the back-seat occupant.

52. *Rapid extrication* is a special rescue removal procedure used to promptly extricate a patient from a vehicle wreck. The first step is to manually stabilize the patient's head. The first piece of equipment needed is/are:
    a. straps.
    b. head blocks.
    c. a long backboard.
    d. a rigid cervical collar.

53. Once the rescuers are in place with the proper equipment, the rapid extrication technique is used to remove an unstable patient from the vehicle in a manner:
    a. that takes less than 30 seconds.
    b. with the least risk of cervical movement.
    c. with the least risk of injury for the rescuers.
    d. that does not make the patient uncomfortable.

54. Performing a rapid extrication with the least possible extension, flexion, or rotation of the patient's spinal column requires:
    a. a minimum of two rescuers.
    b. rescuers who have practiced the rapid extrication technique.
    c. the patient to be unconscious and in critical condition.
    d. a short-board device, straps, tape, and a long backboard.

55. Two skaters collided hard during a hockey game and one did not get up. The skater who is down is the goalie, and he is complaining of neck pain and a loss of sensation in his legs. When you and your partner attempt to place his head in a neutral position, prior to removing his helmet, he complains of increased pain. Which immobilization technique is appropriate for this patient?
    a. Immobilize him in the position found, with his helmet on.
    b. Immobilize him in the position found, with his helmet off.
    c. Make another attempt to bring his C-spine into a neutral position.
    d. Cut away his uniform and the straps prior removing his helmet and placing a cervical collar.

56. A football player was knocked unconscious at a scrimmage. When you arrive at his side, he is awake and lying on the ground with a coach holding manual stabilization of his head. The patient is in uniform and still has his helmet on. He is confused, has an open airway and adequate breathing and pulse. Distal PMS is good in all extremities. Which immobilization technique is appropriate for this patient?
    a. Immobilize him to a long backboard with his helmet on.
    b. Remove his helmet and immobilize him to a long backboard.
    c. Remove his helmet and shoulder pads before immobilizing him.
    d. Apply a collar with the helmet in place and immobilize him to a long backboard.

57. A football helmet that has a _____ can easily be removed to access the airway, without removing the helmet from the player.
    a. shield
    b. jaw pad
    c. chin strap
    d. face guard

58. Which of the following sports utilizes helmets that may have a feature called a *jaw pad,* which must be removed before the helmet is removed?
    a. bicycling
    b. football
    c. motorcycling
    d. auto racing

59. Many _____ helmets are described as full-faced because of the rigid portion of the helmet that extends fully around the chin.
    a. skiing
    b. football
    c. baseball
    d. lacrosse

60. When removing the helmet of a football player who is also wearing protective shoulder pads and needs to be immobilized to a long backboard, the EMT-B:
    a. will need the help of the football coach or trainer.
    b. is taking a great risk and may cause further damage.
    c. first applies a cervical collar before removing the helmet.
    d. will need to pad behind the head to avoid extension of the neck.

61. Many types of sports helmets can be left on the patient even if the patient needs to be immobilized. The reason for this is:
    a. the type of material they are made of.
    b. the helmets fit snugly to the head, making it easy to immobilize.
    c. the helmet manufacturers recommend leaving the helmet in place.
    d. that many of these helmets have special attachment points for immobilization.

62. When removing a full-faced helmet from a supine patient who has a possible spinal injury, the EMT-B should:
    a. cut all the straps before removing the helmet.
    b. use the same method as with an open-faced helmet.
    c. insert one hand inside over the face to avoid mashing the nose.
    d. tilt the helmet slightly, without moving the neck, to avoid mashing the nose.

63. You and your partner are removing a helmet from a supine patient who has a possible head injury and difficulty breathing. While you stabilize the patient's head, using both hands, your partner should:
    a. secure a cervical collar on the patient.
    b. cut all the straps before removing the helmet.
    c. use two hands to stretch the sides of the helmet by pulling outward.
    d. place one hand under the neck and support the head in the occipital region.

64. Your ambulance has a special assignment to stand by at the Funny Car auto races that are in town for the night. While you are standing by, track officials wave you out to the driver of a vehicle that rolled on the track. He is still in the vehicle, which is upright, but he has been knocked out. Blood is dripping down his face, so you decide to remove his helmet to assess him. For this patient, it is appropriate to:
    a. not remove the helmet.
    b. remove the helmet with the patient in the vehicle.
    c. rapidly extricate him and then remove the helmet.
    d. wait until the patient is in the ambulance and then remove the helmet.

65. You are dispatched to a motorcycle collision. You arrive to find the rider, face down, off the side of the road in the grass. He is unconscious with shallow breathing, blood is draining from his mouth, and he has a weak distal pulse. You opt to remove his helmet to better assess the airway. The appropriate way to remove the helmet is to:
    a. logroll the patient onto his back and then remove the helmet.
    b. remove the helmet while this patient is still in the prone position.
    c. remove the helmet after the patient is secured to a long backboard.
    d. remove the helmet after the patient has been moved into the ambulance.

66. After removing a helmet from a patient who has a suspected spinal injury, the EMT-B should continue to maintain cervical stabilization by:
    a. padding beneath the patient's head and the surface he is lying on.
    b. performing a jaw-thrust maneuver and supporting the patient's mandible as needed.
    c. holding manual stabilization of the head until the patient is fully secured to a long backboard.
    d. placing one hand on each side of the patient's head until a cervical collar is applied to the patient.

67. When removing a helmet from an unconscious patient, the EMT-B stabilizing the head will place one hand on each side of the helmet and:
    a. instruct the patient to open her mouth.
    b. instruct the helper to apply the cervical collar.
    c. support the patient's mandible with the EMT-B's fingers.
    d. do nothing until the helper has applied the cervical collar.

68. Which of the following statements is most correct about stabilizing a patient's head with a helmet in place?
    a. It is easier to stabilize the head when the helmet is left on.
    b. It is more difficult than stabilizing the head without a helmet.
    c. The face shield or guard should be lifted up during stabilization.
    d. Proper stabilization cannot be achieved with the helmet left on.

69. One major difference between stabilizing a patient's head with and without a helmet is:
    a. hand placement.
    b. when to apply the cervical collar.
    c. when to assess and reassess distal PMS.
    d. when to secure the head to the long backboard.

70. When a patient is suspected of having a cervical spine injury, the entire spine is immobilized with a long backboard because:
    a. this is the most stable position for the spinal column.
    b. this position will help reduce excess pressure on the cord.
    c. many secondary spinal injuries are preventable with proper immobilization to a long backboard.
    d. all of the above.

71. Why is the long backboard the ideal device for splinting the entire spine when a cervical injury is suspected?
    a. No collar totally eliminates neck movement.
    b. The long backboard splints the spine as if it were a long bone.
    c. It would be difficulty to hold manual stabilization throughout the entire call.
    d. All of the above.

72. You are transporting a patient who is immobilized to a long backboard. She complains of nausea and suddenly vomits. Which straps do you unfasten so that you can roll the patient on her side, while still maintaining spinal immobilization?
    a. none of the straps should be unfastened
    b. the strap holding the cervical collar in place
    c. the stretcher straps holding the long backboard in place
    d. the straps securing the patient to the long backboard

73. During the rapid extrication of a patient onto a long backboard, once the patient is supine on the board, the board is centered on the stretcher and the patient is secured with straps:
    a. from the stretcher only.
    b. attached to the long backboard only.
    c. from the stretcher and then the straps from the long backboard.
    d. attached to the long backboard first and then the stretcher straps.

74. The rationale for using a short spine immobilization device when moving a patient from the sitting to the supine position is to protect and immobilize the entire spine immediately and:
    a. to build trust and confidence with the patient.
    b. to keep the patient from talking on the cell phone.
    c. to prevent the patient from going into spinal shock.
    d. continuously until the patient is secured to the long backboard.

75. The short spine board device is used to immobilize and:
    a. secure the patient's entire body before the patient is moved.
    b. effectively prevent any further pain for the patient.
    c. extricate patients who are found seated in an automobile.
    d. rapidly correct any misalignment of the spine resulting from the collision.

76. In which of the following patients might the use of rapid extrication make the difference between life and death?
    a. decompensated shock
    b. impaled object in the eye
    c. penetrating injury to the arm
    d. open fracture of the lower leg

77. The use of the rapid extrication technique on a patient who is stable may:
    a. cause nausea for the patient.
    b. increase the risk of further spinal injury.
    c. cause increased pressure on the abdomen.
    d. allow the patient to better follow your instructions during the move.

78. On the site at a construction project, a worker was struck in the head by a falling object. The object struck his hard hat and left a dent. The patient is alert, ambulatory, and denies any injury, but when you palpate his cervical spine he has tenderness. You decide to immobilize and transport him for evaluation. What method do you use?
    a. Immobilize the patient with the hard hat on.
    b. Remove the hard hat and perform a standing takedown.
    c. Remove the hard hat and instruct the patient to sit down on the long backboard.
    d. Any of these above methods is appropriate.

79. Which of the following is an indication for leaving a helmet on a patient?
    a. removal will not cause further injury
    b. there is adequate head movement within the helmet
    c. there is no face shield that flips up to allow access to the face
    d. proper immobilization can be accomplished with the helmet on

80. A helmet should be removed from the patient's head in all of the following situations, except:
    a. respiratory or cardiac arrest.
    b. the patient is hyperventilating.
    c. you are unable to adequately assess the airway.
    d. proper immobilization cannot be performed with the helmet on.

Chapter 28 Answer Form

	A	B	C	D			A	B	C	D
1.	❏	❏	❏	❏		33.	❏	❏	❏	❏
2.	❏	❏	❏	❏		34.	❏	❏	❏	❏
3.	❏	❏	❏	❏		35.	❏	❏	❏	❏
4.	❏	❏	❏	❏		36.	❏	❏	❏	❏
5.	❏	❏	❏	❏		37.	❏	❏	❏	❏
6.	❏	❏	❏	❏		38.	❏	❏	❏	❏
7.	❏	❏	❏	❏		39.	❏	❏	❏	❏
8.	❏	❏	❏	❏		40.	❏	❏	❏	❏
9.	❏	❏	❏	❏		41.	❏	❏	❏	❏
10.	❏	❏	❏	❏		42.	❏	❏	❏	❏
11.	❏	❏	❏	❏		43.	❏	❏	❏	❏
12.	❏	❏	❏	❏		44.	❏	❏	❏	❏
13.	❏	❏	❏	❏		45.	❏	❏	❏	❏
14.	❏	❏	❏	❏		46.	❏	❏	❏	❏
15.	❏	❏	❏	❏		47.	❏	❏	❏	❏
16.	❏	❏	❏	❏		48.	❏	❏	❏	❏
17.	❏	❏	❏	❏		49.	❏	❏	❏	❏
18.	❏	❏	❏	❏		50.	❏	❏	❏	❏
19.	❏	❏	❏	❏		51.	❏	❏	❏	❏
20.	❏	❏	❏	❏		52.	❏	❏	❏	❏
21.	❏	❏	❏	❏		53.	❏	❏	❏	❏
22.	❏	❏	❏	❏		54.	❏	❏	❏	❏
23.	❏	❏	❏	❏		55.	❏	❏	❏	❏
24.	❏	❏	❏	❏		56.	❏	❏	❏	❏
25.	❏	❏	❏	❏		57.	❏	❏	❏	❏
26.	❏	❏	❏	❏		58.	❏	❏	❏	❏
27.	❏	❏	❏	❏		59.	❏	❏	❏	❏
28.	❏	❏	❏	❏		60.	❏	❏	❏	❏
29.	❏	❏	❏	❏		61.	❏	❏	❏	❏
30.	❏	❏	❏	❏		62.	❏	❏	❏	❏
31.	❏	❏	❏	❏		63.	❏	❏	❏	❏
32.	❏	❏	❏	❏		64.	❏	❏	❏	❏

	A	B	C	D			A	B	C	D
65.	❏	❏	❏	❏		73.	❏	❏	❏	❏
66.	❏	❏	❏	❏		74.	❏	❏	❏	❏
67.	❏	❏	❏	❏		75.	❏	❏	❏	❏
68.	❏	❏	❏	❏		76.	❏	❏	❏	❏
69.	❏	❏	❏	❏		77.	❏	❏	❏	❏
70.	❏	❏	❏	❏		78.	❏	❏	❏	❏
71.	❏	❏	❏	❏		79.	❏	❏	❏	❏
72.	❏	❏	❏	❏		80.	❏	❏	❏	❏

Infants and Children

CHAPTER

29

Infants and Children

1. A respiratory rate of 20 to 30 breaths per minute is normal in each of the following age groups, except:
   a. toddlers.
   b. preschool.
   c. school-age.
   d. adolescents.

2. The basics of language are normally mastered by:
   a. infancy.
   b. 36 months.
   c. school-age.
   d. preschool age.

3. During the first year of life, the heart rate of an infant slows to an average of _____ beats per minute.
   a. 120
   b. 140
   c. 160
   d. 180

4. The normal respiratory rate for adolescents is _____ breaths per minute.
   a. 12 to 20
   b. 20 to 30
   c. 25 to 35
   d. 30 to 40

5. In which developmental age group do children lose their primary teeth?
   a. toddler
   b. preschool
   c. school-age
   d. adolescent

6. Which developmental age group has the highest metabolic and oxygen consumption rates?
   a. infants
   b. children
   c. adolescents
   d. adults

7. Proportionate to each age group, which has the most prevalent normal weight gain?
   a. infants
   b. children
   c. adults
   d. the elderly

8. The respiratory system of the infant is different from that of an older child or an adult in that the:
   a. lung tissue is less fragile.
   b. lung capacity is increased.
   c. accessory muscles are immature and fatigue easily.
   d. chest wall is more rigid, causing diaphragmatic breathing.

9. _____ is a sign of respiratory distress that is observed in children, but rarely seen in adults.
   a. Grunting
   b. Coughing
   c. Choking
   d. Wheezing

10. Which of the following signs of respiratory distress indicates the most severe distress in a child?
    a. grunting and crying
    b. stridor and coughing
    c. wheezing and sneezing
    d. slow and gasping breaths

11. The most prominent indicator that a child is progressing from respiratory distress to respiratory failure is:
    a. changing skin color.
    b. increasing respiratory rate.
    c. use of accessory muscles.
    d. decreasing level of consciousness.

12. The small airways of the pediatric patient are prone to obstructions from:
    a. secretions.
    b. head position.
    c. foreign bodies.
    d. all of the above.

13. When a child 1 to 3 years of age has a sudden onset of respiratory distress or stridor, the EMT-B should first suspect:
    a. croup.
    b. epiglottitis.
    c. secretions.
    d. an aspirated foreign body.

14. A respiratory emergency that presents with great difficulty exhaling, and may occur in any pediatric age group, is:
    a. croup.
    b. asthma.
    c. epiglottitis.
    d. pneumonia.

15. You are helping to teach a CPR class, and your station is foreign body airway obstruction in the unresponsive child with no injuries. When you teach your students to open the airway, you demonstrate the:
    a. jaw-thrust maneuver.
    b. cross-finger technique.
    c. tongue jaw-lift maneuver.
    d. head-tilt chin-lift maneuver.

16. While on duty, you stop for lunch at a fast-food restaurant. As you enter, you hear a woman cry for help and see a crowd gathering around a child who appears to be unconscious in his mother's arms. When you approach and ask what happened, the mother tells you that her 6-year-old son was choking on a mouthful of french fries before he passed out. The next step you take is to:
    a. perform a finger sweep.
    b. attempt to ventilate the child.
    c. position the child supine on the floor.
    d. reposition the head and chin and attempt to ventilate.

17. (Continuing with the preceding question) You are unable to ventilate the child, because of the obstruction, so you perform abdominal thrusts and attempt to ventilate again. You do this several times without success as your partner notifies dispatch and requests ALS to the scene. What steps do you take next?
    a. Continue with abdominal thrusts.
    b. Attempt back blows and chest thrusts.
    c. Check for a pulse; if no pulse is present, begin CPR.
    d. Perform a finger sweep, reposition the head, and attempt to ventilate.

18. It is time to recertify in CPR, and you are practicing foreign body airway obstruction on an infant mannequin. After you confirm that the infant cannot make a sound or breathe, and is not moving, the next step you take is to perform:
    a. a tongue-jaw lift.
    b. a finger sweep.
    c. five back blows.
    d. five chest thrusts.

19. You have been dispatched for an asthma attack. Your initial impression of the 5-year-old male patient is severe respiratory distress. The child looks pale and exhausted, and is working hard to breathe. You calmly give him oxygen and get ready to assist his ventilations and ask your partner to call:
    a. the child's pediatrician to get confirmation of a history of asthma.
    b. medical control for an order to assist with a bronchodilator treatment.
    c. medical control for an order to assist with an anti-inflammatory treatment.
    d. the child's pediatrician to determine if this type of event has happened before.

20. A first-time mother of a 10-week-old infant calls EMS because her baby is not acting right. The baby appears to be struggling to breathe and the mother states that the baby did not want to drink her bottle. You assess the baby and find that her nose is congested with mucus, and you hear congestion in her breathing. The next step you take is to suction the:
    a. nose with a bulb syringe.
    b. mouth with a bulb syringe.
    c. nose with a rigid-tip catheter.
    d. mouth with a rigid-tip catheter.

21. The parents of a 3-year-old boy called EMS because the boy awoke crying, scared, and complaining that he cannot breathe. The boy is alert, tugging at his neck, and crying when you approach. His skin is very warm and pale. You suspect that he has croup when you hear his barking cough. The primary approach to the management of this patient is:
    a. to avoid alarming or agitating the child.
    b. rapid transport, oxygen, and call for ALS.
    c. to assist ventilation with a BVM and call for ALS.
    d. to allow one of the parents to help you assist ventilations.

22. A 2-year old has been sick for 24 hours with diarrhea and vomiting. Her airway is clear and breath sounds are adequate, but the respiration rate is fast. Her brachial pulse is 150 and regular. Skin CTC is pale, warm, and dry, and capillary refill is 5 seconds. You suspect:
    a. no shock.
    b. bronchiolitis.
    c. compensated shock
    d. decompensated shock.

23. A 6-month-old infant was discharged from the hospital three days ago for dehydration. Since she has been home, she had not fed well and is fussy. The mother took her temperature and found that it is 101°F. The infant has nasal flaring and grunting, and she is working hard to breathe. Skin CTC is cyanotic, warm, and dry. The child has signs and symptoms of:
    a. respiratory failure.
    b. respiratory distress.
    c. compensated shock.
    d. decompensated shock.

24. You arrive at a day care center for a seizure call. The patient is 18 months old and is sleepy. The airway is clear, breathing is adequate, and the skin is warm and moist. The caregiver reports seeing the child have a seizure that lasted approximately a minute. There is no history of seizures with this patient, but the child was given acetaminophen for a fever this morning. You suspect a febrile seizure and
    a. dehydration.
    b. adequate perfusion.
    c. compensated hypoperfusion.
    d. decompensated hypoperfusion.

25. Which of the following is an indirect measure of end-organ perfusion?
    a. urine output
    b. capillary refill
    c. mental status
    d. distal versus proximal pulses

26. One of your partners is assessing the vital signs of a sick baby while you obtain a history from the mother. What piece of information does she provide to you that suggests the baby may have inadequate end-organ perfusion?
    a. The baby was born premature.
    b. The baby is using fewer diapers than normal.
    c. The baby has been crying and fussing for hours.
    d. The last temperature taken on the baby was 101.1°F

27. When assessing the perfusion in a child, which of the following findings suggests that cardiac output is less than adequate?
    a. systolic BP of 90 mm Hg
    b. pink mucous membranes
    c. capillary refill less than 2 seconds
    d. cool extremities in a warm setting

28. The EMT-B who is assessing and treating a very sick child can reduce the chance of cardiac arrest and significantly increase the chance of recovery by:
    a. providing rapid transport to the nearest hospital.
    b. recognizing respiratory distress and treating it appropriately.
    c. recognizing the signs of child abuse and reporting it appropriately.
    d. obtaining a focused history from the parent prior to transporting the patient.

29. Which of the following is the primary cause of cardiac arrest in children?
    a. suicide
    b. toxic ingestion
    c. infection/sepsis
    d. respiratory arrest

30. The mother of a 10-day-old infant calls 9-1-1 because the baby is unresponsive after a possible seizure. En route to the call, you consider the most common possible causes of seizure in babies, and recall that a seizure caused by _____ is often the most straightforward to manage in the prehospital setting.
    a. fever
    b. toxic ingestion
    c. congenital defect
    d. trauma from childbirth

31. You are assessing an 11-year-old child who is postictal from his first seizure. The child is sleepy, breathing slowly and shallowly, and is hot and moist to the touch. The caregiver states that the child stayed home from school today because of a fever, aches, and pains. You suspect the cause of the seizure is:
    a. trauma.
    b. epilepsy.
    c. infection.
    d. brain tumor.

32. The causes of seizures vary for each age group, but the one cause that remains common in all pediatric age groups is:
    a. trauma.
    b. congenital.
    c. drug related.
    d. alcohol related.

33. The family of a special-needs child calls EMS because their 4-year-old is in status epilepticus and his anti-seizure medication is not working today. The patient is seizing in his bed when you arrive. Special care steps for this patient include:

    a. do not transport; call ALS and suction while waiting.
    b. suction, high-flow oxygen, and rapid transport.
    c. high-flow oxygen and calling the pediatrician for specific instructions.
    d. high-flow oxygen, cooling, and bringing the caregiver with you to the ED.

34. The school nurse called EMS because one of the students with a history of epilepsy experienced a seizure in class. When you arrive, the 8-year-old female is alert and resting. The nurse tells you that the patient may have missed taking her antiseizure medication and that it has happened before. The parents have been notified and will meet you at the hospital. The next step in the care of this patient is:

    a. supportive care with attention to the airway.
    b. removal of any excess clothing to keep the child from overheating.
    c. searching the patient for a Medic Alert tag identifying her as an epileptic.
    d. to call medical control and ask for permission to assist the patient in taking her antiseizure medication.

35. The parents of a 24-month-old are very upset and describe seeing their baby have a seizure that lasted for approximately 2 minutes. They said the baby stopped breathing. Your initial assessment shows that the child is sleepy, but is breathing adequately. The child has been sick with cold symptoms since last night. The next step in the care of the child is to:

    a. insert an OPA.
    b. remove the child's clothing.
    c. administer high-flow oxygen.
    d. administer acetaminophen for the fever.

36. Because of their disproportionate sizes, the _____ are injured more frequently in children than in adults.

    a. chest and abdomen
    b. head and abdomen
    c. head, face, and neck
    d. airway and abdomen

37. An infant who experiences a fall from a height of three times her own is more likely to suffer a _____ injury than a child or adult falling from a proportionate height.

    a. head
    b. chest
    c. extremity
    d. abdominal

38. Children are at high risk for injury to internal organs of the chest in a traumatic event, because:

    a. of the lack of use of child restraints in motor vehicles.
    b. of the improper use of child restraints in motor vehicles.
    c. their developing bones are not as strong as mature bones.
    d. injury from child abuse injury is more prevalent in the chest area.

39. The use of an OPA in an unconscious infant with traumatic injury is:

    a. never recommend.
    b. inserted the same as for an adult.
    c. appropriate in the absence of a gag reflex.
    d. appropriate in the presence of a gag reflex.

40. A 6-year-old was knocked off his bike by a vehicle that was backing up. The child was wearing a helmet, which was removed by a first responder to clear the airway. Spinal stabilization is being maintained. The child is unconscious, has labored breathing, and his abdomen appears to be distended. Which management step do you begin first?

    a. Assist ventilations.
    b. Perform a detailed physical exam.
    c. Immobilize to a long backboard.
    d. Remove his clothing and perform a rapid trauma exam.

41. A family of five traveling in a minivan was involved in a high-speed rollover collision. You have been assigned to assess the youngest member of the family, who is a 2-year-old still in a car seat. The child appears to be stable and has no distress, but the MOI is significant enough to warrant transport for evaluation. You will transport the patient:

    a. immobilized in the car seat.
    b. immobilized to a short spine board.
    c. in the car seat without immobilization.
    d. on your stretcher with no immobilization.

42. Which of the following findings is not associated with signs of sexual abuse of a child?

    a. hearing or speech deficit
    b. difficulty walking or sitting
    c. anxious child who avoids eye contact
    d. child who is uncooperative with certain aspects of an assessment

43. A baby with mouth and gum lacerations may suggest abuse with an MOI of:

    a. improper nourishment.
    b. shaken baby syndrome.
    c. a bottle being shoved too hard, repeatedly, into the mouth.
    d. chewing on an electrical cord in the absence of parental supervision.

44. You are documenting findings related to a possible child abuse situation. Which of the following observations would be inappropriate to document?
    a. evidence of alcohol use
    b. your opinion about the caretaker's character
    c. family members giving different accounts of the MOI
    d. an MOI that does not fit the situation found on scene

45. When managing a pediatric patient who may be a victim of child abuse, EMT-Bs should report their findings to the:
    a. ED staff.
    b. caregiver or parent.
    c. national registry for victims of abuse.
    d. relative who is not living with the patient.

46. When documenting a call that involves suspected child abuse, the EMT-B is the ideal health care provider to:
    a. identify inappropriate interaction with the caregiver or parent.
    b. provide information about the family's constant switching of hospitals.
    c. provide information about the condition of the child's home environment.
    d. all of the above.

47. Which of the following statements is most correct regarding child abuse?
    a. Child abuse is a crime.
    b. Not every EMT-B is required to report suspected child abuse.
    c. When abuse is suspected, the initial assessment of the child is modified.
    d. Some form of alcohol or drug use is always associated with child abuse.

48. You and your partner have arrived at the hospital with a 10-year-old male who is your partner's cousin. The patient was the victim of a near-drowning and is still unresponsive upon arrival at the ED. Before you go back into service, you should first:
    a. get a probable diagnosis from the ED physician.
    b. talk about the call with your partner and assess his reaction.
    c. notify your supervisor to take your partner out of service for the day.
    d. notify your supervisor about the relation of the patient to your partner.

49. Which of the following statements about the need for debriefing following a difficult infant or child emergency call is correct?
    a. Some EMT-Bs do not need an organized debriefing session.
    b. EMT-Bs should talk about the call with the medical director, if possible.
    c. EMT-Bs should talk about the call with the other crew members as soon as possible.
    d. All of the above.

50. After arriving at the ED with a 4-month-old who is in cardiac arrest, you give report and begin documenting the call. After being at the hospital for a while, the initial feedback from the staff is that SIDS may be the cause of death. You and your crew are feeling upset about the call. What is one of the most effective things you can do first to help debrief from this call?
    a. Talk to your crew.
    b. Talk to the parents.
    c. Go home for the remainder of the shift.
    d. Go back to work to take your mind off this call.

51. Which of the following statements is most correct about the special considerations for taking pediatric vital signs?
    a. Most adult emergency medical equipment will fit pediatric patients.
    b. The EMT-B should memorize the normal BP values for each age group.
    c. An adult BP cuff can be used to obtain an accurate BP on a young child.
    d. The EMT-B should use a reference for vital sign values instead of memorization.

52. To rapidly determine the severity of an illness or injury of a pediatric patient, the EMT-B must:
    a. keep the child from crying.
    b. approach the patient the same as he would an adult.
    c. perform an age-appropriate initial assessment and physical exam.
    d. consider the use of immobilization for the uncooperative infant or young child.

53. In which age group should the EMT-B begin to involve the child in the history-taking process?
    a. toddler
    b. preschool
    c. grade school
    d. adolescent

54. You have been dispatched for a cardiac arrest call. The patient is an 8-month-old infant who was last seen awake in the middle of the night. At 7:00 a.m., the infant was found blue, warm, apneic, and pulseless. The family is crying and you find it difficult to obtain any addition information. CPR is begun and you attend to the feelings of the family by:

    a. removing the child to the ambulance.

    b. reinforcing that the treatment of the child is your first priority.

    c. telling them that you need them to give you the child's medical history.

    d. explaining that nothing can be done for the child at this time.

55. You are splinting the arm of a 5-year-old girl who has a painful, swollen, and deformed wrist. The father is very anxious and is asking a lot of questions. While you splint the arm, you:

    a. are thinking that this is a possible act of child abuse.

    b. honestly explain the procedure and keep him informed.

    c. ask him to step out of the room, as he is upsetting the child.

    d. stop what you are doing and ask him let you care for the child without interruption.

56. A mother called EMS when her 3-year-old daughter fell off the couch and cut her scalp on the coffee table. When you get there, the mother is crying and tells you that it is all her fault, because she was out of the room when the child fell and injured her head. You quickly see that the injury is superficial, with bleeding that has already stopped. The mother is still really upset, so you:

    a. allow her to assist you in the treatment.

    b. call the police to investigate the incident.

    c. consider that she may be guilty of neglect.

    d. reassure her that the bleeding is controlled and permit her to observe.

57. It would not be uncommon for an EMT-B who is a parent to _____ caring for an ill or injured pediatric patient.

    a. burn out after

    b. feel nothing at all

    c. feel emotional stress in

    d. avoid whenever possible

58. By remaining calm and reassuring the parents of a sick or injured child will:

    a. support the child's environmental needs.

    b. help to establish trust with both the parents and the patient.

    c. reinforce the parents' perceived loss of control of the situation.

    d. help the EMT-B understand his own emotional response to the call.

59. When managing a complex pediatric call, each of the following considerations is paramount, except:

    a. avoiding overwhelming the patient.

    b. having the correctly sized equipment ready and available.

    c. the need to examine the patient while the child is in the parent's arms.

    d. assigning a crew member to inform and deal with the parents or caregiver.

60. When assessing and interviewing a teenager in the presence of her parents, the EMT-B should:

    a. not take sides in disputes with the parents.

    b. consider using a Broslow tape or other pediatric reference.

    c. ask the parents to leave while the patient is being examined.

    d. approach this patient exactly the same as he would an adult.

61. Which cause of cardiac arrest is more common in adults than children or infants?

    a. trauma

    b. toxic ingestion

    c. airway obstruction

    d. myocardial infarction

62. At 22:30, your crew is dispatched on a call for a 4-year-old male who is having difficulty breathing. At the residence, a nervous father flags you down and brings you inside to his son, who is crying in high-pitched, squeaking sounds. The father says the boy woke up crying and stated that he could not breathe. The boy has been sick with a viral infection and cold symptoms for several days. There is no history of asthma or other respiratory disease, although this happened once before about a year ago. They had to call the ambulance then, too. The boy is tugging at his throat and nasal flaring is prominent. In addition to administering oxygen, what is going to be a key approach to the management plan for this patient?

    a. providing aggressive ventilation assistance using a BVM

    b. transporting the child safely strapped into his own car seat

    c. inspecting the inside of the patient's mouth and throat if possible

    d. letting the patient stay in a position of comfort with minimal disturbance

63. (Continuing with the preceding question) Your partner, with the help of the father, administers oxygen to the patient. You obtain vital signs carefully, without upsetting the child. It is cool outside and you have the father cover the child with a blanket and proceed to the ambulance. The transport time is short and the patient improves significantly on the ride in. What do you suspect is the cause of the respiratory distress?

    a. croup
    b. epiglottitis
    c. bronchiolitis
    d. new onset of asthma

64. A mother of a 4-month-old infant calls EMS because her child is sick. The mother reports that the child has been fussy, has not been feeding well, and has been vomiting. She laid the infant down for a nap and now is unable to arouse her. The patient does not appear to respond to your touch. The airway is open, she has a rapid respiratory rate, her skin is pale and dry, her extremities are cool, she has no peripheral pulses, and capillary refill time is 6 seconds. What do these signs indicate?

    a. hypoperfusion
    b. physical abuse
    c. respiratory failure
    d. respiratory distress

65. (Continuing with the preceding question) You call dispatch and request an ALS intercept. Next, you administer high-flow oxygen and prepare the patient for transport. What additional care will you provide until ALS can meet you?

    a. Hyperventilate with an infant-sized BVM.
    b. Suction the patient, elevate her legs, and attach the AED.
    c. Administer oxygen, provide warmth, and begin rapid transport.
    d. Apply hot packs to the extremities, cover the head, and begin rapid transport.

Chapter 29 Answer Form

	A	B	C	D		A	B	C	D
1.	❏	❏	❏	❏	29.	❏	❏	❏	❏
2.	❏	❏	❏	❏	30.	❏	❏	❏	❏
3.	❏	❏	❏	❏	31.	❏	❏	❏	❏
4.	❏	❏	❏	❏	32.	❏	❏	❏	❏
5.	❏	❏	❏	❏	33.	❏	❏	❏	❏
6.	❏	❏	❏	❏	34.	❏	❏	❏	❏
7.	❏	❏	❏	❏	35.	❏	❏	❏	❏
8.	❏	❏	❏	❏	36.	❏	❏	❏	❏
9.	❏	❏	❏	❏	37.	❏	❏	❏	❏
10.	❏	❏	❏	❏	38.	❏	❏	❏	❏
11.	❏	❏	❏	❏	39.	❏	❏	❏	❏
12.	❏	❏	❏	❏	40.	❏	❏	❏	❏
13.	❏	❏	❏	❏	41.	❏	❏	❏	❏
14.	❏	❏	❏	❏	42.	❏	❏	❏	❏
15.	❏	❏	❏	❏	43.	❏	❏	❏	❏
16.	❏	❏	❏	❏	44.	❏	❏	❏	❏
17.	❏	❏	❏	❏	45.	❏	❏	❏	❏
18.	❏	❏	❏	❏	46.	❏	❏	❏	❏
19.	❏	❏	❏	❏	47.	❏	❏	❏	❏
20.	❏	❏	❏	❏	48.	❏	❏	❏	❏
21.	❏	❏	❏	❏	49.	❏	❏	❏	❏
22.	❏	❏	❏	❏	50.	❏	❏	❏	❏
23.	❏	❏	❏	❏	51.	❏	❏	❏	❏
24.	❏	❏	❏	❏	52.	❏	❏	❏	❏
25.	❏	❏	❏	❏	53.	❏	❏	❏	❏
26.	❏	❏	❏	❏	54.	❏	❏	❏	❏
27.	❏	❏	❏	❏	55.	❏	❏	❏	❏
28.	❏	❏	❏	❏	56.	❏	❏	❏	❏

	A	B	C	D
57.	❏	❏	❏	❏
58.	❏	❏	❏	❏
59.	❏	❏	❏	❏
60.	❏	❏	❏	❏
61.	❏	❏	❏	❏

	A	B	C	D
62.	❏	❏	❏	❏
63.	❏	❏	❏	❏
64.	❏	❏	❏	❏
65.	❏	❏	❏	❏

Operations

CHAPTER

30

Ambulance Operations

1. It is your turn to perform the daily check of the extrication equipment located on your agency's emergency vehicle. As you go through the equipment, which of the following items appear out of place?
   a. ropes
   b. penlight
   c. Stokes rescue basket
   d. socket set with sockets

2. Pillows, blankets, stethoscopes, penlights, and disposable gloves are all examples of _____ equipment.
   a. first aid
   b. splinting
   c. portable nonmedical
   d. miscellaneous patient care

3. In the daily inspection of your vehicle mechanical systems, which of the following items is not a component of that inspection?
   a. oil level
   b. fuel level
   c. brake test
   d. stretcher mount

4. Replacing equipment on the ambulance and completing an inventory of equipment are tasks typically performed in each of the following phases of an ambulance call, except:
   a. at the scene.
   b. at the hospital.
   c. the daily shift inspection.
   d. in the station after the call.

5. During which phase of an ambulance call would the EMT-B typically obtain permission to treat a patient?
   a. at the scene
   b. after the call
   c. at the hospital
   d. en route to the scene

6. When responding to the scene of a MVC, the EMT-B should consider which of the following guidelines first?
   a. Use lights and siren only if the need exists.
   b. Notify the hospital with necessary patient information.
   c. Know the type of equipment needed and where it is stored.
   d. Listen for a status report from a first responder on the scene.

7. According to vehicle and traffic regulations, emergency vehicles may use lights and sirens to respond:
   a. to a drill.
   b. when returning from a call.
   c. to a medical emergency.
   d. during driver training on the road.

8. While you are transporting a patient, your ambulance is struck by another vehicle at an intersection. The driver of the ambulance must:
   a. continue to the ED if the patient is critical or unstable.
   b. continue, but she must notify the police through the dispatcher.
   c. stop to assess damage, render aid, and exchange information.
   d. stop to assess damage; if there is none, she can continue.

9. You are responding to a high-priority call on a divided highway. The motorist in front of you is not yielding the right of way. The proper action to take now is to:
   a. follow the vehicle while using excessive siren tones.
   b. wait for a safe location to pass the vehicle on the left.
   c. flash your high beams continuously until the driver moves to the right.
   d. edge up to the vehicle's rear bumper so he can better see your lights.

10. Your ambulance is transporting a high-priority patient to the ED when you notice that a family member is driving right behind your ambulance with his flashers on. The family member has just followed your ambulance through an intersection with a red light. What action is appropriate at this point?
   a. Continue driving and do nothing about the family member.
   b. Turn off your lights and siren and continue to the hospital in a safe manner.
   c. Continue driving and notify your dispatcher about the illegal driving actions of the family member.
   d. Stop the ambulance and discourage the family member from using the ambulance as an escort.

11. You and your partner have just completed an emergency vehicle operator course (EVOC). Having completed this course means that you both have:
   a. taken extra effort to ensure safe driving practices.
   b. authorization to drive all types of emergency vehicles.
   c. special immunity from lawsuits resulting from motor vehicle collisions involving your emergency vehicle.
   d. learned all the vehicle and transportation laws associated with the operation of emergency vehicles.

12. According to most state laws, whenever the driver of an ambulance exercises privileges during an emergency response, that driver:
   a. is held to a higher standard in the eyes of the law.
   b. assumes the burden of driving with due regard for others.
   c. has the added responsibility of ensuring that no one is injured because of his driving.
   d. all of the above.

13. While driving the ambulance to a low-priority call, an animal runs out in the road directly in your path. Which of the following actions is appropriate for this situation?
   a. Turn on your siren to encourage the animal to move.
   b. Base your reaction on your speed and the size of the animal.
   c. Decelerate suddenly while swerving to avoid the animal.
   d. Flash your headlights several times to encourage the animal to move.

14. The first priority of the ambulance operator is to:
   a. operate the vehicle safely.
   b. transport the patient to the ED.
   c. rapidly transport the patient and crew to the hospital.
   d. learn all the vehicle and transportation laws in her state.

15. Which of the following is not considered a distraction for the operator of an ambulance?
   a. drowsiness
   b. smoking while driving
   c. wearing contact lenses
   d. incomplete dispatch information

16. A request for an escort should be considered:
   a. only if the escort is a police car.
   b. very rarely, because it is so dangerous.
   c. only if the escort is another ambulance.
   d. if you are unable to locate the patient's location.

17. Using another emergency vehicle as an escort to the hospital is dangerous for:
   a. the patient.
   b. the EMT-B driver.
   c. other drivers on the road.
   d. all of the above.

18. When two emergency vehicles are responding to high-priority calls, and are within view of each other:
   a. one operator should shut off the siren.
   b. both operators should shut off the sirens.
   c. the operators should use different siren modes.
   d. one operator should use the horn instead of the siren.

19. Part of the EMT-B's driving responsibilities is exercising due regard for the safety of others. An example of this is:
   a. allowing other motorists enough time to clear a path.
   b. deciding which priority to use to transport the patient to the ED.
   c. conserving fuel and reducing vehicle wear by using slow startup and stopping procedures.
   d. notifying the dispatcher that your patient needs alternative transportation if the ambulance breaks down.

20. Which of the following points is not typically considered when determining if an ambulance operator was using due regard in the use of signaling equipment?
   a. What type of signal was given?
   b. Was the signaling equipment used?
   c. Was the signaling equipment routinely inspected?
   d. Was it necessary to use the signaling equipment?

21. "A reasonable and careful person performing similar duties and under the same circumstances would act in the same manner" is an accepted definition of:
   a. due regard.
   b. emergency privileges.
   c. OSHA regulation 1910.
   d. Good Samaritan privileges.

22. The shift supervisor has asked you to train a new EMT-B. To start, you review with the new EMT-B what information is essential to respond to a call. You include all the pertinent factors for these procedures and place the highest emphasis on:
    a. arriving safely.
    b. address information.
    c. nature of illness or injury.
    d. responder mode using lights and sirens.

23. The time between the receipt of a call by the dispatcher and the time the call is given to the unit to respond is called the:
    a. queue time.
    b. public access time.
    c. system-ready phase.
    d. prearrival instruction phase.

24. Dispatch has given you a call for an unconscious patient in a large motel. You are told that the caller is someone who is calling for the patient, but is not in direct contact with the patient. This type of call is a _____ party caller.
    a. first-
    b. second-
    c. third-
    d. fourth-

25. The enhanced 911 system helps to increase rapidity of response to an emergency call by:
    a. providing computer displays of the caller's telephone number and location.
    b. identifying the actual room where the call was made in a large building.
    c. providing instant callback capability in case a caller hangs up too fast.
    d. all of the above.

26. During the early part of your shift, the dispatcher notifies you that there is a problem with the _____. This problem means that portable radios will not be powerful enough to reach the base station from some locations.
    a. repeater
    b. telemetry
    c. simplex system
    d. multiple system

27. Which of the following factors can significantly delay the response to a call in a 9-1-1 system?
    a. the caller's chief complaint
    b. the caller is a first-party caller
    c. the caller is using a cell phone
    d. time for the prearrival instructions

28. While taking a shower, a very large lady fell in the tub and was unable to get out on her own. Her only injury is a possible ankle sprain. With the help of additional crew members, you are able to get her out of the tub. The house is a bungalow with little space to move around. Which device is best to assist her outside of the house with?
    a. Reeves
    b. stretcher
    c. stair chair
    d. Stokes rescue basket

29. (Continuing with the preceding question) During the move out of the house, the patient complained of severe pain in her ankle. After you get outside and before you can load her into the ambulance, she says that she feels like she is going to pass out—and then she does. Now which device is the most appropriate to move the patient with?
    a. Reeves
    b. stretcher
    c. stair chair
    d. long backboard

30. You are assessing a 48-year-old, severely overweight female who injured herself when she tripped and fell. She is lying on the floor on her side and refuses to roll onto her back because of the increased pain when she moves. After completing a focused physical exam, you determine that she has a possible hip fracture or dislocation and decide to move her to the ambulance by using a:
    a. stretcher.
    b. stair chair.
    c. long backboard and stretcher.
    d. traction splint, long backboard, and stretcher.

31. (Continuing with the preceding question) You have discovered the patient lying on the floor on her side with a possible hip fracture or dislocation. The device you have chosen to move the patient to the ambulance with:
    a. will serve as a splint for the possible fracture or dislocation.
    b. is appropriate because no additional splinting is required with this type of injury.
    c. is appropriate, but the patient will need to be splinted with another device once she is inside the ambulance.
    d. is appropriate because the patient will be splinted and can be moved right into the ambulance without any additional equipment.

32. An elderly patient with moderate respiratory distress due to congestive heart failure lives in a small apartment on the first floor. She is sitting on the couch in the living room near the front door. A stretcher will not fit into the apartment, so you choose to move her out to the ambulance by:
    a. stair chair.
    b. laying her in a Reeves stretcher.
    c. carrying her on your long backboard.
    d. having her walk outside and sit on the stretcher outside.

33. Noting the official transfer of a patient to a nurse or physician on your patient care report:
    a. protects you from litigation.
    b. helps document that you did not abandon the patient.
    c. ensures that the patient's personal belongings will not get lost.
    d. guarantees a quick turnaround so you can get back into service.

34. The timely completion of a patient care report (PCR), using accurate and complete information with no misspelled words, will:
    a. impress the ED staff.
    b. impede the continuity of patient care.
    c. provide professional data for evaluation of quality of care.
    d. ensure that the EMT-B will never be involved in litigation.

35. The typical patient care report (PCR) includes information that will be used for which of the following functions?
    a. administrative recordkeeping
    b. legal tool to protect the patient
    c. personnel assignment record
    d. equipment maintenance record

36. The steps taken to prepare your ambulance for the next response are:
    a. required by OSHA.
    b. key to the safety and health of you and your crew.
    c. necessary for the safety and health of your patient.
    d. vital for the safety and health of you, your crew, and the patient.

37. Once a patient is transferred to the hospital and paperwork is completed, the crew should prepare as quickly as possible for the next response by:
    a. quickly getting back to the station to restock and clean the vehicle.
    b. cleaning and restocking the ambulance before notifying the dispatcher of availability.
    c. notifying the dispatcher of availability, making a list of restock items, and returning to the station.
    d. checking the fuel, washing the ambulance, and notifying the dispatcher of availability.

38. The patient you just transferred to the ED vomited in your ambulance during the transport. There is a spill on the floor and the ambulance smells bad. You take which steps to clean and disinfect this type of mess?
    a. Use a disposable towel first, then use soap and water and let it air-dry.
    b. Open all the doors, don gloves, use a disposable towel first, and then wipe the surface with a germicidal solution and air-dry.
    c. Document the spill, notify dispatch that you are out of service, and begin sterilization procedures.
    d. Turn on the ambulance and let the AC and vents run, don gloves and wipe the surface with germicidal solution, then close all the doors and spray a deodorizer inside.

39. During the last call, you had an infectious exposure. Which of the following steps is necessary only on high-exposure calls before returning to service?
    a. Wash the area of contact thoroughly.
    b. Change your entire uniform, including socks and shoes.
    c. Document the situation in which the exposure occurred.
    d. Describe the actions taken to reduce chances of infection.

40. Which of the following steps is out of place for the completion of a call and return to service?
    a. washing your hands
    b. verifying proper immunization boosters
    c. giving a verbal report on the patient
    d. transferring the patient's personal belongings

41. It is your turn to clean the equipment used on the last call and return it to the ambulance. The long backboard that was used has blood on it, so you get it ready to go back into service by:
    a. cleaning it with soap and water.
    b. sterilizing it while at the hospital.
    c. disinfecting it with a germicidal cleaner.
    d. hosing it down with water and wiping it with a disposable towel.

42. The product you are using to clean equipment after a call states on the label that it will kill most bacteria, some viruses, and some fungi, but not *Mycobacterium tuberculosis* or bacterial spores. This level of cleaning is:
    a. sterilization.
    b. low-level disinfection.
    c. high-level disinfection.
    d. intermediate-level disinfection.

43. _____ is a process that kills all forms of microbial life on medical instruments.
    a. Cleaning
    b. Sterilization
    c. High-level disinfection
    d. Intermediate-level disinfection

44. The process of removing dirt from the surface of an object using soap and water is called:
    a. cleaning.
    b. sanitizing.
    c. sterilization.
    d. disinfection.

45. The cleanup of a blood spill on the floor of the ambulance begins with removing moist blood with a paper towel, followed by a:
    a. high-level disinfection with hot water.
    b. soap-and-water mopping and air-drying.
    c. towel wipedown with a sanitizer and AC drying.
    d. wipedown with a spray disinfectant and air-drying.

46. When using a plastic spray bottle of concentrated household bleach as a disinfectant for cleaning, the usual recommended dilution in water is:
    a. 1:1.
    b. 1:10.
    c. 1:100.
    d. 1:1000.

47. During cleanup and restock after a call, you have reusable equipment that must be decontaminated from urine and vomit. You should place those items in a _____ bag.
    a. red
    b. clear
    c. yellow
    d. orange

48. Proper verbal report of patient information, upon arrival at the ED, is necessary to:
    a. get a patient properly registered.
    b. rapidly locate a specialty physician.
    c. have a bed ready for the patient upon arrival at the ED.
    d. help prevent any confusion that may potentially be harmful to the patient.

49. The EMT-B's reporting of patient information, with regard to assisting the patient with his nitroglycerin, is very specific. Which of the following items is included on the written report rather than the verbal report?
    a. patient's response to the medication
    b. the prescribed name on the medication
    c. dose, route, and time of administration
    d. the person who assisted with the administration

50. The patient information included in the typical radio report to the ED:
    a. is a courtesy and not mandatory.
    b. helps prepare the ED for the patient's arrival.
    c. enables the patient to prepare for arrival at the ED.
    d. allows other EMS agencies to be aware of busy hospitals.

51. Basic ambulance maintenance, such as oil and filter changes, are typically the responsibility of the:
    a. EMT-B.
    b. junior EMS responder.
    c. senior EMS responder.
    d. agency's vehicle mechanic.

52. The primary purpose of completing a daily ambulance checklist is to:
    a. have the unit prepared to respond to a call.
    b. prevent or reduce the risk of lawsuits.
    c. help the crew learn the location of the medical equipment.
    d. help the crew learn the location of the nonmedical equipment.

53. Air medical transport has been requested to the scene of a serious MVC with multiple patients. The head-on collision occurred on a high-speed road at night. Both drivers and one passenger are dead. A front-seat passenger in his early twenties has a head injury with altered mental status. One passenger who was ejected is in cardiac arrest, with CPR in progress. There is a toddler in a car seat who appears uninjured and a 10-year-old with a possible fractured forearm and ankle. Which patient has the highest priority for air medical transport?
    a. toddler
    b. cardiac arrest
    c. head injury with AMS
    d. 10-year-old with extremity injuries

54. (Continuing with the preceding question) A landing zone is being set up in a field 50 yards from the collision. Command has been notified that the helicopter is small, that it can take one patient, and that the ETA is 5 minutes. This aircraft will require a landing zone that is:

a. 50 × 50 feet
b. 60 × 60 feet
c. 60 × 60 yards
d. 100 × 100 feet

55. You and your partner have been assigned to do a long-distance transport of a stable patient who requires constant oxygen by non-rebreather mask at 10 lpm. The transport will take 2 hours. The onboard oxygen tank is an M cylinder with 1,500 psi. Using the following formula, estimate the time in minutes you have available with the current onboard tank.

$$\frac{1{,}500 \times 1.56}{10 \ (\text{lpm})} \ \text{(cylinder constant for an M tank)}$$

a. 96 minutes
b. 234 minutes
c. 960 minutes
d. 2,340 minutes

Chapter 30 Answer Form

	A	B	C	D		A	B	C	D
1.	❏	❏	❏	❏	29.	❏	❏	❏	❏
2.	❏	❏	❏	❏	30.	❏	❏	❏	❏
3.	❏	❏	❏	❏	31.	❏	❏	❏	❏
4.	❏	❏	❏	❏	32.	❏	❏	❏	❏
5.	❏	❏	❏	❏	33.	❏	❏	❏	❏
6.	❏	❏	❏	❏	34.	❏	❏	❏	❏
7.	❏	❏	❏	❏	35.	❏	❏	❏	❏
8.	❏	❏	❏	❏	36.	❏	❏	❏	❏
9.	❏	❏	❏	❏	37.	❏	❏	❏	❏
10.	❏	❏	❏	❏	38.	❏	❏	❏	❏
11.	❏	❏	❏	❏	39.	❏	❏	❏	❏
12.	❏	❏	❏	❏	40.	❏	❏	❏	❏
13.	❏	❏	❏	❏	41.	❏	❏	❏	❏
14.	❏	❏	❏	❏	42.	❏	❏	❏	❏
15.	❏	❏	❏	❏	43.	❏	❏	❏	❏
16.	❏	❏	❏	❏	44.	❏	❏	❏	❏
17.	❏	❏	❏	❏	45.	❏	❏	❏	❏
18.	❏	❏	❏	❏	46.	❏	❏	❏	❏
19.	❏	❏	❏	❏	47.	❏	❏	❏	❏
20.	❏	❏	❏	❏	48.	❏	❏	❏	❏
21.	❏	❏	❏	❏	49.	❏	❏	❏	❏
22.	❏	❏	❏	❏	50.	❏	❏	❏	❏
23.	❏	❏	❏	❏	51.	❏	❏	❏	❏
24.	❏	❏	❏	❏	52.	❏	❏	❏	❏
25.	❏	❏	❏	❏	53.	❏	❏	❏	❏
26.	❏	❏	❏	❏	54.	❏	❏	❏	❏
27.	❏	❏	❏	❏	55.	❏	❏	❏	❏
28.	❏	❏	❏	❏					

CHAPTER

31

Gaining Access

1. Extrication is a process in which actions are taken to free a patient entrapped in a:
   a. tunnel.
   b. vehicle.
   c. swimming pool.
   d. any of the above.

2. The purpose of extrication is to:
   a. ensure the safely of the rescuer and the patient.
   b. remove a patient from entrapment without causing further injury.
   c. develop specialized teams with skills for different types of rescues.
   d. have an effective preplan that includes specific equipment for various rescues.

3. _____ is a rescue term associated with the removal of parts or debris from around a patient in an effort to free that patient from a vehicle compartment or structure.
   a. Recovery
   b. Hazard control
   c. Disentanglement
   d. Rapid extrication

4. With the proper training and equipment, the EMT-B may participate in which phases of a rescue?
   a. size-up and hazard control
   b. gaining access to the patient
   c. disentanglement and patient packaging
   d. any of the above

5. In a rescue operation, the next step after gaining access to a patient is:
   a. disentanglement.
   b. patient packaging.
   c. body recovery and stabilization.
   d. medical assessment and treatment.

6. Rescue awareness for the EMT-B means that she has enough knowledge to:
   a. recognize when a patient is stable or unstable.
   b. recognize when it is not safe to gain access to a patient.
   c. gain access to a patient for treatment purposes in any circumstance.
   d. gain access to a patient for assessment purposes in any circumstance.

7. While working in or near water, the EMT-B should use _____ as part of the minimum personal safety equipment.
   a. a rope rescue bag
   b. turnout coat/pants
   c. a personal flotation device (PFD)
   d. self-contained breathing apparatus

8. Which of the following items is not part of the minimum level of protective equipment for the EMT-B at the scene of a rescue operation?
   a. helmet
   b. level A hazmat
   c. turnout coat/pants
   d. hearing and eye protection

9. Personal protective equipment for the EMT-B in a rescue situation is:
   a. the typical BSI equipment plus a helmet.
   b. the same for all types of rescues.
   c. highly specialized and has been developed just for EMS providers.
   d. more extensive than the typical gloves, eye shield, and mask worn for BSI.

10. The phase of extrication that includes estimating the severity of injuries and the patient transport needs is the _____ phase.
    a. scene size-up
    b. transportation
    c. disentanglement
    d. medical treatment

11. As the first ambulance to arrive at the scene of an extrication involving a hazardous material, you complete a scene size-up, notify dispatch, and begin any possible hazard control. The EMT-B's approach to hazard control should be limited to:
    a. creating a safe perimeter.
    b. attempting to contain the substance involved.
    c. keeping reporters away from the danger zone.
    d. rapidly getting any victims who can walk out of the area.

12. The final component or phase of a extrication for the EMT-B is the:
    a. overhaul.
    b. cleanup.
    c. transportation.
    d. patient packaging.

13. You have been dispatched with the fire department for two people stuck in an elevator. When you arrive, you learn that the power is out because of an electrical fire in the building. There is a smoke condition and the building is being evacuated. What can you do to protect the two victims in the elevator?
    a. Tape a sheet over the outside of the elevator door.
    b. Stay by the elevator and provide supportive instructions.
    c. Stand by until the fire department has extricated the victims.
    d. Attempt to pass oxygen tubing through the floor of the elevator.

14. A victim is entangled in debris at a construction site after a small explosion caused the collapse of a floor. The fire department is on the scene attempting to gain access to the patient. While the firefighters are working, you observe the patient from a point nearby and see that there is crumbing concrete falling on and near the victim. What equipment from the ambulance can you offer to shield the patient?
    a. sheets
    b. towels
    c. blankets
    d. backboards

15. Your partner has gained access to the driver of a motor vehicle, who is trapped with his legs pinned, and is stabilizing the patient's cervical spine. The rescue crew with the fire department is about to break the glass in the door before prying the door off with a power tool. What item can you give your partner to protect the patient from the glass?
    a. a short backboard
    b. a disposable blanket
    c. an aluminized fire blanket
    d. any of these items will work

16. _____ is the type of terrain that can become dangerous, because of difficult footing, when carrying a patient in a basket.
    a. Low angle
    b. High angle
    c. Short angle
    d. Vertical rescue

17. Once a vehicle is determined to be in a stable position, the first attempt to gain access to a patient in that vehicle should be to:
    a. locate an unlocked door.
    b. force open the door nearest to the patient.
    c. force open the door farthest from the patient.
    d. locate an unlocked door farthest from the patient.

18. A teenager is stranded on a large rock in fast-running water approximately 25 feet from the shore. A special rescue team has been called and you are awaiting its arrival. What can you do until the rescue team arrives?
    a. There is really nothing to do at this point.
    b. Attempt to throw a rope out to the victim.
    c. Throw a personal flotation device (PFD) to the victim.
    d. Attempt to rescue the victim while wearing a personal flotation device (PFD).

19. When the EMT-B is attempting to gain access to a patient through the doors of a vehicle that was involved in a collision, she should first try all doors. If she cannot gain access through a door, then she should try gaining access:
    a. by forcing open the trunk or rear hatch.
    b. by breaking the windshield with a pry bar.
    c. through the window nearest to the patient.
    d. through the window furthest from the patient.

20. The driver of a vehicle that was involved in a collision in an intersection is uninjured but unable to open her door. It is an older vehicle, and all the doors are manually locked from the inside. You ask her to try to roll down a window so that you can get inside to stay with her until the fire department can get her out. This type of access is:

    a. noninvasive.
    b. simple access.
    c. complex access.
    d. disentanglement.

21. The fire department is attempting to gain access into a motor vehicle that has extensive damage. None of the doors will open easily, and the firefighters have broken the glass in the rear window to allow access to the patient. This type of entry into the vehicle is referred to as:

    a. simple access.
    b. horizontal entry.
    c. complex access.
    d. disentanglement.

22. Arriving at the scene of a motor vehicle collision, you see a car on its hood. The fire department has stabilized the vehicle with cribbing and now it is safe to attempt to gain access to the patient. The rear driver's-side door opens enough for you to climb in. This type of access is referred to as:

    a. simple access.
    b. complex access.
    c. disentanglement.
    d. upside-down entry.

23. Ropes, an exposure suit, and a personal flotation device (PFD) are the equipment needed for which type of rescue?

    a. low-angle
    b. ice or water
    c. confined-space
    d. hazardous materials

24. What resource can the EMT-B utilize in the ambulance to identify hazardous materials from a distance?

    a. NFPA 704 placard system
    b. UN numbers and DOT placards
    c. North American Emergency Response Guidebook
    d. any of the above

25. Which of the following factors would significantly change the treatment of a patient involved in a rescue effort, making treatment different from that of any other patient?

    a. the patient's past medical history
    b. lengthy time before access to the patient
    c. any past experience the patient may have had with a rescue
    d. the amount of psychological support needed for the patient

26. The potentially greatest hazard for the EMT-B working at the scene of a collision is:

    a. the traffic.
    b. fire or explosion.
    c. glass and sharp metal edges.
    d. exposure to leaking fluids such as fuel and oil.

27. The roof supports of an automobile are identified as A, B, C, or D posts. Which post supports the roof at the windshield?

    a. A
    b. B
    c. C
    d. D

28. _____ radiation is the form of radiation particles that can infiltrate the body and cause internal and external injury, making it the most dangerous form of radiation.

    a. Alpha
    b. Beta
    c. Delta
    d. Gamma

29. Identification placards for chemicals list the properties of potential hazards associated with the chemical and include all of the following, except:

    a. reactivity.
    b. flammability.
    c. health hazards.
    d. infiltration ranges.

30. Confined spaces are deceiving and can present a great threat to a rescuer because:

    a. these spaces may contain very little oxygen.
    b. employees infrequently work in and around them.
    c. OSHA requires a work-site permit to work in them.
    d. many EMT-Bs are too large to gain access to them.

Chapter 31 Answer Form

	A	B	C	D			A	B	C	D
1.	❏	❏	❏	❏		16.	❏	❏	❏	❏
2.	❏	❏	❏	❏		17.	❏	❏	❏	❏
3.	❏	❏	❏	❏		18.	❏	❏	❏	❏
4.	❏	❏	❏	❏		19.	❏	❏	❏	❏
5.	❏	❏	❏	❏		20.	❏	❏	❏	❏
6.	❏	❏	❏	❏		21.	❏	❏	❏	❏
7.	❏	❏	❏	❏		22.	❏	❏	❏	❏
8.	❏	❏	❏	❏		23.	❏	❏	❏	❏
9.	❏	❏	❏	❏		24.	❏	❏	❏	❏
10.	❏	❏	❏	❏		25.	❏	❏	❏	❏
11.	❏	❏	❏	❏		26.	❏	❏	❏	❏
12.	❏	❏	❏	❏		27.	❏	❏	❏	❏
13.	❏	❏	❏	❏		28.	❏	❏	❏	❏
14.	❏	❏	❏	❏		29.	❏	❏	❏	❏
15.	❏	❏	❏	❏		30.	❏	❏	❏	❏

CHAPTER

32

Overviews

1. The amount of responsibility an EMT-B typically has at the scene of a hazmat incident is determined by:
   a. dispatch.
   b. the most experienced EMS provider on the scene.
   c. the local hazmat plan and level of hazmat training the EMT-B has.
   d. how many patients are involved and the type of chemical involved.

2. Of the following tasks, which must the EMT-B do first upon arrival at a scene with a potential hazmat?
   a. Perform triage.
   b. Complete a scene size-up.
   c. Establish a decon corridor.
   d. Assume the role of safety officer.

3. The role of the EMT-B as a first responder to the scene of a hazmat incident is to:
   a. determine what type of hazmat specialist will be needed.
   b. keep herself and the crew from being exposed or injured.
   c. identify the chemical substance involved using the NFPA 704 placard system.
   d. determine the type of decontamination procedure that will be needed.

4. Ensuring bystander safety at the scene of an MCI is the primary responsibility of the:
   a. police.
   b. safety officer.
   c. incident commander.
   d. senior EMT-B or paramedic.

5. Establishing safety zones should be completed _____ a hazmat operation.
   a. in the later phase of
   b. in the early phase of
   c. in the cleanup phase of
   d. after hazmat specialist arrives at

6. To keep bystanders safe at or near a hazmat operation, the EMT-B should first:
   a. establish safety zones.
   b. call for the police to assist.
   c. call for the fire department to assist.
   d. assign the task to the safety officer.

7. You believe that a product with a flammability hazard is present at the scene. Your partner goes to the ambulance and brings back a hazmat resource guide, which states that a flammability hazard may have any of the following warnings, except:
   a. may be fatal if inhaled.
   b. may cause fire or explosion.
   c. may ignite other combustible materials.
   d. may be ignited by heat, sparks, or flames.

8. After responding to a low-priority call for a sick person, you quickly discover that there are two others in the residence with the same symptoms as the patient, but to a lesser degree. All three have headache, nausea, and dizziness and you suspect possible inhalation poisoning. The next action you take is to:
   a. establish safety zones.
   b. get everyone out of the residence.
   c. open all the windows in the residence.
   d. attempt to identify the poisonous substance.

9. On the scene of a call for a sick person, you suspect that there is a hazard in the basement. The patient had been working down there for an hour when he developed a cough, watery eyes, and nausea. You are upstairs and do not have any resources immediately available to help with information about the substance he was working with. At this point you:
   a. search the residence for the MSDS.
   b. interrogate the patient and family members.
   c. call dispatch and request a hazmat response.
   d. go into the basement to find the packaging label for the substance.

10. When approaching the scene of a hazmat incident, the ambulance needs to stay clear of all spills, vapors, fumes, and smoke. This is usually achieved by:
    a. parking at least 500 feet from the scene.
    b. parking behind the largest fire apparatus.
    c. approaching and parking downwind of the scene.
    d. approaching and parking upwind and uphill of the scene, if possible.

11. As an EMT-B trained to the hazmat awareness level, your duties are to:
    a. recognize a hazmat and carry out basic confinement.
    b. recognize a hazmat, back off, and call for the appropriate help.
    c. select and don appropriate PPE, then carry out basic control and containment.
    d. establish incident command and assign duties to incoming rescue personnel.

12. Dispatch has put out a call for a 30-year-old male with possible exposure to a hazardous material. Before you arrive at the scene, an updated report from dispatch informs you that the material was liquid chlorine and that it was splashed in the patient's face. When you arrive, as you perform a scene size-up your first priority is to:
    a. determine the need for additional resources.
    b. avoid any exposure to yourself and your crew.
    c. assess for any risks of primary or secondary contamination of the patient.
    d. assess for any risks of primary or secondary contamination of other responders.

13. When arriving at the scene of a hazmat incident in progress, the ambulance should report and stage in the_____ zone.
    a. hot
    b. cold
    c. warm
    d. control

14. You are assisting in the decontamination of a patient who accidentally splashed diesel fuel on his head, face, chest, and extremities. The first step you took was to instruct the patient to remove his clothing and then pour water on himself. This step is referred to as _____ decontamination.
    a. self
    b. gross
    c. tertiary
    d. secondary

15. During a hazmat incident, a treatment sector (group) is established so that EMS can:
    a. dress and actively monitor the teams working in the hot zone.
    b. monitor the hazmat team before and after entry into the hot zone.
    c. determine what type of decontamination is appropriate for the incident.
    d. directly report any irregularities on the part of the hazmat team to the incident commander.

16. _____ is the process of removing hazardous materials from exposed persons and equipment at a hazmat incident.
    a. Corrosion
    b. Extrication
    c. Degradation
    d. Decontamination

17. An early-morning fire in an apartment complex has 36 residents out on the street watching their homes being destroyed. Many of the residents were asleep when the fire started, and nearly half of them are coughing or complaining of a burning sensation in the throat. Until proven otherwise, EMS should suspect that:
    a. there may still be residents in the building.
    b. one of the residents is most likely an arsonist.
    c. there is a possibility of carbon monoxide poisoning in all the victims of this fire.
    d. many of these victims may have seizures within an hour.

18. Your unit was dispatched to stand by at a tire fire in a junkyard. You have been staged a quarter-mile away. From there you can see that the fire is significant and that black smoke is rising in extremely large clouds. With residential housing surrounding three sides of the junkyard, which of the following environmental factors could create an immediate hazard for these residents?
    a. rain
    b. snow
    c. lightning
    d. wind direction

19. Dispatch sends you down to Pier 3 for an injured worker. When you arrive, you discover that the victim is pinned by a piece of iron and a second person was injured while attempting to free the first victim. This incident is now a/an:
    a. hazmat.
    b. confined space rescue.
    c. multiple-casualty incident (MCI).
    d. extrication with two patients on scene.

20. It is 2300 hours and you are responding to a private residence for an alcohol overdose. Police are on the scene when you arrive; they advise you that there was a party with teenage drinking. As you size up the scene, it is apparent that several teenagers are highly intoxicated. You immediately advise dispatch to send two additional ambulances and declare this to be a/an:

    a. rescue operation.
    b. EMS sector (branch).
    c. multiple-casualty incident (MCI).
    d. prolonged and involved incident involving minors.

21. At 0700 hours, it is a foggy morning and you are dispatched to a motor vehicle collision. When you arrive and complete a scene size-up, you find a bus on its side with the unresponsive driver still inside, but no additional passengers. A second vehicle is involved, and there are four occupants with various complaints of injury. This incident is a:

    a. hazmat incident.
    b. confined space rescue.
    c. complicated extrication.
    d. multiple-casualty incident (MCI).

22. The EMT-B who establishes command at a large incident will determine how many sector (group) functions to establish based on:

    a. the level of his training.
    b. how many sector (group) vests are available.
    c. the number of patients each hospital can accept.
    d. the complexity of the incident and the number of staff.

23. The first EMS unit to arrive at a scene involving several patients is typically the one that:

    a. establishes EMS command.
    b. notifies dispatch of the first-in size-up report.
    c. locates police and fire officers to establish unified command.
    d. all of the above.

24. Your assignment at the scene of a multiple-casualty incident is to oversee the treatment of patients who have been triaged. This assignment is designated:

    a. treatment officer.
    b. medical command.
    c. staging sector (group).
    d. treatment sector (group).

25. When you have more than one patient to manage, you need to determine which one is more severely injured or ill. This is referred to as:

    a. triage.
    b. patient identification.
    c. rapid physical examination.
    d. patient discovery and classification.

26. As the second ambulance arriving on scene at a large office building, which has begun evacuation of its employees because of an unusual odor, you are assigned the detail of triage tagging. This phase is important because:

    a. it helps to eliminate the need to repeatedly reassess each patient.
    b. using triage tags eliminates the need for nonemergency treatment.
    c. using triage tags eliminates the need for rapid emergency treatment.
    d. the first ambulance to arrive is too busy with other assignments on the scene.

27. Typically, the only treatment completed on a patient in the triage stage of a multiple-casualty incident is:

    a. splinting for children.
    b. CPR for a cardiac arrest.
    c. opening a patient's airway.
    d. none; no treatment is done during the triage stage.

28. The EMT-B must be able to recognize when a disaster is developing, so that she can quickly adapt to meet the special considerations for that disaster. Therefore, she knows that a disaster is caused by:

    a. chemical leak.
    b. disease outbreak.
    c. natural forces such as a hurricane or flooding.
    d. any of the above.

29. The role of the EMT-B in a disaster operation is to:

    a. follow the national disaster plan.
    b. provide medical and psychological support to those who need it.
    c. get involved in the preplanning and training for disaster operations.
    d. acknowledge Homeland Security (HLS) efforts and work with HLS teams.

30. The EMT-B can better understand what his role may be in disaster operations by:

    a. becoming involved in preplanning and training.
    b. realizing that there is really no way to prepare for major disasters.
    c. obtaining the highest level of medical training affordable.
    d. talking to as many people as possible who have been in disasters.

31. An incident has become large enough to require the resources of agencies outside of the community. Communication among all the resources will:

    a. work best when plain English only is used.
    b. be designated by the incident commander.
    c. use the common "disaster system" terminology.
    d. use the code system of the originating jurisdiction.

32. Before a disaster that could involve numerous victims occurs, many communities preplan and train for various possibilities. These plans use a tool called _____, which manages personnel and resources during a multiple-casualty incident.

    a. Homeland Security (HLS)
    b. incident management system (IMS)
    c. disaster and rescue operations (DRO)
    d. environmental disaster management (EDM)

33. The larger a multiple-casualty incident (MCI) is, the more functional components may be required. With enough resources, the incident commander can utilize up to four components, which include:

    a. fire, police, media, and mutual aid.
    b. treatment, transport, logistics, and finance.
    c. operations, planning, logistics, and finance.
    d. operations, logistics, treatment, and transport.

34. Many emergency departments will _____ before they accept a hazmat patient, even when that patient was decontaminated at the scene.

    a. contact the hazmat team specialist
    b. ask you to decontaminate the patient again
    c. take the patient through their own decontamination procedures
    d. have the local fire department respond to inspect a patient for contamination

35. To prevent unnecessary contamination of EMS equipment at the scene of a hazmat incident, the EMT-B should:

    a. use only disposable items.
    b. use only the equipment of the hazmat team.
    c. stage equipment in the cold zone of an operation.
    d. not use any equipment until the patients have been decontaminated.

36. To help prevent contamination of the ambulance by a patient who has been exposed to a hazardous material, during the decontamination phase the:

    a. patient's clothing must be removed in the hot or warm zones.
    b. trained hazmat personnel will give the patient special instructions.
    c. EMT-B will follow special instructions given by the trained hazmat chief.
    d. patient will be wrapped in a special sealed blanket and an oxygen mask applied.

37. As a proactive EMT-B, you have been reviewing the local MCI plan. Now you want to learn more about the areas in your community where hazardous materials are stored in large quantities and the location of possible sites for an incident. Therefore, you:

    a. research at the local library.
    b. contact the local or state office of OSHA.
    c. get all the information from research online.
    d. go to the local fire department for the information.

38. The EMT-B can review the local MCI plan by:

    a. getting the plan from the chief officer.
    b. attending mutual-aid MCI training days.
    c. attending continuing education on the subject in the community.
    d. all of the above.

39. Which of the following is not in the category of weapons of mass destruction (WMD)?

    a. fire
    b. chemical
    c. explosive
    d. biological and nuclear

40. When reporting to an incident involving weapons of mass destruction (WMD), the EMT-B's role includes:

    a. establishing command and performing a scene size-up.
    b. reporting to command and then to an assigned sector (group).
    c. providing the initial scene report to dispatch and requesting additional resources.
    d. identifying yourself and your level of training to the transportation sector officer.

41. EMS and fire are dispatched for a fire alarm at a dance club. When you arrive, there is a crowd standing outside the building and the police and fire departments are on the scene. The club manager reports that a spotlight over the stage started smoking and set off the fire alarm; the crowd panicked and a few customers were injured while exiting the building. You grab your triage tags and begin to get a count of the number of patients, and you start sorting them to determine which ones will need immediate emergency care. After an initial triage, which of the following patients can be considered a P-3, green, or categorized with minor injuries?

    a. 23-year-old female having an asthma attack from smoke inhalation
    b. 43-year-old female complaining of headache, nausea, and vomiting
    c. 44-year-old female with a nosebleed and a possible fractured nose
    d. 28-year-old male with a swollen and deformed ankle and abrasions on both hands

42. (Continuing with the preceding question) Which patient is most in need of immediate emergency care?

    a. 23-year-old female having an asthma attack from smoke inhalation
    b. 43-year-old female complaining of headache, nausea, and vomiting
    c. 44-year-old female with a nosebleed and a possible fractured nose
    d. 28-year-old male with a swollen and deformed ankle and abrasions on both hands

43. Your unit has been dispatched to a local produce farm for a patient who has abdominal pain. Two hours after beginning work today, a 19-year-old male began complaining of severe abdominal cramps and nausea, and he has a new skin irritation with redness and itching on both arms and his neck. Shortly after arriving, you discover that there are multiple patients on the scene, with similar symptoms, who are all going to require transport for evaluation. Three more patients are complaining of headache, eye irritation, sore throat, nausea, and dizziness. What is the next action to take?

   a. Triage and tag each patient, then request the appropriate number of ambulances.
   b. Notify dispatch that you are declaring an MCI with a hazmat exposure.
   c. Avoid any contamination of yourself and your crew by retreating to the ambulance to wait for additional resources.
   d. Avoid any further possible contamination by identifying a decontamination area, and begin washing the patients.

44. A medical emergency that creates a number of patients and places excessive demands on personnel and available equipment is referred to as a/an:

   a. disaster.
   b. mass-casualty incident.
   c. multiple-casualty incident.
   d. incident management system.

45. Plenty of resources have been dispatched to a motel fire, but your ambulance is the first unit to arrive. Flames and smoke are visible, and you quickly identify two victims in a third-floor window who are trapped by the fire. You should attempt a rescue only when:

   a. the victims are children, elderly, or disabled.
   b. the victims will perish before the fire department arrives.
   c. you are trained to do so and have the proper equipment.
   d. you should never attempt such a rescue, as it is the job of the fire department.

Chapter 32 Answer Form

	A	B	C	D
1.	❏	❏	❏	❏
2.	❏	❏	❏	❏
3.	❏	❏	❏	❏
4.	❏	❏	❏	❏
5.	❏	❏	❏	❏
6.	❏	❏	❏	❏
7.	❏	❏	❏	❏
8.	❏	❏	❏	❏
9.	❏	❏	❏	❏
10.	❏	❏	❏	❏
11.	❏	❏	❏	❏
12.	❏	❏	❏	❏
13.	❏	❏	❏	❏
14.	❏	❏	❏	❏
15.	❏	❏	❏	❏
16.	❏	❏	❏	❏
17.	❏	❏	❏	❏
18.	❏	❏	❏	❏
19.	❏	❏	❏	❏
20.	❏	❏	❏	❏
21.	❏	❏	❏	❏
22.	❏	❏	❏	❏
23.	❏	❏	❏	❏

	A	B	C	D
24.	❏	❏	❏	❏
25.	❏	❏	❏	❏
26.	❏	❏	❏	❏
27.	❏	❏	❏	❏
28.	❏	❏	❏	❏
29.	❏	❏	❏	❏
30.	❏	❏	❏	❏
31.	❏	❏	❏	❏
32.	❏	❏	❏	❏
33.	❏	❏	❏	❏
34.	❏	❏	❏	❏
35.	❏	❏	❏	❏
36.	❏	❏	❏	❏
37.	❏	❏	❏	❏
38.	❏	❏	❏	❏
39.	❏	❏	❏	❏
40.	❏	❏	❏	❏
41.	❏	❏	❏	❏
42.	❏	❏	❏	❏
43.	❏	❏	❏	❏
44.	❏	❏	❏	❏
45.	❏	❏	❏	❏

Advanced Airway

CHAPTER 33

Advanced Airway

1. The right and left lungs are separated in the chest by the:
   a. vallecula.
   b. mediastinum.
   c. glottic opening.
   d. mainstem bronchi.

2. During an intubation, the EMT-B will visualize which of the following landmark structures?
   a. epiglottis
   b. cricoid cartilage
   c. thyroid cartilage
   d. mainstem bronchi

3. The true vocal cords lie _____ the false vocal cords.
   a. within
   b. anterior to
   c. posterior to
   d. 5 cm under

4. Unlike the adult airway, the smallest circumference of the infant's airway proportionately is/are the:
   a. lungs.
   b. nares.
   c. mouth.
   d. cricoid ring.

5. Until the age of _____, the position of an unresponsive patient's head is especially important during airway maintenance, to avoid blocking the airway structures.
   a. 8
   b. 10
   c. 16
   d. 18

6. Compared to the adult, the trachea of the infant and child is:
   a. stiffer.
   b. longer.
   c. straighter.
   d. more flexible.

7. _____ reflex is a reliable indication that a patient is unable to protect her own airway.
   a. A positive gag
   b. Loss of the gag
   c. A positive cough
   d. Loss of the sneezing

8. You are managing an unresponsive patient and attempt to establish a patent airway by performing a head-tilt, chin-lift maneuver. There is no need to suction, so the next step is to:
   a. insert an oral airway.
   b. obtain an SpO2 reading.
   c. hyperventilate the patient.
   d. intubate with a large ET tube.

9. In the patient with potential or actual airway compromise, the EMT-B must first _____ before attempting any advanced airway techniques.
   a. remove any foreign bodies
   b. correctly position the head and neck
   c. suction secretions, blood, or vomitus as needed
   d. all of the above.

10. Placing an oropharyngeal airway incorrectly into the mouth of an infant can easily cause bleeding, because of the infant's:
    a. large-sized head.
    b. highly vascular tissues.
    c. undeveloped gag reflex.
    d. undeveloped cough reflex.

11. Managing a patient's airway with simple or advanced techniques is a messy skill and always requires:
    a. suction.
    b. body substance isolation.
    c. the use of sterile procedures.
    d. the use of endotracheal tubes.

12. An unresponsive patient who is seizing has clenched teeth and abnormal respirations. Which of the following airway adjuncts would be appropriate for this patient?
    a. oral intubation
    b. French catheter
    c. oropharyngeal airway
    d. nasopharyngeal airway

13. When ventilating an unresponsive apneic patient with a BVM, the EMT-B should squeeze in _____ cc without oxygen connected and squeeze in _____ cc with oxygen connected.
    a. 600, 800
    b. 800, 600
    c. 1,000, 800
    d. 1,200, 1,000

14. When a patient's chest does not appear to be rising and falling adequately, it is appropriate to use which of the following oxygen delivery devices first?
    a. nasal cannula at 6 lpm
    b. positive pressure ventilation
    c. automatic transport ventilator
    d. high-flow oxygen by non-rebreather mask

15. Placing an endotracheal tube into the airway requires the rescuer to stop ventilations for a brief time, which can pose the risk of hypoxia. Therefore, it is recommended that the patient be _____ before attempting the procedure.
    a. suctioned
    b. medicated
    c. hyperventilated
    d. hyperoxygenated

16. You have a patient who is in need of a nasogastric tube. First you assemble the equipment and determine which nostril appears more patent, and then you:
    a. measure and mark the tube.
    b. lubricate the distal end of the tube.
    c. lubricate the proximal end of the tube.
    d. document the tube size and which nostril has been selected.

17. Each of the following patients is showing signs of gastric distention. Which one has an indication for nasogastric tube insertion?
    a. an 18-month-old with croup
    b. an unresponsive infant who is vomiting
    c. a 4-year-old unresponsive child with facial trauma
    d. a 2-year-old with drooling and suspected epiglottitis

18. The nasogastric tube has several uses; however, the most common indication that the EMT-B will have for its use is to:
    a. lavage ingested poisons in the stomach.
    b. inject medications directly into the stomach.
    c. relieve gastric distention in an infant or child.
    d. remove blood associated with intestinal bleeding.

19. When checking to see if the nasogastric tube is correctly placed, the EMT-B will attach a syringe to the tube, aspirate the gastric contents, and then:
    a. tape the tube securely in place and document the procedure.
    b. connect low-flow suction to the tube and continue to aspirate.
    c. document the size of the tube, the time inserted, and verification of placement.
    d. inject air while listening with a stethoscope for gurgling over the epigastric area.

20. Ideally, the application of Sellick's maneuver during BLS or ALS airway management should be performed by:
    a. the EMT-B attempting the intubation.
    b. the EMT-B assisting with ventilations.
    c. an EMT-B dedicated to no other tasks.
    d. the most senior EMT-B on the scene.

21. Sellick's maneuver can be used to ease endotracheal tube placement and to decrease the chances of regurgitation, but incorrectly performed it can:
    a. cause aspiration.
    b. occlude the airway.
    c. close off the esophagus.
    d. fracture the Adam's apple.

22. You have just arrived on the scene where an elderly female is unresponsive. The family suspects she may have taken too much of her pain medication by accident. Her respirations are slow and shallow; pulse rate is 60, strong and regular; you have not obtained a BP yet. You begin to assist her ventilations with a BVM and find that you are unable to make a good mask seal because her dentures are out. What can you do to improve ventilations?
    a. Squeeze the bag faster.
    b. Squeeze the bag harder.
    c. Use two hands to make the mask seal.
    d. Reinsert the dentures and try to ventilate again.

23. Dispatch has sent you to a call for an unconscious patient with a possible alcohol overdose. Your initial assessment of the patient upon arrival is that of a male in his thirties who is unresponsive, with snoring respirations, and smells of alcohol. Which of the following is a consideration for attempting an orotracheal intubation on this patient?
   a. You are able to insert an oropharyngeal airway.
   b. You are trained and approved to intubate a patient as needed.
   c. You are unable to insert a nasopharyngeal airway due to gagging.
   d. The patient's vital signs are adequate, but you are unable to awaken him.

24. You are adequately ventilating an apneic patient with a BVM. He has a strong, regular pulse rate of 72 and a blood pressure of 140/80. When you are deciding whether to intubate, which of the following factors would make you consider holding off on intubating?
   a. a long transport
   b. the patient is vomiting
   c. the transport to the ED is 5 minutes
   d. the patient's stomach is becoming distended

25. The equipment needed to verify tube placement after an orotracheal intubation attempt includes:
   a. suction, stethoscope, and direct visualization.
   b. 10 cc syringe, stethoscope, and an end-tidal CO_2 device.
   c. stethoscope and esophageal detection or end-tidal CO_2 device.
   d. tracheal tube-securing device, 10 cc syringe, and stethoscope.

26. The minimum personal protective equipment recommended for performing any advanced airway procedure includes:
   a. gloves.
   b. gloves, eye protection, and gown.
   c. eye protection, face mask, and gown.
   d. gloves, eye protection, and face mask.

27. Which of the following pieces of equipment is not typically used for an orotracheal intubation?
   a. suction unit
   b. 10 cc syringe
   c. lidocaine gel lubricant
   d. esophageal detection device

28. Before inserting a curved laryngoscope blade into the mouth of a patient, the EMT-B must:
   a. ensure that the patient has a pulse.
   b. check to see that the light is working.
   c. ensure that the patient is unconscious.
   d. select the correct size tube restraint for the ETT.

29. Which of the following blade(s) would you select for an intubation if you wanted to lift the epiglottis to visualize the vocal cords?
   a. Miller
   b. McIntosh
   c. Wisconsin
   d. either straight or curved

30. The blade that is designed to be placed into the vallecula is the _____ blade.
   a. Miller
   b. Flagg
   c. curved
   d. straight

31. To allow the EMT-B to view the vocal cords, the distal tip of the straight blade is designed to fit:
   a. in the trachea.
   b. in the vallecula.
   c. over the epiglottis.
   d. under the epiglottis.

32. Because of the anatomical differences in infants and children, the _____ blade is preferred and recommended by the American Heart Association.
   a. straight
   b. curved
   c. fiberoptic
   d. disposable

33. When using _____ blade, the procedure is to insert the blade into the right side of the mouth and then sweep the tongue up and to the left.
   a. a straight
   b. any type of
   c. the curved
   d. a fiberoptic

34. During an orotracheal intubation, once the endotracheal tube has been passed through the vocal cords, the next step is to:
   a. remove the stylet.
   b. ventilate with a BVM.
   c. secure the tube in place.
   d. attach the end-tidal CO_2 device.

35. The stylet used in an orotracheal intubation is placed inside the endotracheal tube:
   a. no further than the Murphy eye.
   b. 2 inches before the tip of the tube.
   c. until it extends just beyond the bevel of the tube.
   d. until it extends to the very end of the tip of the tube.

36. The reason for using a stylet for orotracheal intubation is:
   a. to prevent right mainstem intubation.
   b. to give the tube shape and stability.
   c. for proper measurement and placement.
   d. that it makes visualization of the cords easier.

37. When preparing to perform an orotracheal intubation, in addition to selecting the proper size tube, the EMT-B should also:
   a. select one tube that is larger.
   b. have an extra one of the same size ready.
   c. select one tube that is smaller and one that is larger.
   d. have an extra one of the same size and one larger size ready.

38. The patient you are caring for is in cardiac arrest. He is 66 years old with an average height and weight. You do not expect that this will be a difficult intubation. The first size tube you select for this patient is:
   a. 7.0 mm i.d.
   b. 8.0 mm i.d.
   c. 9.0 mm i.d.
   d. 10.0 mm i.d.

39. You are selecting an endotracheal tube for an adult woman on whom you anticipate a difficult airway and complications. The first size tube you decide to use is _____ mm i.d.
   a. 6.0
   b. 7.0
   c. 8.0
   d. 9.0

40. While assisting with a childbirth, you determine that the fetus is full term and that the mother has had pre-natal care. You do not expect any problems until the bag of waters breaks and thick meconium is present. Thinking ahead, you ask your partner to set up the intubation kit and pull out the _____ size tubes.
   a. 3.0 cuffed
   b. 3.5 cuffed
   c. 2.0 uncuffed
   d. 3.0 uncuffed

41. You are helping your partner select the correct size endotracheal tube for a 2-year-old child. Using the formula 4 + (age of the child in years/4), you select size _____ mm i.d.
   a. 2.5
   b. 3.0
   c. 4.5
   d. 6.0

42. The 4-year-old patient you are treating is in severe respiratory distress and you anticipate the need for possible orotracheal intubation. You cannot recall the formula for sizing the tube, so you:
   a. use the pediatric length-based reference tape.
   b. select a tube with the inside diameter of the child's largest nare.
   c. select a tube with the outside diameter of the child's smallest finger.
   d. do any of the above.

43. A major complication associated with moving a patient who has been intubated is:
   a. the pilot balloon tends to deflate.
   b. the tube moves out of the trachea.
   c. the tube moves out of the esophagus.
   d. there is an increased risk of vomiting.

44. You have successfully intubated an adult male who is in cardiac arrest. Tube placement was confirmed by auscultation and with the use of an esophageal detection device. En route to the hospital, you notice that the pilot balloon on the tube is deflated, so the next action you take is to:
   a. remove the tube and insert a new one.
   b. use the 10 cc syringe and inflate it again.
   c. remove the tube and ventilate with a BVM.
   d. make no changes unless there are no breath sounds.

45. During an intubation attempt on an unconscious patient, it is common for the heart to _____, especially in children.
   a. speed up
   b. slow down
   c. stop beating
   d. go into ventricular fibrillation

46. An endotracheal tube that has been placed in the right mainstem bronchi will:
   a. ventilate only the left lung.
   b. ventilate only the right lung.
   c. cause bruising on the carina.
   d. stimulate the gag reflex and cause vomiting.

47. When placing an endotracheal tube into a child, you insert the tube to a depth:
   a. below the carina.
   b. using the centimeter markings on the tube.
   c. recommended on your pediatric reference chart.
   d. that results in equal breath sounds with ventilations.

48. You must select the appropriate tube for a infant or child. An uncuffed tube is recommended for the patient who is less than _____ year(s) old.
   a. 1
   b. 3
   c. 5
   d. 8

49. A baby that is born premature is very likely to need assisted ventilations and possibly intubation. The appropriate size tube for the premature infant is _____ mm i.d.
   a. 1.0
   b. 1.5
   c. 2.0
   d. 3.0

50. During an intubation attempt, the laryngoscope handle is:
    a. held in the left hand.
    b. held in the right hand.
    c. supported by the palm and forearm.
    d. suspended between the thumb and forefinger.

51. Before intubating a patient who does not have a suspected cervical injury, the head should be placed in the _____ position.
    a. flexed
    b. sniffing
    c. in-line head-tilt
    d. hyperextended

52. During an intubation attempt, the time between stopping and restarting ventilations should be no longer than:
    a. 15 seconds.
    b. 30 seconds.
    c. 60 seconds.
    d. 90 seconds.

53. The infant's vocal cords are located more anteriorly than an adult's. This explains why a:
    a. curved blade is easier to use than a straight.
    b. curved blade is harder to use than a straight blade.
    c. curved blade is preferred during intubation of an infant.
    d. curved blade is more likely to traumatize the oropharynx.

54. The major difference between intubating an adult and intubating an infant is:
    a. size of all the equipment.
    b. the use of Sellick's maneuver.
    c. increased risk of vomiting in children.
    d. level of training of the person performing the skill.

55. The position of an infant's head during endotracheal intubation is:
    a. sniffing position.
    b. a mild extension.
    c. the same as with an adult with cervical trauma.
    d. the same as with an adult with no cervical trauma.

56. You are en route to the hospital with an unresponsive patient who was intubated at the scene. The patient suddenly begins to deteriorate rapidly. What steps should you take next?
    a. Quickly hyperventilate the patient.
    b. Immediately check tube placement.
    c. Deflate and remove the tube, then reintubate.
    d. Suction the tube, as it has probably clogged up.

57. During an intubation attempt, the first indication that the tube has been placed in the correct location is:
    a. the confirmation of equal breath sounds.
    b. no breath sounds over the epigastric area.
    c. the free pull of the esophageal detection device.
    d. visualization of the tube passing through the vocal cords.

58. Which of the following is an indication that an unintentional esophageal intubation has occurred?
    a. The patient vomits.
    b. The BVM is difficult to squeeze.
    c. The abdomen appears to be sunken in.
    d. The chest is rising and falling on one side only.

59. An unrecognized esophageal intubation is a severe complication because:
    a. it can be lethal.
    b. the patient will gag.
    c. the patient will vomit.
    d. it creates the need for suctioning.

60. If the EMT-B suspects that an endotracheal tube is placed in the esophagus, he should:
    a. unplug the pulse oximeter.
    b. hyperventilate the patient.
    c. hyperoxygenate the patient.
    d. deflate the cuff and remove the tube.

61. To minimize the risk of dislodging an endotracheal tube, the EMT-B should secure the tube well and:
    a. immobilize the head.
    b. document the procedure.
    c. avoid suctioning the mouth.
    d. never remove the BVM once it is attached.

62. Before securing a tube in place, the EMT-B should note, and later document, the:
    a. length of the tube used.
    b. type of PPE used for the procedure.
    c. centimeter mark at the level of the patient's teeth.
    d. size of syringe used to inflate the pilot bulb on the tube.

63. When a commercial device is not available for securing an endotracheal tube in place, the EMT-B can use:
    a. manual stabilization.
    b. tape and an OPA for a bite block.
    c. cervical collar to stabilize the head and neck.
    d. tape and a rigid-tip suction catheter for a bite block.

64. You are caring for a 26-year-old asthmatic who is in severe respiratory distress. She is not getting better even with high-flow oxygen and bronchodilator treatment. Now you begin to assist her ventilations and consider the possibility of intubation if she does not improve. At this point it would be appropriate to:
    a. discuss the possibility of intubation with the patient.
    b. obtain the patient's consent for intubation if needed.
    c. explain everything you are doing to the patient.
    d. all of the above.

65. A 40-year-old male collapsed in cardiac arrest in his home. Your unit was very close when the call came in, and you arrive to find that the patient is not breathing and has no pulse. The frantic family reports that he has no past medical history of cardiac problems. His wife sees you use the AED to shock the patient and watches as you assemble a Combitube to manage the airway. She becomes even more anxious at the sight of the equipment. What should you do next?
    a. Ask the police to take her into another room.
    b. Explain what you are doing and why you are doing it.
    c. Put the Combitube away and ventilate the patient with a BVM.
    d. Ignore her and continue with your airway management and CPR.

66. When a child needs positive pressure ventilation for a prolonged period of time, the ideal advanced airway procedure is:
    a. Combitube.
    b. endotracheal intubation.
    c. BVM ventilation.
    d. Laryngeal Mask Airway (LMA).

67. Which of the following is not considered an advantage of managing an airway with endotracheal intubation?
    a. It is an easy skill to perform.
    b. It provides the best control of the airway.
    c. Blood and vomit in the upper airway are prevented from getting into the lower airway.
    d. Keeping a face-mask seal is more difficult than bagging a tube during a long transport.

68. The primary advantage of the use of a Combitube over an endotracheal tube is:
    a. one size fits all.
    b. it is easier to ventilate with.
    c. that placement does not require visualization of the vocal cords.
    d. that training is minimal and no retraining or practice is necessary.

69. The responsibility for EMTs performing advanced airway procedures lies primarily and fundamentally with:
    a. regional hospitals.
    b. state EMS department.
    c. local EMS training facility.
    d. EMS service medical director.

70. The EMT-B who is trained to perform advanced airway procedures is:
    a. an asset to a community with little or no ALS.
    b. an advantage in an EMS system with EMT-B trained responders.
    c. in certain situations, able to improve a patient's chances in a life-or-death situation.
    d. all of the above.

71. The use of a stylet during orotracheal intubation is especially helpful in each of the following cases, except:
    a. in intubations of trauma patients.
    b. in warm temperatures.
    c. an intubation in a newborn.
    d. in patients with unusual airway anatomy.

72. The stylet is a piece of equipment used in orotracheal intubation. It helps the EMT-B doing the intubation to:
    a. better control placement of the distal tip of the tube.
    b. identify the centimeter marker on the endotracheal tube.
    c. secure the tube after confirming the correct placement of the tube.
    d. keep the tube from being placed in the esophagus or right mainstem bronchi.

73. If for any reason a patient requires extubation, the EMT-B will need to have _____ ready.
    a. suction
    b. a stylet
    c. a pulse oximeter
    d. scissors and tape

74. Inserting a laryngoscope blade into the larynx may cause:
    a. the tongue to swell.
    b. the heart rate to speed up.
    c. soft-tissue injury and bleeding.
    d. the blood pressure to increase.

75. When first confirming breath sounds, it is common for the tube to be placed in the _____, creating unilateral breath sounds.
    a. stomach
    b. esophagus
    c. left mainstem
    d. right mainstem

76. Once the endotracheal tube is placed through the vocal cords, the EMT-B must quickly confirm adequate breath sounds in order to:
    a. monitor SpO2 readings.
    b. secure the tube in place.
    c. monitor EtCO2 readings.
    d. rule out an esophageal intubation.

77. To rapidly recognize proper placement of an endotracheal tube, the EMT-B should first verify absence of breath sounds over the:
    a. left lung.
    b. trachea.
    c. right lung.
    d. epigastric area.

78. The centimeter markings on an endotracheal tube are used while securing the tube to:
    a. estimate the need for tracheal suctioning.
    b. measure the distance between the mouth and carina.
    c. determine the need for additional securing measures.
    d. mark correct placement and identify any movement thereafter.

79. When an endotracheal tube is not secured properly, the primary complication that is likely to occur is that the tube:
    a. will move out of the trachea.
    b. may move out of the esophagus.
    c. will move deeper into the trachea.
    d. may become an airway obstruction.

80. Securing an endotracheal tube in place may require the use of an OPA, which is used to:
    a. serve as a bite block.
    b. help open the oropharynx.
    c. keep the tongue off the tube.
    d. create an opening in which to suction.

Chapter 33 Answer Form

	A	B	C	D		A	B	C	D
1.	❑	❑	❑	❑	33.	❑	❑	❑	❑
2.	❑	❑	❑	❑	34.	❑	❑	❑	❑
3.	❑	❑	❑	❑	35.	❑	❑	❑	❑
4.	❑	❑	❑	❑	36.	❑	❑	❑	❑
5.	❑	❑	❑	❑	37.	❑	❑	❑	❑
6.	❑	❑	❑	❑	38.	❑	❑	❑	❑
7.	❑	❑	❑	❑	39.	❑	❑	❑	❑
8.	❑	❑	❑	❑	40.	❑	❑	❑	❑
9.	❑	❑	❑	❑	41.	❑	❑	❑	❑
10.	❑	❑	❑	❑	42.	❑	❑	❑	❑
11.	❑	❑	❑	❑	43.	❑	❑	❑	❑
12.	❑	❑	❑	❑	44.	❑	❑	❑	❑
13.	❑	❑	❑	❑	45.	❑	❑	❑	❑
14.	❑	❑	❑	❑	46.	❑	❑	❑	❑
15.	❑	❑	❑	❑	47.	❑	❑	❑	❑
16.	❑	❑	❑	❑	48.	❑	❑	❑	❑
17.	❑	❑	❑	❑	49.	❑	❑	❑	❑
18.	❑	❑	❑	❑	50.	❑	❑	❑	❑
19.	❑	❑	❑	❑	51.	❑	❑	❑	❑
20.	❑	❑	❑	❑	52.	❑	❑	❑	❑
21.	❑	❑	❑	❑	53.	❑	❑	❑	❑
22.	❑	❑	❑	❑	54.	❑	❑	❑	❑
23.	❑	❑	❑	❑	55.	❑	❑	❑	❑
24.	❑	❑	❑	❑	56.	❑	❑	❑	❑
25.	❑	❑	❑	❑	57.	❑	❑	❑	❑
26.	❑	❑	❑	❑	58.	❑	❑	❑	❑
27.	❑	❑	❑	❑	59.	❑	❑	❑	❑
28.	❑	❑	❑	❑	60.	❑	❑	❑	❑
29.	❑	❑	❑	❑	61.	❑	❑	❑	❑
30.	❑	❑	❑	❑	62.	❑	❑	❑	❑
31.	❑	❑	❑	❑	63.	❑	❑	❑	❑
32.	❑	❑	❑	❑	64.	❑	❑	❑	❑

	A	B	C	D		A	B	C	D
65.	❏	❏	❏	❏	73.	❏	❏	❏	❏
66.	❏	❏	❏	❏	74.	❏	❏	❏	❏
67.	❏	❏	❏	❏	75.	❏	❏	❏	❏
68.	❏	❏	❏	❏	76.	❏	❏	❏	❏
69.	❏	❏	❏	❏	77.	❏	❏	❏	❏
70.	❏	❏	❏	❏	78.	❏	❏	❏	❏
71.	❏	❏	❏	❏	79.	❏	❏	❏	❏
72.	❏	❏	❏	❏	80.	❏	❏	❏	❏

Appendix A: Answer Key with Rationales

Chapter 1: Introduction to Emergency Medical Care

1. d. An EMS system is a network of services working together to provide patient care at the scene, during transport, and until the patient is received at the emergency department (ED).

2. c. Access to EMS with a cell phone is not any faster than with a landline. In fact, in many cases cell phone use has caused significant delay with deleterious results. However, improvements are being made, such as use of modified GPS locators.

3. a. First responder, EMT-B (basic), EMT-I (intermediate), and EMT-P (paramedic) are the four levels of prehospital emergency responders recognized by the National Registry of Emergency Medical Technicians (NREMT).

4. c. In 1978, doctor Jeff Clawson introduced EMD, a system that involves prearrival instructions and dispatch according to medical priority protocols.

5. b. EMD is emergency medical dispatch, and a dental technician is not part of ED staff. These are examples of health care professions or allied health personnel.

6. b. In nonmedical workplace sites, the first responder is typically the first trained person to arrive at a patient's side to provide care for an acute illness or injury. Nurses are common in the workplace, although it is not as common to staff a nurse 24/7 or have the nurse leave an office to response at the site of a workplace accident.

7. a. Additional examples of advocating for your patients are protecting their confidentiality and not allowing your personal biases to affect patient care.

8. d. A deficit in color vision would not hinder one's ability to take an EMT-B certifying exam, maintain emergency equipment, or keep good documentation. However, color recognition is important to the emergency vehicle operator.

9. a. Activating EMS is typically done by the public; issuing standing orders is done by a physician;

registering with NAEMT is an option, not a responsibility.

10. c. Honesty, integrity, and sympathy are all great traits for persons employed in the field of emergency medicine (as well as for life in general), but each has a slightly different meaning.

11. c. When responding to any scene, the number one priority is your personal safety and the safety of your crew.

12. b. Personal safety includes maintaining good health. The components of good health or wellness are proper nutrition and keeping mentally and physically fit. This includes keeping immunizations up to date.

13. d. Recognizing potential or actual dangers and hazards at the scene is paramount for the EMT-B, yet identifying every single one at every scene is not possible for anyone.

14. b. The issuance of certification or licensure based on prior training in another state is referred to as *reciprocity*.

15. d. Placing the needs of your patients, including protecting their personal belongings while patients are in your care, is an example of patient advocacy.

16. a. The process called *continuous quality improvement* is designed to uncover problems through the practice of reviewing and auditing, and to provide solutions to those problems within an EMS system.

17. a. *Protocols* are guidelines for the management of specific patient problems.

18. a. Training is one of the areas that continuous quality improvement recognizes as a source of potential problems and an area that can be improved.

19. b. The primary role of the medical director is to ensure quality patient care.

20. c. Written protocols are also referred to as *offline* or *indirect medical control*.

21. b. *Online* or *direct medical control* is the ability to obtain real-time direction and orders.

22. c. A medical director of an EMS agency has authority over patient care, and the EMS provider in that agency is acting as a designated agent or an extension of the physician.

23. d. The PCR contains patient information and administrative information such as patient demographics, run times, and dispatch information.

24. d. Local, regional, and state authorities can authorize the policies and procedures used by an EMS system.

25. d. PHTLS is a 16-hour course and is not a state EMT-B certifying exam.

Chapter 2: Well-Being of the EMT-B

1. d. Avoiding and/or relieving the effects of chronic stress can be accomplished through numerous methods.

2. a. Talking with crew members enables emergency personnel to vent feelings and facilitates an understanding of stressful situations.

3. a. The stress generated by involvement in trauma, death, disaster, and crime scenes can cause delayed stress reactions for the EMT-B. This stress commonly leads to burnout.

4. c. Many medical emergencies call for the EMT-B to provide supportive care for the family members on the scene or at the hospital. This is especially true when death or near-death is a likely outcome. Supportive care includes listening and answering questions as best as you can without providing false hope.

5. d. The stages of the grieving process are: shock, denial, anger, bargaining, depression, and acceptance. As EMTs, you and your co-workers, as well as terminal patients and their family members, may experience grief from death and dying. The EMT-B is expected to be able to recognize the stages of grieving and allow those experiencing grief to express their feelings.

6. c. Denial is a defense mechanism. It is the inability or refusal to believe the reality of the event and is part of the normal grieving process.

7. b. When family or caretakers are inconsolable despite efforts to explain the reality of the current situation, the EMT-B must see this as part of the grieving process and provide some form of support. Getting the patient out of sight in the ambulance allows some people a brief opportunity to begin to realize what is happening. This is a form of support.

8. a. *Acceptance* is the realization of fate and obtaining a reasonable level of comfort with the anticipated outcome or loss.

9. c. Many terminally ill patients experience the stages of the grieving process. Until you talk to them, you will not be able to know which stage they are experiencing. The approach to take with any terminally ill patient is to make her as comfortable as possible, maintain her dignity, and show respect at all times.

10. d. Your family's unhappiness typically adds to the stress in your life. Addressing these concerns is important and should not be ignored.

11. b. Getting a call near the end of the shift and not getting out on time is the nature of this stressful business. Although it is not always possible, you should avoid scheduling anything close to the end of a shift. This is one way to avoid placing additional stress on yourself, your friends, and your family.

12. d. An unhappy spouse is another stress factor; this unhappiness should be addressed promptly to avoid more serious stress reactions and, ultimately, burnout.

13. d. The stress experienced during a critical incident and the effects from the incident will be different for each EMT-B. The way a person handles stress is directly affected by previous exposures to stress and the coping mechanisms that person has developed.

14. c. The symptoms described are indications of excessive stress.

15. a. Fatigue is a common indication of excessive stress and occurs in part as a result of lack of sleep. Getting plenty of rest is one technique for reducing stress.

16. b. Self-medication may include the use of alcohol, drugs, or a combination. It may be dangerous and is not a recommended technique for reducing stress.

17. a. Examples of environmental stress related to EMS include siren noise, inclement weather, confined workspaces, rapid scene response, and life-and-death decision making.

18. d. Physical conditioning improves brain function, metabolism, personal appearance, and self-image. The more physically fit a person is, the better equipped she is to handle stress.

19. b. The EMT-B must think safety first. When 9-1-1 is activated in the middle of the night, it would be normal and expected for a light to be turned on at the caller's residence. No lights could mean that the caller is blind or unable to turn the lights on, but it could also mean that a crime has occurred or is still in progress.

20. c. Think safety first. Have dispatch send the police, if they are not there already. Do not turn your back on the patient. Keep an exit open and guarded by a crew member. Be prepared to leave quickly.

21. b. An icy walkway can be managed easily with rock salt. The fire department will stabilize a vehicle that is leaking fuel, and the police are needed to handle violence and other crime scenes.

22. d. BSI is a method of protecting against disease transmission by pathogens in blood or other body fluids.

23. c. Handwashing after every patient contact and after each call is the responsibility of the individual EMT-B and every health care provider.

24. a. Once an exposure has been reported, it is the employer's responsibility to arrange for you to be evaluated by a health care professional as soon as possible. The agency's exposure control plan includes having this policy in writing, and it must be available for the employee to review and understand.

25. c. Hepatitis is a bloodborne pathogen and staph is transmitted by direct contact or touch.

26. d. The immunizations currently recommended for the EMT-B are: chickenpox, hepatitis B, influenza, Lyme disease, measles, mumps, polio, rubella, tetanus, and diphtheria. After September 11, 2001, many military personal were required to get the smallpox immunization. Smallpox immunization for the general public is available but is not strongly recommended.

27. a. For geographical locations with higher-than-average numbers of known TB cases, screening is recommended twice a year.

28. b. At a minimum, gloves should be considered for any patient contact. The more information you have about the patient, the more PPE you may find necessary.

29. b. The current recommendations for the use of PPE for bacterial meningitis with a transmission mode of oral and nasal secretions are to wear gloves and a surgical mask, followed by handwashing after patient contact.

30. b. The current recommendations for the use of PPE for whooping cough with a transmission mode of respiratory secretions and airborne droplets are to wear gloves and a surgical mask, followed by handwashing after patient contact.

31. a. The EMT-B's primary responsibility is personal safety. Even when working at a scene with an established safety officer, police officer, or EMS supervisor, the EMT-B must make her own safety the top priority.

32. d. It is one of the EMT-B's responsibilities to attempt to keep bystanders from becoming victims at a scene with hazards.

33. b. Preventing exposure of another ill or injured patient, yourself, or a crew member is the reason for properly cleaning and decontaminating equipment as soon as possible.

34. d. Dressing the part of a professional is important, but many agencies have a policy on uniforms that leaves little choice. Routinely demonstrating good sense in taking protective measures against infectious disease is a great trait for a coach or mentor.

35. c. Talking about using PPE is one thing, but actually having the students put it on is better, especially during initial training.

Chapter 3: Medical, Legal, and Ethical Issues

1. c. State law identifies the actions and care that the EMT-B is legally permitted to perform.

2. a. When documenting, the EMT-B should always try to use objective language and not make judgments.

3. d. The driver of an emergency vehicle must exercise *due regard,* which means that "a reasonably careful person performing similar duties and under the same circumstances would act in the same manner."

4. a. EMT-B certification or licensure is granted by the state. Reciprocity can occur for certification or licensure, and is typically granted based on the type of training and/or experience the applicant has.

5. b. The DNR is signed by a patient and his physician. When a patient is not capable of signing, his legal custodian can sign for him.

6. b. Advance directives, such as a DNR or living will, are legal documents that contain instructions on treatment and the patient's wishes and are drawn up before an event to which they would apply has occurred.

7. d. A durable power of attorney or health care proxy allows a person to designate an agent to act when the person is unable to make decisions himself.

8. c. A *living will* is a document that states the type of life-saving medical treatment a patient wants or does not want to be used in case of terminal illness, coma, or persistent vegetative state. These decisions are typically made in the hospital setting.

9. c. For patients of legal age or emancipated minors who are able to make reasoned decisions, the EMT-B must obtain consent to treat, either verbally (most often the case), nonverbally, or in writing. That same patient can revoke consent at any time.

10. d. There are many acceptable ways to ask for consent.

11. a. When an adult patient with severe mental disability requires life-saving treatment, implied consent is

the rule. When the problem is not life-threatening, consent must be obtained from the patient's guardian.

12. c. For patients of legal age or emancipated minors who are able to make reasoned decisions, the EMT-B must obtain express consent.

13. b. Implied consent, also called the *emergency doctrine,* is the type of consent that remains in effect for as long as the patient requires life-saving treatment.

14. d. The emergency doctrine, also called *implied consent,* is the type of consent that remains in effect for as long as the patient requires life-saving treatment.

15. b. Implied consent, also called the *emergency doctrine,* is the type of consent that remains in effect for as long as the patient requires life-saving treatment.

16. c. A person makes a threat or gesture of suicide to ask for help rather than die. Any patient who has expressed the intent to harm himself needs help and must be transported for a psychological evaluation.

17. a. A pediatric patient who is experiencing a life-threatening condition with no parent present is treated under implied consent.

18. d. A minor who is married, pregnant, or a parent, and living on his or her own; or who is in the armed forces, is considered emancipated and can legally give consent for or refuse care. The definition of emancipated minor varies by state. Be familiar with your state's definition of an emancipated minor.

19. b. A minor who is married, pregnant, or a parent, and living on his or her own; or who is in the armed forces, is considered emancipated. The definition of emancipated minor varies by state. Be familiar with your state's definition of an emancipated minor.

20. a. Consent to treat a minor must be obtained from a parent or legal guardian, unless the illness or injury is life-threatening, in which case consent is implied.

21. d. A competent adult may refuse care or any part of care. The EMT-B should explain the possible dangers associated with refusing, carefully document the refusal, and have the patient sign the refusal.

22. d. A minor cannot legally refuse treatment for a life-threatening injury. Treatment for a non-life-threatening injury requires the consent or refusal of a parent or legal guardian.

23. c. There are specific conditions that preclude a patient from refusing care (e.g., mentally incompetent adult, minor, an unresponsive patient, a patient with an altered mental status).

24. b. When a competent adult refuses care or transport and you feel this may cause further harm, consider trying to get a family member or friend to stay with him or transport him.

25. c. A competent adult may refuse care or any part of care. The EMT-B should explain the possible dangers associated with refusing, carefully document the refusal, and have the patient sign the refusal.

26. a. *Negligence* is deviation from the accepted standard of care (typically as a result of carelessness or inattentiveness).

27. c. Once a patient–provider relationship has been established, the EMT-B must stay with the patient until that patient can be turned over to another health care provider with an equal or higher level of training.

28. a. The EMT-B was assaulted. Some states or jurisdictions have made it a serious crime to assault or strike an EMS provider while he is in the course of his duties.

29. a. Transporting a patient without permission or detaining a patient without his consent or legal authority is considered false imprisonment or kidnapping. This is one of the reasons why it is so important to get consent before taking a patient to the hospital.

30. a. Touching a competent adult patient without consent may be considered assault or battery.

31. b. A duty to act is a legal responsibility to provide service to the patient. The EMT-B's first priority is personal safety, and he may delay action if there is a safety issue.

32. d. When you are off duty or out of your jurisdiction, your ability to practice may be limited by the lack of medical control. The safest approach when faced with a life-threatening medical emergency or injury outside your medical control region is to limit your care to life-saving BLS treatment as a first responder.

33. d. The EMT-B's legal and primary responsibilities concern patients, the public, and the agency's medical director.

34. c. State and local laws do vary as to "duty to act." For example, in some states the EMT-B must stop to assist an ill or injured person even when the EMT-B is not on duty.

35. a. To maintain the patient–EMS provider relationship, information about the patient's history, the assessment findings, and treatment rendered must remain confidential.

36. c. The release of patient information requires written permission from the patient or the patient's legal guardian.

37. b. *Slander* is an act in which a person's character or reputation is injured by the false or malicious spoken words of another person, such as when spreading rumors.

38. b. The law in each state requires mandatory child abuse reporting. The method of reporting and to whom the suspected abuse is reported varies from state to state.

39. a. The EMS provider has an ethical, but not legal, responsibility to resuscitate any potential organ donor so that others may benefit from the organs.

40. d. The EMT-B can identify a potential organ donor by an organ donor card, by a signature or sticker on a

driver's license indicating such, and/or by a family member providing the information.

41. c. A potential organ donor should be treated the same as any other patient requiring emergency care. In addition, the EMT-B should contact medical control and advise of the potential for organ donation.

42. a. A potential organ donor should be treated the same as any other patient requiring emergency care. In addition, the EMT-B should contact medical control and advise of the potential for organ donation.

43. a. The knot is evidence and should not be untied or even handled, if possible. The correct approach is to make a clean cut with a sharp knife at least 6 inches from the knot.

44. a. The body should be left in the position found. Many EMS and police agencies require that an EKG be obtained, and this can be done without moving the patient.

45. c. The EMT-B must not allow the victim to remove any clothing or bathe, and (if possible) not to use the bathroom. The ED will use a rape kit to obtain evidence samples from the victim's body and clothing.

46. d. As with any documentation, only objective information should be included. Your suspicions are subjective and should not be included in documentation.

47. b. Animal bites; abuse, and injuries as a result of a crime are all examples of calls that are typically reportable in most states.

48. a. Most states make it mandatory for the EMT-B to report violent crimes such as rape and abuse. Failure to do so may result in criminal charges and/or disciplinary action against the EMT-B.

49. b. Patient care comes first. Advising the ED of your suspicions right away and not waiting is appropriate, though. Documentation should include only objective information.

50. c. Assault and battery is a criminal offense.

Chapter 4: The Human Body

1. c. In the anatomical position, the body is standing erect, facing forward, with arms down and palms facing forward.

2. a. *Plane* is the surface of an object split down the middle.

3. a. The cervical spine is comprised of 7 vertebrae; the thoracic has 12, the lumbar has 5, the sacrum has 5, and the coccyx has 3 to 5 fused.

4. b. *Bilateral* refers to two sides; *proximal* means close to; *superior* is above.

5. c. *Supine* means lying on the back; *prone* means lying face down; *lateral* means the side; *anatomical* position is standing facing forward.

6. c. The quadrants of the abdomen are named for the location on the body: upper left and right, and lower left and right.

7. c. The esophagus lies directly in the midline of the body. The stomach is in the ULQ, the heart is near the midline, and the large intestine lies in all four quadrants of the abdomen.

8. b. *Midshaft* describes the location of the middle of a long bone.

9. d. Mid-axillary describes the location under the armpit (axilla) and the vertical middle line. The two vertical lines on either side of the mid-axillary line are the anterior-axillary and posterior-axillary lines.

10. c. The cervical spine is located in the posterior (back) of the neck.

11. d. The pharynx is the cavity or space just in back of the mouth into which the nostrils, esophagus, and trachea open. The glottis is a slit-like opening between the vocal cords. The nares are the openings of the nose, and sinuses are any of several cavities in the skull.

12. a. The larynx, located in the upper part of the trachea, contains the vocal cords.

13. d. The epiglottis is a thin plate of flexible tissue that protects (covers) the airway during swallowing.

14. a. Alveoli are small sacs in the lungs. During inspiration, they fill with air; a gas exchange between oxygen and carbon dioxide then takes place within the pulmonary capillaries, and carbon dioxide is released during exhalation.

15. b. The end expiratory pressure in the lungs is negative.

16. c. The primary muscles used for breathing are the diaphragm, a sheet of muscle between the chest and abdominal cavities, and the intercostal muscles, the muscles between the ribs.

17. d. The prefix *pneumo* is used for terms relating to air, breathing, and the lungs.

18. c. During inhalation, the diaphragm and the intercostals contract. The diaphragm also moves downward.

19. d. The lungs adhere to the chest wall with a tension surface created by serous fluid, similar to the way two sheets of glass would stick together if a few drops of water were trapped between them.

20. a. The respiratory system is comprised of the organs that are responsible for gas exchange. Oxygen moves into the cells and carbon dioxide moves out.

21. b. Heart sounds are created by the opening and closing of heart valves, which occurs with contraction and relaxation of the heart muscle.

22. a. The throbbing sensation, or *pulse,* that can be felt in the arteries is caused by contraction of the heart.

23. b. Blood returns to the heart by way of the vena cava, the largest vein in the body. The superior vena cava receives blood from the upper body and the inferior vena cava receives blood from the lower body.

24. b. Blood flows into the heart by passing through the tricuspid valves, then through the pulmonary valve into the lungs, and then out of the heart by way of the bicuspid and aortic valves.

25. c. The pulmonary artery carries blood from the right ventricle to the lungs. It is the only artery that carries deoxygenated blood.

26. d. Plasma contains serum, the fluid portion of blood that contains minerals, salts, and proteins.

27. c. At birth, both ventricles are about the same size. As an infant matures, the left ventricle becomes larger and more muscular.

28. b. The coronary arteries supply the heart with blood. The pulmonary arteries supply the lungs, the carotid arteries supply the brain and head, and the superior vena cava is a vein.

29. c. The peripheral or distal circulation supplies the extremities with blood.

30. a. *Infarct* and *necrosis* both mean dead tissue.

31. d. When working properly, the pulmonic valve should prevent any backflow of blood from the pulmonary artery back into the right ventricle.

32. a. The tibial pulse is felt in the back of the lower leg. The femoral pulse can be palpated on the upper inside thigh, the dorsalis pedis on the top of the foot, and the brachial pulse in the inside upper arm.

33. a. Deoxygenated blood is returned to the heart by veins.

34. b. An *embolism* is an obstruction in a blood vessel caused by a blood clot or other substance. *Varicose* describes a swollen vein, *edema* is an abnormal accumulation of fluid, and *palpation* is touching.

35. d. Special cells in the heart muscle generate electrical impulses that are transmitted (conducted) through the heart to stimulate contractions. This electrical activity can be seen on an electrocardiogram or ECG.

36. a. Bones, cartilage, ligaments, and tendons are all forms of connective tissue. Bones are different from other connective tissues in that they are hardened by calcium.

37. b. Cartilage allows smooth movement at the joints.

38. c. An uncomplicated fracture of the tibia, fibula, or humerus can result in a blood loss of 500 mL over the first two hours, whereas a femur fracture can cause a 1,000-mL loss.

39. b. A sprain is a sudden and sometimes severe twisting of a joint with stretching or tearing of ligaments.

40. a. A knee dislocation can completely disrupt the blood supply to the lower leg when the tibia is displaced to the posterior, compressing the posterior tibial artery. The elbow, when dislocated, can threaten the brachial artery and blood supply to the arm.

41. b. All ribs attach to the spine in the back. In the front, pairs 1 through 10 attach to the sternum with cartilage, but the last two pairs do not articulate with anything. This makes it difficult to fracture these ribs; however, they can cause serious injury to the underlying organs of the upper abdominal quadrants (e.g., lungs, liver, and spleen).

42. d. *Masticate* means to chew; a *machete* is a large knife; *crunch* could be the noise of a bone fracturing (though it is not a medical term). *Crepitation* is the term for broken bone ends rubbing against each other.

43. d. Smooth muscle is found in the lower airways, blood vessels, and intestines. Smooth muscle can relax or contract to alter the inner lumen diameter of the vessels.

44. d. The ilium, pubis, and ischium are parts of the pelvis and the acetabulum is the socket on the external surface of the pelvis that receives the head of the femur.

45. b. The three divisions of the sternum from top to bottom are the manubrium, sternum, and xiphoid process.

46. c. A heart attack occurs when heart muscle dies from lack of oxygenation. Stroke, seizure, and spinal cord injury (SCI) occur as a result of an event affecting the brain, spinal cord, or both.

47. d. The CNS includes the brain, brain stem, and spinal cord. The peripheral nervous system (PNS) includes everything outside of the CNS.

48. d. The release of hormones into the blood is influenced by the autonomic nervous system (ANS).

49. d. The nervous system is subdivided into voluntary and involuntary. The autonomic nervous system manages the involuntary nervous system and glands and is further subdivided into the sympathetic and parasympathetic nervous systems.

50. b. Sensory nerves carry impulses from the brain to the body and from the body back to the brain. Specifically, afferent neurons carry impulses from the body to the brain and efferent neurons carry impulses from the brain to the body.

51. a. The autonomic nervous system manages the involuntary nervous system and glands and is further subdivided into the sympathetic and parasympathetic nervous systems. When the sympathetic nervous system is stimulated, the heart rate increases.

52. a. Skin is an organ that covers the entire body. It is the largest organ of the human body and accounts for about 15 percent of body weight.

53. a. The second layer of skin, the dermis, contains blood vessels, sensory nerves, sweat glands, oil glands, and hair follicles.

54. d. The subcutaneous layer is the third layer of skin. It contains fat, soft tissue, blood vessels, and nerves. The thickness varies on different parts of the body.

55. c. The epidermis contains four layers, except for the palms of the hands and the soles of the feet where the epidermis is thicker.

56. c. The endocrine system produces secretions (hormones) that are released and distributed by way of the bloodstream.

57. b. The pancreas produces insulin; the adrenal glands produce epinephrine and norepinephrine; the thyroid releases hormones that regulate metabolism, growth, and development; gonads produce hormones for reproduction and sex attributes.

58. a. The ovaries and testes (or gonads) collectively produce sex attributes and reproductive hormones.

59. b. Diabetes mellitus is a chronic disease of the endocrine system. The number of people affected by this disease is growing in alarming numbers each year and so are the EMS calls related to diabetic emergencies.

60. a. Kidneys do not produce or release hormones. The pituitary is the master gland, the thymus produces hormones that help in the development of the immune system, and the adrenal glands produce epinephrine and norepinephrine.

Chapter 5: Baseline Vital Signs and SAMPLE History

1. d. Look (sight), listen (hearing), and feel (touch). All these senses are used to assess a patient's vital signs.

2. b. Temperature is often referred as the fourth vital sign. It is an especially important vital sign in children and the elderly. ECG and pulse oximetry readings are diagnostics rather than vital signs.

3. c. Infants use their abdominal muscles for breathing because their chest wall muscles are immature. Watching the belly rise and fall is an easy way to obtain the breathing rate of an infant without touching or disturbing the child.

4. b. Counting the respiratory rate while palpating a pulse is common method for obtaining an unguarded breathing rate.

5. d. The terms *rate, quality,* and *effort* are used to describe a patient's breathing and also are used in documentation and to give report to other health care providers.

6. a. *Labored, shallow,* and *absent* are terms commonly associated with description of a patient's respiratory effort.

7. a. *Retractions* is a term associated with the accessory muscles of breathing. It is used to describe the increased physical work of breathing, rather than the sound of noisy breathing.

8. d. *Severe respiratory distress* is defined as increased work of breathing with signs of inadequate oxygenation. Any of the conditions described in the other answers, combined with labored breathing, indicates severe respiratory distress.

9. d. A sustained rapid heart rate with signs of shock (e.g., moist and pale skin) is a serious finding. A slow heart rate in a nondistressed, healthy person is a normal finding. A rate of 160 for a crying newborn is normal, as is a slightly elevated heart rate in a toddler with a fever.

10. c. Palpating the umbilical stump is the quickest and easiest method for obtaining a pulse in the newly born. The pulse should be obtained at 1 and 5 minutes after birth as part of the APGAR score used for assessing the newly born.

11. c. The radial pulse on any patient is palpated distally on the lateral (thumb) side of the forearm.

12. c. The loss of distal pulses in a pediatric patient is a finding associated with poor perfusion or cold temperatures. When the ambient temperature is warm, consider poor perfusion and look for other findings associated with poor perfusion, such as decreased mental status, bradycardia, and respiratory failure.

13. d. The apical (apex or point of the heart) pulse is typically auscultated on the chest over the heart. In some patients, especially newborns and infants, the apical pulse may be palpated.

14. b. An irregular pulse should be assessed for one full minute to obtain an accurate rate. An irregular pulse does not necessarily indicate shock, and an irregular pulse will be the same on both sides. The term *pulse deficit* is associated with an ECG showing an electrical rate that is faster than the pulse rate.

15. a. Flushed skin is caused by vasodilation, jaundice or yellow skin is associated with liver dysfunction, and blood vessel constriction causes skin to become pale and cool rather than hot.

16. d. D-CAP-BTLS stands for deformity, contusion, abrasion, puncture/penetration, burn, tenderness, laceration, and swelling. These are all possible findings associated with the skin. The SAMPLE and OPQRST mnemonics are used for obtaining a focused history and information about pain, respectively. HAZMAT is an abbreviation of *hazardous materials.*

17. c. Evaluation of skin CTC is a direct measure of a patient's circulatory status.

18. a. Pressing on the skin or nail bed will initially cause it to blanch; it should return to normal color within 2 seconds after release of pressure. A capillary refill time of more than 2 seconds is considered abnormal.

19. b. Deoxygenated blood and tissues will appear cyanotic (bluish). Flushed, hot, and clammy are terms associated with vasodilation, and jaundice (yellowing) is associated with liver dysfunction.

20. b. Jaundice is typically seen first in the eyes, where normally they are white. Later, yellowing can be seen in the skin and nail beds.

21. a. An extremity that is red and hot to the touch suggests a local infection. Diabetics are prone to poor distal circulation and vascular disease, which puts them at increased risk for wounds, ulcers, and infections in the lower extremities.

22. d. Persons who are experiencing a new onset of fever are most likely to feel hot, and they could feel dry or moist if they have been sweating. Cool and clammy or cold and moist indicate poor perfusion, whereas warm and pink is normal.

23. b. The longer an extremity has had impaired circulation, the cooler you can expect it to feel.

24. d. Newly developed deep frostbite will cause severely impaired blood flow to the affected area. You can expect the skin to look white or waxy and feel cold and hard to the touch. Discolorations, including black, come later on.

25. a. Severe anaphylactic reaction is shock. The skin CTC will be pale, cool, and moist.

26. b. Infants have great circulation, so, in the absence of cool or cold ambient temperatures, a capillary refill time of more than 2 seconds is considered an abnormal finding, suggesting a problem with perfusion.

27. a. Infants have great circulation; this is why skin signs, including capillary refill, are very reliable assessment findings.

28. c. Shading both eyes from the ambient light will allow the pupils to dilate in response to the darkness. This is an appropriate method for stimulating a pupillary reaction.

29. a. The size of the pupil is measured in millimeters. Many pocket guides and references include a scale to help measure the exact pupil size in millimeters.

30. a. One of the normal responses of the pupils is to dilate or constrict simultaneously, even if a stimulus is given to only one. This is called the *sympathetic response*.

31. b. In bright ambient light, the optic nerve will constrict the pupils to minimize the amount of light allowed into the eyes.

32. a. A small percentage of the population has unequal pupils as a normal status. Before making any treatment decisions based on abnormal physical findings, remember to first ask the patient if this is normal for her.

33. b. It is very common for elderly patients to fall when they are suffering the effects of a stroke. The fall combined with a new onset of unequal pupils makes the possibility of stroke one of the first things to consider with this patient. Head injury, infection, and medication problems are other possibilities.

34. d. A concussion, fright, and pink eye do not cause a nonreactive response to light. A blinded eye or an artificial eye would have a nonreactive response to light. Remember to first ask the patient if this is normal for him.

35. d. Obtaining an accurate blood pressure with both systolic and diastolic readings is always preferred, in order to establish trends and make good treatment decisions. When this cannot be accomplished because of loud ambient noise, it is reasonable to take a blood pressure by palpation.

36. a. The diastolic reading is the last sound heard. Cardiac output is determined by heart rate times stroke volume, and stroke volume cannot be measured in the prehospital setting.

37. a. The systolic blood pressure is the pressure created within the walls of the arteries when the ventricles (predominately the left) of the heart contract and eject blood out through the aorta.

38. b. The systolic blood pressure is the pressure created within the walls of the arteries when the ventricles (predominately the left) of the heart contract and eject blood out through the aorta.

39. c. The diastolic blood pressure is the pressure created within the walls of the arteries when the ventricles (predominately the left) of the heart are refilling with blood.

40. d. Mercury/glass sphygmomanometers are antiquated now, but the unit of measure mm Hg (millimeters of mercury) is still used today with electronic and tympanic BP devices.

41. a. A blood pressure can be taken in other locations on the body (e.g., calf).

42. a. A blood pressure obtained by auscultation is more accurate and no more difficult than obtaining the BP by palpation.

43. d. The "E" in SAMPLE is a reminder to inquire about the events leading up to the current call for 9-1-1.

44. d. When it is not possible to get a reliable SAMPLE history from the patient, the EMT-B should attempt to obtain one from family, a caretaker, the patient's personal physician, or anyone else who may have knowledge of the patient's medical history.

45. b. A *symptom* is something the patient tells you about and a *sign* is a finding you detect.

46. b. A *symptom* is something the patient tells you about and a *sign* is a finding you detect.

47. d. *Trending* is the process of obtaining a baseline assessment, repeating the assessment multiple times, and using the information to determine whether the patient is getting better, worse, or not changing. Trending is an important tool in patient care.

48. c. Time and manpower permitting, vital signs should be obtained every 5 minutes on an unstable patient and every 15 minutes on a stable patient.

49. b. In many cases, patients are told to place the Vial of Life in the refrigerator for EMS and other health care professionals (home health aides or nurses) to use as needed.

50. d. The EMT-B often has a unique perspective in that he can see the way a patient lives at home. When there is evidence that a person is not able to adequately manage activities of daily living, whether due to a condition of new onset or a deterioration of a chronic problem, the EMT-B has an ethical obligation to report this information to the ED. Some communities have services that the EMT-B can refer to the patient to in an effort to help improve home living conditions.

Chapter 6: Lifting and Moving Patients

1. a. In an effort to avoid injury, the principles and practices of safe and proper lifting techniques should be practiced every day, on the job or off.

2. b. *Supination* means to turn or move to a face-up position; *proprioception* is the body's awareness of itself in respect to its surroundings; *hydraulics* refers to practical applications of liquid in motion.

3. a. Keeping the back straight and locked with lifting is an example of good body mechanics.

4. b. Keeping the weight close to the body is another example of good body mechanics.

5. a. The higher the center of gravity, the easier it becomes to tip the load.

6. b. The four-person lift is not always possible or necessary, and therefore is not commonly used. The lift-in stretcher with one EMT-B on each side is still utilized with older model stretchers, but is not common anymore. Today, numerous roll-in-type stretchers are available and used to help reduce the risk of back injury.

7. d. The age and weight of a patient are important factors in considering which type of carrying device to use, but a suspected spinal injury is the most critical factor. A carrying device with spinal immobilization is needed to protect a patient from further spinal injury.

8. c. Patients who are apneic, pulseless, or have a suspected spinal injury should be moved with a long backboard. A patient contaminated with hazardous materials can ambulate if possible, or will be carried on a long backboard through a decontamination area.

9. b. Another example of good body mechanics is to avoid leaning to the opposite side when carrying an object with one hand.

10. c. The actions in each of the other answers require two hands to perform.

11. c. Securing a patient to a carrying device before moving her up or down stairs significantly helps to reduce the risk of injury to both rescuers and patient.

12. c. Most basements have a stairway access. Using a stair chair for a conscious patient is ideal for this type of move. Moving a patient on stairs using a reeves, stretcher, or long backboard may cause the patient to slide on the device, creating stress for the patient and possible injury to the rescuers who must compensate for the slippage.

13. d. Twisting while lifting, reaching, or moving is dangerous and is never recommended.

14. a. Keeping the load close to the body when reaching and lifting is an example of good body mechanics.

15. d. When reaching is necessary, keep the back straight and locked, the distance to reach short, and the time spent reaching very short.

16. c. When reaching is necessary, keep the back straight and locked, the distance to reach short, and the time spent reaching very short.

17. c. Good body mechanics for lifting include keeping the weight of the load close to the body.

18. a. Pulling or pushing anything while reaching overhead is dangerous and is not an example of good body mechanics.

19. b. *Urgent* and *nonurgent* are the two terms typically used to describe moves carried out by the EMT-B. A patient with a rapidly deteriorating condition would warrant an urgent move.

20. d. In the absence of a suspected spinal injury, most EMT-Bs will allow the patient to assume a position of comfort.

21. a. *Urgent* and *nonurgent* are the two terms typically used to describe moves carried out by the EMT-B. A patient who is at risk or has a rapidly deteriorating condition would warrant an urgent move.

22. c. Rapidly moving this patient out of the hot environment is appropriate management. A seizing patient lying on the floor, an entrapped patient in a stable vehicle with a non-life-threatening injury, and an infant crying in a car seat are all relatively safe and do not require urgent moves.

23. d. The question describes a device called a *flexible* or *Reeves* stretcher.

24. b. The question describes a scoop stretcher.

25. b. The logroll, basket stretcher, and short spine board can be employed without causing further injury to a patient with a suspected spinal injury.

Chapter 7: Airway

1. c. The carina, bronchi, and bronchioles are part of the lower airways.

2. d. The epiglottis is a cartilage flap, the diaphragm is a large muscle that separates the chest and abdomen, and alveoli sacs are located inside the lungs.

3. a. Oxygenated blood from the lungs returns to the heart by way of the left atrium; from there it is pumped into the left ventricle and out into the body.

4. c. The carina and bronchi are well down into the lower airway. The diaphragm is a muscle of breathing located between the abdomen and chest cavities, and is not part of the airway.

5. c. Prolonged exhalations are associated with air trapping (as seen in patients with chronic lung disease) and grunting is an abnormal sound that occurs primarily in infants and small toddlers when the child breathes out against a partially closed epiglottis. Grunting is usually a sign of respiratory distress.

6. d. The EMT-B will assess by looking for signs of distress such as the use of accessory muscles to breathe, irregular breathing patterns, and poor skin color. Then he will listen for audible abnormal breath sounds, auscultate the lungs, and feel for skin temperature and abnormal chest wall movement.

7. d. The pulse oximeter tool is not reliable for every patient in every situation. Look at the patient too. Slow deep and snoring respirations are normal during sleep.

8. b. Follow the ABCs: make sure the airway is open and will remain open, then assess breathing and circulation. With a conscious patient, this usually means just watching to see that the patient is able to maintain his own airway.

9. b. COPD is chronic lung disease, epistaxis is a nosebleed, and diaphoresis is sweating.

10. a. Position the head and open the airway with a chin lift. It is fast, easy, and noninvasive.

11. b. If an unresponsive patient is not supine initially, place him in this position as soon as possible to prevent him from falling. The patient can be moved to a long backboard afterward. If the patient is maintaining his airway, then the recovery position is appropriate. A prone or face-down position is not appropriate. The patient may suffocate and you will not be able to fully assess him.

12. d. The head-tilt chin-lift maneuver is not appropriate for a patient with a suspected cervical injury. Use the jaw-thrust maneuver instead.

13. c. Open the airway using the head-tilt chin-lift maneuver to assess the airway and listen for breathing.

14. a. For the patient with a suspected head injury, cervical injury must be suspected as well. Maintain manual stabilization of the spine and use the jaw-thrust maneuver to open the airway.

15. d. Cervical stabilization must be maintained until the patient is immobilized on a long backboard. The jaw-thrust maneuver should be used to open and maintain the airway. If the patient loses his gag reflex, an oropharyngeal airway (OPA) should be inserted.

16. d. The jaw-thrust maneuver is a technique used to jut the jaw forward without moving the cervical spine. This is accomplished by the EMT-B placing his fingers on the angle of the patient's jaw just below the ears and pushing the lower jawbone forward.

17. c. The jaw-thrust maneuver is a technique used to jut the jaw forward without moving the cervical spine.

18. d. By placing both elbows on the same surface as the patient's head, the EMT-B can stabilize the cervical spine while opening the airway.

19. c. Rigid-tip catheters are not designed to remove large objects such as chunks of food, teeth, or foreign bodies.

20. d. Aspiration is detrimental for any patient. Aspiration causes an immediate problem by creating an airway obstruction and later by causing respiratory infection, permanent lung tissue damage, and in some cases death.

21. a. A rigid-tip catheter is easy to manipulate within the upper airway. The soft-tip or French catheters are better for endotracheal suctioning.

22. c. To avoid depleting a patient of the residual tidal volume, suctioning should be performed after inserting the catheter and while the catheter is being drawn out. Suction for no more than 15 seconds at a time.

23. d. Suctioning is a messy procedure that carries a high risk of exposure for the EMT-B. At a minimum, anyone who is near the airway while suctioning is being performed should be wearing gloves, eye protection, and a mask.

24. a. Oxygen delivery is stopped during suctioning. The patient should be suctioned for no more than 15 seconds at a time.

25. a. A good mask seal covers both the nose and the mouth of the patient.

26. c. The rescuer needs to be able to see the patient's airway to observe for vomitus, blood, or other secretions to prevent possible aspiration.

27. b. An adult BVM can deliver approximately 1,200 mL of air when fully squeezed with two hands. Blowing through a face mask, an adult could deliver a larger volume if needed.

28. a. The recommendation for ventilating a child is to deliver each ventilation over 1 to 1½ seconds without an oxygen source.

29. b. To avoid any movement of the cervical spine while ventilating a patient with a BVM, one rescuer should ventilate and one rescuer should maintain stabilization of the head and neck.

30. a. The jaw-thrust maneuver is used on patients with suspected or actual cervical injury.

31. c. Using a BVM requires two hands and often two rescuers. BVMs are disposable and do not require cleaning. Larger volumes of air can be provided through a pocket face mask.

32. c. BVMs are available in adult, child, infant, and premature neonate sizes.

33. a. Nasal prongs are part of the nasal cannula.

34. c. Obtaining a proper mask seal often takes two hands.

35. a. Hyperventilation is no longer recommended. The patient should be hyperoxygenated with ventilations provided once every 5 seconds and the BVM connected to a high-flow oxygen source.

36. d. Before providing ventilations, the airway should be suctioned and an airway adjunct inserted as needed.

37. a. Improved skin color is a sign of improved oxygenation. Rapid breathing, patient resistance, or air movement out of the mouth and nose do not indicate anything about the adequacy of the ventilations.

38. d. Each of the answers is a sign or indication that the ventilations being provided are adequate.

39. c. Auscultating lung sounds during ventilations is the most reliable method of assuring that ventilations are adequate. Pulse oximetry readings can be unreliable and the filling of the reservoir bag only means that the bag is full. Good compliance during squeezing is one indication that ventilations are adequate, but listening directly to the lungs is more reliable.

40. a. Check to see if an airway adjunct has been inserted properly. The tongue is the most common cause of airway obstruction in any patient.

41. a. An inadequate mask seal will cause leaking. It is common for one rescuer ventilating with a BVM to have a problem making a good mask seal.

42. c. Decreased or absent lung sounds, no chest rise, and difficulty squeezing the bag are clear indications that ventilations are inadequate and some adjustments should be made quickly.

43. a. The use of a FROPVD can cause a pneumothorax and gastric distention. However, an audible alarm will sound when the relief valve is activated.

44. d. The device does have to be cleaned, the parts are not inexpensive, and the device does use a lot of oxygen.

45. d. Gastric distention and barotrauma (pneumothorax) are major disadvantages to the use of the FROPVD.

46. b. The rate is 1½ to 2 seconds for adults and 1 to 1½ seconds for infants and children. With an oxygen source attached, deliver the ventilation over 1 second for all patients.

47. b. A partial stoma means that the patient's airway is still partially open through the oropharynx and during ventilations the openings must be sealed to prevent a leak.

48. d. Mucus plugs and thick secretions can cause an obstruction, which is often the reason EMS is called.

49. d. The length of the distance from the center of the patient's lips to the angle of the jaw is approximately the same distance as from the lips to the back of the throat.

50. a. Properly sized OPAs are designed to keep the tongue from blocking the airway. If the OPA is too small, it will not keep the tongue from obstructing the airway; if it is too large, it will become an obstruction itself.

51. b. Absence of a gag reflex is the indication for use of an OPA. Seizing patients often have clenched teeth, so a nasopharyngeal airway (NPA) is better for them.

52. c. A lubricant is needed to insert an NPA, and a water-soluble jelly is preferred. Petroleum jelly is harmful to lung tissue.

53. a. The NPA cannot be used on patients with significantly deviated septums, nasal trauma, or infants.

54. b. The length from the tip of the patient's nose to the tip of the earlobe is approximately the same length as from the nares to the back of the throat.

55. a. All oxygen cylinders must be hydrostatically tested on a regular basis.

56. c. The oxygen cylinder only stores oxygen; the BVM, pocket face mask, and pressure regulator are oxygen delivery devices.

57. d. Suction and airway adjuncts are not considered components of an oxygen delivery system.

58. a. The patient receives oxygen from both the reservoir bag and the supply line (oxygen tubing).

59. d. Patients with apnea, respiratory arrest, and cardiac arrest require assisted ventilations.

60. c. The non-rebreather mask (NRB) delivers approximately a 90 percent concentration of oxygen.

61. c. There is a mask made to fit over stomas; however, a NRB can be placed over the stoma and is the preferred oxygen delivery device for a stoma patient with respiratory distress.

62. c. There is no need to distress a patient further by trying to force a face mask on. When a patient adamantly refuses a mask, administer oxygen with a nasal cannula.

63. d. A sick, crying child gets blow-by oxygen; a newly born with poor respiratory effort one minute after birth gets assisted ventilations; a woman in active labor with nausea gets a cannula. Until the reason for the fainting is discovered, the

COPD patient gets high-flow oxygen by NRB if tolerated.

64. c. Unless the patient is injured or has a serious condition that requires extra oxygenation, the patient can be left on the same liter flow as found.

65. d. Severe hypoxia, mouth breathing, and poor respiratory effort are relative contraindications for use of a nasal cannula.

66. b. The nasal cannula is easy to use, is more comfortable than a face mask, and does not cause nausea or require weaning.

67. b. For the unresponsive patient with a gag reflex, an NPA is the appropriate airway adjunct. The patient requires assisted ventilations once every 5 seconds. Hyperventilation is no longer recommended; hyperoxygenate instead.

68. c. Cricoid pressure or Sellick's maneuver is commonly used during an intubation attempt to better visualize the patient's vocal cords.

69. a. Shallow respirations, tenderness on the chest, and the mechanism of injury (MOI) suggest that the patient may have rib fractures in addition to the chest bruising. Shallow respirations are a form of guarding that occurs because of the pain that is present with each breath.

70. b. With the possibility of injured ribs, the chest should be splinted. Administer high-flow oxygen and coach the patient to improve ventilations by taking a deep breath regularly.

71. c. You can expect the SpO2 reading to be high, but most likely it would be inaccurate. CO binds to hemoglobin 200 times better than oxygen, which means that some portion of the blood will be better oxygenated than the rest. The pulse oximeter does not give a reading on this distinction. It only measures the portion of blood with the highest readings.

72. a. The most obvious answer is the best answer. The longer the exposure, the more severe you would expect the symptoms to be.

73. b. Stridor is an abnormal breath sound associated with obstruction. The patient is getting air in, but the cyanosis indicates that not enough oxygen is reaching the tissues.

74. a. For a partial obstruction with poor air exchange, the patient needs help clearing the obstruction. Perform the Heimlich maneuver.

75. c. The patient is trying to blow off excess acid (Kussmaul's respirations), as indicated by the abnormal respiratory pattern of deep and rapid hyperventilation.

Chapter 8: Scene Size-Up

1. d. It is the EMT-B's responsibility to complete a scene size-up and ascertain what type of BSI is needed, recognize actual or potential safety issues, and attempt to identify the MOI, NOI, or both.

2. b. The EMT-B should first maintain a high suspicion of danger for this scenario. You would expect a resident who has called EMS late at night to have a light on, unless the resident is blind or the call was made by a third party.

3. d. The symptoms of headache and nausea reported by each household resident suggest the possibility of the flu, food poisoning, or carbon monoxide poisoning. CO poisoning must be ruled out quickly and corrected if necessary. Call the fire department to obtain CO readings.

4. b. When there are downed power lines at the scene of a MVC, the EMT-B must assume that they are live and very dangerous. Automobiles are grounded, so the occupants are safe as long as they stay inside the vehicle.

5. a. Based on the dispatch information, a minimum level of protection will include the use of gloves. Once at the scene, the EMT-B can decide what additional PPE is needed.

6. a. Pets can be a significant hazard for responders. The EMT-B may be attacked by a pet that is trying to protect its owner, or the EMT-B may be distracted from completing an assessment or obtaining information at the scene, or the pet could be injured if it is underfoot during the patient move.

7. b. As the saying goes, lightning does not strike twice in the same place. Each of the other scenes is dangerous and requires properly trained support to manage the scene. Even when the EMT-B is trained to manage any of the other scenarios, the situation with the patient struck by lightning would still be the safest.

8. b. First make sure that the vehicle is turned off, that it is shifted into park, and that the parking brake is applied. This will prevent the vehicle from moving accidentally while you are gaining access to the patient. Letting the air out of the tires is another fast and easy way to stabilize a vehicle and should be considered after ensuring that the engine is off. The use of seat belts or unlocked doors does not affect stabilization of the vehicle.

9. c. Stabilizing an overturned vehicle with cribbing (e.g., blocks of wood) is the appropriate step to take before the fire department arrives. Attempting to move the vehicle could further injure the vehicle occupants or even the responders.

10. b. A burn is a traumatic injury or MOI rather than an illness or NOI.

11. a. The primary injuries you would expect to find from this type of MOI involve the head, face, and neck. Injuries to the chest, abdomen, or extremities would be secondary injuries.

12. b. When a child pedestrian is struck by an automobile, the classic injury pattern seen is a blow to the torso, followed by a blow to the legs, and then a head injury when the head is slammed on the hood or the ground.

13. a. Initially, the couple must be kept separated to prevent another escalation. They both need medical attention, but should not be transported in the same ambulance.

14. c. With only one unconscious patient visible and a broken-out windshield, there is no way of knowing if there were any passengers. It is necessary to search the area for other victims.

15. b. The incident commander (IC) will need an accurate count of patients to determine what additional resources will be needed. The triage officer should be triaging patients at this point and will continue to do so. You can get the current patient count and get the information back to the IC, allowing the triage officer to finish his task.

16. b. Scene size-up begins with assessing the scene for safety, including BSI precautions, personal safety, crew member safety, and patient and bystander safety. You then determine the MOI/ NOI; count or estimate the number of patients; and finally determine what additional resources (if any) are needed.

17. a. There are a number of ways to manage this situation, none of which should include leaving the spouse alone for any amount of time. When it is not possible to wait for someone to come and stay with the spouse, take the spouse along to the hospital.

18. c. With a two-person crew, one ambulance is needed for each critical patient and one ambulance for the two stable patients, for a total of three ambulances.

19. b. Each responder is responsible for personal safety. You should enter the residence and conduct a scene size-up the same as with any other call. Four eyes are better than two, so when your partner approaches and enters the residence he should also conduct a scene size-up.

20. d. The elements of the scene size-up are dynamic and can change quickly. For example, while you are caring for a patient, the spouse may become so distressed that he develops chest pain—and now there are two patients. Reconsideration of the elements of the scene size-up is ongoing during the time spent on the scene.

21. c. In most cases, the decision to call for additional help or to restrain the patient is made after the initial assessment. The fact that police are on the scene does not guarantee your or your partner's personal safety. During the initial assessment of a patient in this type of scenario, it is practical to assure an unobstructed exit.

22. d. Each state has a mandatory reporting procedure for suspected child abuse or neglect. The specific way to report may vary slightly from state to state, but the initial prehospital approach is the same: get the child to the hospital for care and never confront the parent or caregiver with your suspicions.

23. a. This information must be passed on to the ED so that the patient is not returned home before a home assessment is made and the residence is determined to be safe or improved. Some communities have additional resources available to help residents in this type of situation, and EMS can activate those resources.

24. c. A picture is worth a thousand words. Taking a photograph to the ED is an excellent way to help the physician understand the MOI.

25. a. Working in traffic is one of the most dangerous aspects of the EMS field. Rubbernecking is contagious, and the result has often been fatal for rescuers, because the rubbernecking driver becomes distracted by the collision and does not see the rescuers.

Chapter 9: Initial Assessment

1. d. Forming a general impression of a patient means getting a sense of the patient's level of distress and appraising it as mild, moderate, or severe. Threats to life are typically discovered during the initial assessment, whereas MOI, NOI, and scene safety are assessed during the scene size-up.

2. a. Unless the patient is experiencing an allergic reaction, allergy information is not pertinent to forming a general impression of the patient. It is, however, very helpful in making treatment decisions involving the administration of medications.

3. d. AVPU is used to assess mental status. When you see that a patient is aware of you by her watching you, that patient is considered *alert* (A); if the patient is unaware of your presence and you have to speak to get a response, this is considered *verbal* (V); when the patient requires a physical stimulus, this is considered *painful* (P); *unresponsive* (U) is when the patient does not respond to any stimulus.

4. c. When a physical stimulus is required to draw a response from the patient, the rating is P for painful.

5. d. Unless you know the patient, it is difficult to determine the patient's normal or baseline status. It will be necessary to speak with someone who does know the patient to establish if something is different today.

6. d. Unless the child's state is unresponsive, the most reliable information about the child's baseline behavior will come from a parent or caregiver.

7. b. Drooling and epistaxis (nosebleed) can create potentially serious airway problems in unconscious patients; the concern with active TB is disease transmission. Facial fractures raise an immediate and potentially serious concern about airway problems. The injuries may obstruct the airway with swelling, bleeding, or protruding bones, and injured nerves can paralyze facial muscles.

8. c. Look, listen, and feel are the methods used to assess a patient. You are looking to see if the airway is open. The indication of an open airway is the ability of air to enter and exit. If it is not open, you will look to see if there is an obstruction. When a patient is able to talk, you can assess mental status and respiratory effort. When a patient is unconscious or has an altered mental status, you will need to assess the airway by looking, listening, and feeling.

9. a. Absence of pain in the cervical area following a significant MOI does not mean there is no cervical injury. The patient may be distracted by pain in another location, or just stunned by the event and not aware of a minor pain. It is possible to injure the spine without feeling pain immediately.

10. b. Unless the patient has an altered mental status or loss of consciousness, the patient is usually the most reliable source of information regarding the MOI. Often there are no witnesses and not enough information available from the surroundings (environment).

11. a. *Retractions* are increased use of the accessory muscles for breathing. When retractions are present, the patient is working hard to breathe. Labored speech rather than slow speech is associated with inadequate breathing. Delayed capillary refill and a low pulse oximeter reading are not reliable findings for inadequate breathing.

12. a. Oxygenation and perfusion status are assessed by looking at the skin and checking for a pulse. Look in the mouth and nose for airway patency.

13. c. Breathing is adequate with a clear airway, a rate in the normal range, and good skin CTC. However, seizures often produce a brief period of apnea, so oxygen administration is appropriate during a seizure and for a short time following a seizure.

14. d. The recumbent position is appropriate for an unresponsive patient who has a clear airway with adequate breathing and circulation. In this position, any secretions that develop will drain out of the mouth.

15. b. The child is wheezing and using accessory muscles (nasal flaring) to breathe, and the skin is pale, indicating respiratory distress. The child needs oxygen, but it is key to keep the child calm. Upsetting the child may worsen the condition quickly. Begin by administering blow-by oxygen and allow the parent or caregiver to assist.

16. d. The patient most likely has bruised and/or fractured some ribs. This injury produces pain with each respiration, which causes the patient to take shallow respirations and possibly hypoventilate. Administer oxygen by NRB and coach the patient to take deeper inspirations intermittently.

17. d. Yellow is associated with jaundice; moist skin is associated with warm temperatures, overexertion, a stress reaction, or shock; pale skin could be a result of cold, hypoxia, or shock. Cyanosis is clearly a sign of deoxygenation.

18. b. The patient can tell you whether he feels dyspneic, or you may be able to see when a patient is experiencing dyspnea. *Apnea* is absence of breathing, *tachypnea* is rapid breathing, and *tachycardia* is a rapid heart rate.

19. b. From birth through the first 4 weeks of life, an infant is an obligate nose breather. Secretions or nasal congestion can be a significant airway obstruction at this age.

20. c. Grunting on expiration is abnormal and indicates distress.

21. d. Provision of adequate ventilations begins with making a good mask seal and assuring that the chest rises with each squeeze of the bag. The presence of equal breath sounds and improved color also indicate that ventilations are adequate.

22. a. Infants have softer and more flexible airways, and the lung tissue is fragile. With age, the cartilage in the trachea becomes more rigid. The airway tissues in the elderly shrink and lose normal mucous membrane linings. Years of exposure to pollutants inevitably lead to decreased diffusion of gases through the alveoli and a generalized decrease in lung capacity.

23. d. The features of the pulse that are assessed include presence or absence, rate, regularity, location, and quality. *Quality* is how strong or weak the pulse feels to the examiner.

24. a. The central pulses are the femoral and carotid. The femoral pulse is palpated in the upper thigh in the area or crease between the lower abdomen and leg.

25. a. The brachial artery is palpated by pressing the artery against the bone in the medial aspect of the upper arm.

26. b. The steps in the AHA "quick check" for the professional rescuer include: check for responsiveness; if unresponsive, open the airway and check for breathing; if there is no breathing, give two breaths and check for a carotid pulse.

27. d. Arterial bleeding can be life-threatening and must be managed quickly after ensuring that there is an airway and the patient is breathing.

28. a. When a life-threatening problem is identified, it must be managed quickly after ensuring that there is an airway and the patient is breathing.

29. b. Jaundice manifests as yellow eyes, skin, or certain body fluids; it is caused by excess bilirubin (a yellow pigment produced by the normal breakdown of red blood cells) in the blood.

30. b. Sometimes assessing skin color can be difficult because people come in so many different tones and shades. The sclera of the eyes, the lips, and the nail beds will reveal abnormal skin color (e.g., cyanosis or jaundice) in a person of any color.

31. a. Unless the child has been choking or has aspirated the shampoo, the skin color should be pink, warm, and dry.

32. a. Flushed, hot, and moist skin in an ill patient who has been in warm ambient temperature suggests that he is febrile.

33. b. The elasticity of the skin (turgor) indicates the patient's state of hydration. When the skin is pinched, it should return to its original shape quickly. If the skin remains pinched or the natural contour returns slowly, this is called *tenting* (decreased skin turgor) and indicates dehydration.

34. d. Cold exposure, infection, pain, or fever can produce these findings.

35. b. In the absence of exposure to cold, a capillary refill time of more than 2 seconds is delayed and is considered an abnormal finding in a child.

36. a. Because children usually have excellent circulation, delayed capillary refill indicates a circulation problem (e.g., hypoperfusion).

37. a. The goal of the initial assessment is to find and correct life-threatening conditions, prioritize patient care, and make a transport decision.

38. b. Some patients need the definitive care of an ED or OR quickly. Prioritizing the care for a patient, and making a transport decision, is where the EMT-B can make life-saving decisions for the patient.

39. a. The loss of distal pulses and the finding of a weak central pulse is a clear indication that the blood pressure is very low.

40. b. The airway is open already. Immediate spinal precautions are warranted for this patient because of the MOI and chief complaints.

41. a. When a patient states that he is having difficulty breathing, even though he does not appear to have labored respirations, you must believe him and begin treatment by providing high-flow oxygen. Not treating a patient or incorrectly treating a patient (such as by breathing into a paper bag) may produce serious hypoxia.

42. b. The symptoms are what the patient tells you is concerning him today, and are referred to as the *chief complaint*. Your general impression of the patient, coupled with your objective findings, may support the chief complaint and bring about a field diagnosis.

43. a. It appears that this the patient was asleep. When you awoke her, she answered questions appropriately. Not knowing the date without looking at a calendar is normal for any of us. The patient is alert.

44. b. Begin prioritizing the patient based on the more serious problem. Establish a baseline, reassess, and trend your information. From there you can reprioritize the patient's status.

45. c. The GCS is used to assess the best motor, verbal, and eye-opening responses.

Chapter 10: Focused History and Physical Exam—Trauma Patient

1. c. Many MOIs cause predictable injury patterns. The EMT-B is trained to visualize the forces that were applied to the body and to look for specific injury patterns, even when injury is not immediately visible or apparent or the patient does not complain of any pain.

2. c. Appreciating the severity of an MOI does not mean that the EMT-B will be able to recognize all potential injuries or what the patient's final outcome will be. The EMT-B recognizes shock from findings in the physical exam, not the MOI.

3. a. Getting a complete and accurate history of the incident can help to identify as many as 95 percent of the injuries present.

4. d. The rapid trauma exam is performed on patients with a significant MOI. The patient with a twisted ankle does not need a rapid trauma assessment. Instead, the EMT-B will focus the exam on the isolated extremity injury, unless the MOI was significant.

5. b. An unconscious child who appears to have fallen from a ladder needs a rapid trauma assessment. Each of the other injuries is relatively minor and isolated to an extremity, with no significant MOI.

6. d. Each of answers a, b, and c is correct.

7. c. For the patient involved in a MVC who has no apparent injuries or complaints, but has sustained

tachycardia, the EMT-B must consider the possibility of internal bleeding and treat the patient as a high priority.

8. a. A patient with a significant MOI warrants a rapid trauma assessment to quickly identify any possible life-threatening injuries or injury patterns.

9. c. The rapid trauma assessment is a tool designed to help the EMT-B quickly identify and manage life-threatening injuries, and then make a transport decision. For the critical trauma patient, a short scene time with a rapid transport to the trauma center for definitive care is the goal.

10. b. *Crepitus* is the grinding of fractured bones. To find crepitus in the abdomen, flank, or scalp would be very unusual because there are no bones in these areas.

11. d. The mnemonic D-CAP-BTLS represents deformity, contusion, abrasion, puncture/penetration, burn, tenderness, laceration, and swelling. The SAMPLE and OPQRST mnemonics are used for obtaining a focused history and information about pain respectively. MOI is an abbreviation for *mechanism of injury.*

12. c. Paradoxical movement is associated with flail chest, a fracture consisting of three or more ribs broken in two or more places. The section of ribs will move independently and opposite of the rib cage during inspiration and expiration.

13. b. The medic alert device was a good find and hypoglycemia should be ruled out as soon as possible. However, it is more important to complete the RTA and be thorough in identifying any possible life-threatening conditions, before locating a glucometer or administering oral glucose.

14. c. Prevent the patient from further injury during a seizure by laying him supine; then administer high-flow oxygen. Suctioning a seizing patient is often difficult because of clenched teeth, and the airway should never be pried open. Consider an NPA for seizure patients.

15. d. It is appropriate to stop the RTA and manage a life-threatening injury as soon as it is discovered. For example, if you discover that the patient has stopped breathing while you are assessing the chest for expansion, you would go back to the airway and assist with ventilations.

16. a. For a patient with an isolated extremity injury and no significant MOI, the EMT-B will perform a focused exam on the extremity, assessing for PMS and D-CAP-BTLS.

17. c. For a patient with an isolated extremity injury and no significant MOI, the EMT-B will perform a focused exam on the extremity, assessing for PMS and D-CAP-BTLS.

18. b. The EMT-B will consider the MOI to mentally visualize the forces that were applied to the body and

to look for specific injury patterns; together with the chief complaint, this assessment gives direction as the EMT-B proceeds with the focused history and physical exam.

19. d. The EMT-B should consider causes other than a normally uncooperative disposition for the behavior of a victim of a serious MOI. Consider hypoxia, head injury, hypoglycemia, or shock as the possible cause of the patient's behavior.

20. d. *Crepitus* is the grinding of fractured bones; finding crepitus in the abdomen would be very unusual because there are no bones in the abdomen.

21. a. A baseline set of vital signs is needed next to help establish any trends and to make treatment decisions. The decision to transport immediately is a good one and the DPE can be done en route. Repeating the IA at any time is also good.

22. d. If the shot was at close range, there should be evidence of powder residue. The caliber, gender of the shooter, and shell type, even if found, are not as helpful for determining if a wound is an entry or exit hole.

23. c. Paradoxical movement is associated with flail chest.

24. a. Approximately two liters of blood can be lost in the first two hours from a pelvic injury. To prevent any further damage to internal organs, such as the bladder or rectum, the pelvis should be stabilized quickly. Treat actual and potential life-threatening injuries as they are discovered.

25. d. The EMT-B should perform a focused physical exam based on the patient's chief complaint for a trauma patient with no significant MOI. There is no need to perform a head-to-toe exam on someone with an isolated injury, unless the MOI was significant.

26. b. It is typical for a patient to experience soreness in the days following a MVC. The patient may have an underlying condition of arthritis, osteoporosis, or meningitis that has been aggravated by the new injury, but most likely the pain is from muscle strain.

27. a. The EMT-B should examine the helmet as part of the MOI determination, and take the helmet to the ED. When a helmet shows evidence of damage, the helmet has done its job by keeping the head from absorbing a great deal of mechanical force.

28. c. Recognizing that many MOIs have predictable injury patterns is what gives the EMT-B a high or low "index of suspicion" for potential or actual injuries.

29. d. For the patient with signs of shock, but no external bleeding, following a traumatic MOI, the EMT-B must consider internal bleeding as the problem.

30. a. Life-threatening injuries are managed as soon as they are discovered.

Chapter 11: Focused History and Physical Exam—Medical Patient

1. b. Even though the pain is gone now, the patient's description of pain that was sudden in onset and unlike any pain he had experienced before means that the EMT-B must presume the pain is cardiac until proven otherwise. Make every effort to convince the patient to get evaluated right away.

2. b. Onset, provocation, quality, relief, severity, and time (OPQRST) are the questions related to the history of the present illness or chief complaint.

3. d. Use any source available to you when the patient cannot or will not provide you with the necessary information.

4. b. Feeling tired all the time, increased thirst, and frequent urination are signs and symptoms of a new onset of diabetes.

5. a. A scar in the middle of the chest is consistent with cardiac surgery in most cases. Medication bottles in the refrigerator are usually antibiotics or insulin, and inhalers contain medications to assist breathing.

6. d. The last oral intake and activity at onset are questions relating to the history of the present illness.

7. c. When a patient is unresponsive and there is no witness to the event, the EMT-B must take spinal precautions until a cervical injury can be ruled out.

8. b. The assessment steps for an unresponsive medical patient are to do an initial assessment followed by a rapid physical exam, and then obtain baseline vital signs.

9. a. Airway comes first and gets primary consideration throughout care.

10. b. Fever and/or a new rash are considered infectious and contagious until proven otherwise.

11. d. For conscious patients, the focused history and physical exam are routinely performed concurrently.

12. a. Age is demographic information and not part of the SAMPLE history.

13. c. Complete the physical exam and consider intoxication, but rule out the primary causes of altered mental status such as hypoxia, hypoglycemia, stroke, and trauma.

14. a. Airway comes first and gets primary consideration throughout care.

15. b. The assessment steps for an unresponsive medical patient are to do an initial assessment followed by a rapid physical exam, and then obtain baseline vital signs.

16. b. Limit your questions and ask the most important ones first. Phrase your questions so the patient can answer with a "yes" or "no."

17. b. Each of the remaining questions is very important to the patient's present condition.

18. a. Insulin must be refrigerated.

19. a. First attempt to ask the patient questions. If the patient seems unreliable, then ask someone close to the patient to confirm or refute.

20. c. *Focused history* and *history of present illness or injury* are two expressions used to describe the information about the current event and what led up to it.

21. b. Baseline vital signs are the first complete set of vital signs obtained on a patient. They are used to establish a trend in the patient's condition. The information is then used to make treatment decisions.

22. a. The symptom that is causing the patient the most distress is considered the chief complaint.

23. a. Hypoglycemia and hyperglycemia may cause syncope, but would persist with an altered mental status until the problem was corrected. An AMI in a 60-year-old female could cause syncope followed by weakness without dyspnea or chest pain. However, you would not expect to see vital signs and skin CTC as good as these. Consider stroke or TIA and perform a neurological exam, but do not exclude AMI.

24. a. 9-1-1 was called for a reason. An acute coronary syndrome (ACS) must be ruled out at the ED for patients complaining of chest pain—the sooner the better. Time costs heart muscle, and waiting to see if the pain returns could be a fatal mistake.

25. d. Safety first for the patient. Take any measure necessary to assure that the patient does not get injured during the seizure. Manage the ABCs and call for ALS.

26. c. Pacemakers are surgically inserted under the skin, usually in the upper right or left chest. Automated implantable cardioverter defibrillators (AICDs) are implanted in the abdomen.

27. b. Chest pain and shortness of breath (dyspnea) are often associated symptoms. When a patient has either chest pain or dyspnea, the EMT-B should routinely ask the patient if he is experiencing the other symptom. This information is very helpful in making a differential diagnosis.

28. d. The Vial of Life is a brief health history form that includes patient demographics, past medical history, allergies, medications, contacts, and health insurance information. The form is rolled up and placed in a plastic container and is typically kept in the refrigerator for health care providers to use as needed.

29. b. Jaundice is associated with hepatitis; the mode of transmission for hepatitis is through contact with body fluids. Gloves, eyewear, and handwashing are the recommended protective measures.

30. d. When caring for coughing patients, place a mask on the patient and yourself. The patient's mask can be an oxygen mask if oxygen is needed. You could ask the patient if she is contagious, but you cannot be sure that her information is reliable.

Chapter 12: Detailed Physical Exam

1. a. Allergies are pertinent *medical* information, rather than diagnostic information.

2. c. An assessment for neurological deficits is included in the detailed physical exam. Scene size-up is completed upon arrival at the scene, the patient's age is demographic information, and the administration of oxygen is treatment.

3. a. The DPE is typically performed on a trauma patient with a significant MOI while en route to the hospital, if time and available manpower permit.

4. b. The humerus is the bone of the upper arm. The lower arm contains the radius and ulna, and the lower leg contains the tibia and fibula.

5. c. The pulsing is a finding specific to the abdomen, and could be detected when the patient has an abdominal aortic aneurysm.

6. c. HEENT is a mnemonic for head, eyes, ears, nose, and throat.

7. b. First ask the patient what the patch is for. Many transdermal patches are available with medications for pain, birth control, smoking/nicotine cessation, hormones, and more. It is important to determine exactly what the patch is delivering. If it becomes necessary to remove the patch, use gloves to avoid absorption into your skin.

8. d. None of the injuries is life-threatening; therefore, begin by managing the injury that is most likely causing the most discomfort and may result in permanent damage to a significant organ.

9. c. Unequal pupils are an abnormal finding; however, in a small percentage of the population this condition is normal for them. When any abnormal finding is noted, first ask the patient if this is normal for her.

10. b. The back is often overlooked when a patient is immobilized on a backboard. If the patient's back was not examined before he was immobilized to a backboard, the EMT-B should assess the back by reaching underneath from both sides of the patient.

11. d. After the initial assessment, the EMT-B should focus on the chief complaint and do a focused physical exam of the neck and back, followed by a focused assessment and history for a cause of the fainting.

12. c. The EMT-B should talk to any witness to the event. Of the choices provided, the customer at the checkout would most likely have the most reliable information regarding the loss of consciousness.

13. d. The DPE is typically performed on a trauma patient with a significant MOI, en route to the hospital, with time and manpower permitting.

14. a. Because the DPE is typically performed on a trauma patient with a significant MOI, scene time is often short (10 minutes or less). Therefore, with time and manpower permitting, the DPE is performed en route to the hospital.

15. d. Paradoxical motion is associated with a flail chest injury, JVD is observed only in the neck, and dry mucous membranes may be observed in the mouth and nose.

16. b. The DPE is a more thorough examination of the body and may reveal additional findings that were not noted in the initial assessment or RPE.

17. d. The DPE is usually performed from head to toe in adults and toe to head in young children. However, repeating the exam in the same manner each time, rather than jumping around to various body areas, does help you to avoid missing any areas of the body.

18. c. The order of assessment for the trauma patient with a significant MOI, following the initial assessment, is to perform an RTA, obtain baseline vital signs and SAMPLE history, begin transport, and perform a DPE en route.

19. c. Because time and manpower are often limited, the DPE is typically performed once while en route to the hospital.

20. c. When the MOI warrants the completion of a DPE, the age of the patient is not a factor. In young children, the EMT-B may choose to reverse the order of the DPE by assessing from toe to head. The reason for this direction change is that young children often do not like having their heads, faces, or ears touched, so they may become agitated, making the rest of the assessment difficult.

21. a. A *degloving injury* is when the skin is torn off one or more fingers, as if a glove had been peeled off the hand. Contusion and hematoma are closed injuries, and a crushing injury can be either open or closed.

22. a. Discoloration, such as blood in the white of the eye from a hemorrhage, should be noted in the DPE.

23. c. CSF leaks usually occur through fractures at the base of the skull. Fluid leaks through the nose, down the back of the throat, and into the mouth. The patient may state that she has a salty taste in the mouth. If the eardrum is ruptured, fluid may also leak out through the ears.

24. b. The presence of JVD in the supine position is a normal finding. When the patient is sitting up or is in high Fowler's position, the presence of JVD would be an abnormal finding.

25. a. Assessing in a head-to-toe manner, each body area is reassessed in more detail, including any areas previously assessed or managed earlier.

Chapter 13: Ongoing Assessment

1. a. Abdominal pain with hypotension indicates shock.

2. a. The ongoing assessment is necessary to determine any changes in the patient's condition. The purpose is to assess the effectiveness of your care and to determine the need for changes in treatment priorities. This is done by repeating the initial assessment, baseline vital signs, and the focused physical exam.

3. b. The ongoing assessment is necessary to determine any changes in the patient's condition. The purpose is to assess the effectiveness of your care and to determine the need for changes in treatment priorities.

4. c. The past medical history is important information that should be documented, but it is not part of the ongoing assessment.

5. d. Asking the patient if the pain or cause of distress (e.g., difficulty breathing) is improved, worse, or unchanged is typically what is repeated first and most often in the ongoing assessment.

6. a. The ongoing assessment is necessary to determine any changes in the patient's condition. The purpose is to assess the effectiveness of care and to determine the need for changes in treatment priorities.

7. a. Repeated diagnostic findings, such as pulse oximetry, blood sugar readings, and ECGs, are used to establish trends. Medication compliance and events leading up to the current episode are part of the focused history.

8. a. *Trending* is the process of obtaining a baseline assessment, repeating the assessment multiple times, and using the information to determine whether the patient is getting better, worse, or not changing.

9. c. Decreasing blood pressure associated with internal bleeding is a sign of decompensated shock (hypoperfusion). Additional findings include rapid heart rate, cool and clammy skin, and altered mental status.

10. c. Guarded and shallow respirations are a classic finding associated with fractured ribs, because it hurts to take a breath. Prolonged hypoventilation can cause hypoxia, so the patient must be coached to take deeper breaths despite the pain. Initially the patient will resist and high-flow oxygen is needed to compensate for the guarded breathing.

11. d. Treatment for an isolated extremity injury is splinting. The ongoing assessment includes assessing the adequacy of the splint and reassessing PMS.

12. c. Reassessing a COPD patient who is on high-flow oxygen includes observing for a decreased respiratory drive. In COPD patients, the stimulus to breathe is abnormal and is driven by low oxygen levels. Prolonged administration of high-flow oxygen may cause the patient's respiratory drive to slow down, so the patient must be coached to increase the breathing rate.

13. d. The electrodes from an AED are large and will adhere to even especially hairy chests. Electrodes used to obtain an ECG are smaller and require a smooth surface to properly adhere; thus, shaving is often necessary.

14. c. One of the effects of nitroglycerin is to dilate the coronary arteries. This often causes a drop in blood pressure. Sometimes the blood pressure drops too much, and this condition could worsen the initial cause of chest pain.

15. b. A new complaint of back pain that develops en route to the hospital, while the patient is immobilized to a long backboard, is common. The pain could be caused by the MVC or from lying on the hard board. Loosen the leg straps and allow the patient to flex her knees. This often helps to relieve the pressure on the low back without compromising the cervical spine.

16. c. You must be alert for subtle changes in mental status (e.g., anxiety or confusion), which are the earliest signs of a change in a patient's condition. Changes in lung sounds and skin color can occur quickly, and a drop in blood pressure is a late finding.

17. d. The purpose of the ongoing assessment is to assess the effectiveness of care and to determine the need for changes in treatment priorities.

18. d. Any competent EMS provider may perform the ongoing assessment, and this fact makes the other choices vague. The *most* correct answer is that, with time and manpower permitting, the ongoing assessment should be repeated every 5 minutes for an unstable patient.

19. c. The pressure-bandage and elevation treatments are associated with bleeding control.

20. c. Moving the patient out of a supine position has caused the blood pressure to drop, as evidenced by the paleness and moist skin. The fastest way to correct this condition is to lay the patient flat and elevate his legs.

21. c. The more observations you can obtain, the better information you have to establish a trend. The minimum number of observations needed to begin trending is three.

22. d. The more observations (e.g., serial assessments) you can obtain, the better information you have to establish a trend.

23. b. Treating a life-threatening condition affecting any of the ABCs is the priority, and doing so may not leave time to complete a thorough ongoing assessment. An example would be treating a patient who is in respiratory or cardiac arrest. The rescuers may be fully involved in CPR and not have time to do an ongoing assessment.

24. b. The patient is stable with an isolated extremity injury. Reassessing vital signs every 15 minutes is appropriate for this patient.

25. c. Treatment for an isolated injury is splinting. The ongoing assessment includes assessing the adequacy of the splint and reassessing PMS.

Chapter 14: Communications

1. d. The identifier is the vehicle number or other assigned name and/or number. The use of a personal name is inappropriate.

2. c. State the identifier being called followed by your identifier; for example, "Dispatch, this is Medic 1."

3. c. To avoid stepping on (breaking into) another transmission, listen and wait for clear air space, then proceed to key the microphone.

4. c. EMS providers are trained to present patient information in a standard format. EDs are familiar with that format and expect to hear reports in that format. Deviating from the standard format can cause confusion and missed information.

5. c. EMS providers are trained to present patient information in a standard format. EDs are familiar with that format and expect to hear reports in that format. Deviating from the standard format can cause confusion and missed information.

6. b. The typical medical radio report is presented in the following order: patient's age, sex, chief complaint, severity, emergency treatment provided, and ETA.

7. a. Ineffective communications, whatever the cause, can create a delay in receiving the patient at the hospital, which in turn can cause delay in further emergency care.

8. a. Standard radio operating procedures are designed to improve communications and reduce errors.

9. a. Background noise can significantly affect communications, making a message unclear or completely misunderstood.

10. b. Hospital registration needs patient demographics, chief complaint, and insurance information. More specific medical information is not required for patient registration.

11. b. Verbal report is given both over the radio, while en route, and in person to the next health care provider taking over care of the patient. These reports are followed up with a written report (patient care report or PCR).

12. c. This may vary from system to system, but the EMT-B who is managing the patient is the person best prepared to give report.

13. d. Any of these techniques will improve communication with a patient who has these impairments. Although information from the patient may not be reliable, you can use these techniques to make the patient feel better about the transport.

14. d. Whether you intend it to be or not, standing over someone while you speak is intimidating; avoid doing so whenever possible.

15. d. Children respond to facial expressions. Always keep a smile on when managing children. Getting down to their height is less threatening for them.

16. a. In most cases, all or part of one transmission will get through when two units transmit at the same time.

17. d. The Federal Communications Commission (FCC) is the agency that controls and regulates all radio communications in the United States.

18. d. Slang terms, vulgarity, or any offensive communications should be avoided in all radio transmissions.

19. d. Using a patient's proper name, with the title Mr., Mrs., or Ms., shows respect. If the patient gives permission to use another name, such as a first name or nickname, then it is acceptable to use that name. However, it is disrespectful to use endearing terms such as "dear" or "honey."

20. c. Help the patient put in the hearing aids and use them. Shouting can distort, and not every person who is hearing impaired can read lips or sign.

21. a. Facial expressions, including eye contact, are a universal form of communication.

22. b. You are there to take the patient to the hospital. This is obvious and can be stated without breaching confidentiality or affecting the patient's privacy.
23. c. It is important to relay accurate information to the patient and the patient's family at the scene, without giving false hope or potential outcomes.
24. d. Unless the patient's family members are health care providers who understand medical jargon, the EMT-B should explain things in lay terms.
25. a. The appropriate method for obtaining a medication order is to give the patient's chief complaint, pertinent information about the physical exam and focused history, request the order, and confirm the order back to the physician. If you do not understand any part of the order, you must ask the physician to clarify before administering any medication.

26. a. Dispatch is the official timekeeper for the stages of a call and will acknowledge with a time check after each communication from the ambulance.
27. a. The use of clear and brief communication over the radio is professional, proper, and expected.
28. a. All the information listed in the question is obtained during the scene size-up so that it can be quickly relayed back to dispatch.
29. b. Getting any treatment order recorded is the best way to protect the EMT-B from any possible charges of inaccuracies and to maintain quality assurance.
30. a. It is proper to acknowledge rather than ignore the message. When you cannot provide the information requested immediately, acknowledge the caller with a quick "Stand by."

Chapter 15: Documentation

1. b. The times typically noted on a PCR include: time of dispatch, time en route, time on scene, time off scene, time arriving at the hospital, and time in service.
2. a. Dispatch is the timekeeper and provides all run times.
3. c. Patient discharge instructions are provided by the hospital at time of discharge.
4. c. The items listed are examples of patient demographics.
5. a. The body of the report includes assessment findings, emergency care provided, and reassessment information, which is needed by the next health care provider to continue care of the patient.
6. d. PCR styles vary from agency to agency, and may include boxes to check off and/or a place for narrative. Billing forms require some information about the emergency care provided so that the agency can properly bill for services rendered.
7. b. Military time is used to standardize timekeeping and to minimize time recording errors.
8. b. The GCS score is a cumulative number obtained from the scoring of three factors.
9. c. The patient's ID is demographic information.
10. d. If further assessment of the child reveals no pertinent findings, allow the mother to refuse transport, but recommend follow-up with the child's pediatrician. A person who has been drinking is questionable for competency; a minor needs a parent's consent to refuse treatment; and a victim of violence requires care and mandatory reporting in some states.
11. c. Assessment findings, MOI, treatment recommendations, and implications for refusal should be both discussed with the patient and carefully documented.
12. d. It is a patient's right to refuse all or any part of care. When this occurs, document and ask the patient to

sign off; then continue care as permitted and transport.
13. c. Corrections must be made on all copies, and initials and the date must be placed next to the change. When you cannot obtain all copies, an amended form can be completed with the additional information and then distributed the same as the original.
14. c. A PCR that is incomplete, inaccurate, or illegible gives the impression that proper assessment and care was not provided or was provided incorrectly, and the author is attempting to hide something. This is especially so in a court of law.
15. c. Patient confidentiality is of primary concern for any health care provider, whether information is being transmitted in writing or verbally.
16. b. Reporting requirements as to suspected abuse vary from state to state.
17. a. The reporting of suspected child abuse is mandatory in every state. The specific method of reporting varies from state to state.
18. a. Several types of triage tags, each with different features, are used as the first form of documentation at an MCI.
19. b. The use of medical terminology in charting is appropriate as long as it is used and spelled correctly.
20. b. The correct spelling is "pneumonia."
21. b. Time of administration and assessment findings before and after the administration of any treatment should be carefully documented.
22. a. Radio failure may complicate the call (e.g., by delaying response or care) and should be documented on the PCR. An exposure is documented on a special incident report; SOPs and route of transport are typically not documented on PCRs.

23. b. A PCR that is incomplete, inaccurate, or illegible gives the impression that proper assessment and care were not provided or were provided incorrectly, and that the author is attempting to hide something.

24. d. Another example of a pertinent negative is a patient with shortness of breath, but no chest pain, because the two symptoms are typically present together.

25. c. In 1970, the NHTSA was established with the Department of Transportation to provide leadership to the EMS community and states.

Chapter 16: General Pharmacology

1. c. The National Standard Curriculum states that the EMT-B may administer or use medical control to assist a patient with oxygen, oral glucose, activated charcoal, nitroglycerin, epinephrine auto injector, and meter dose inhalers (e.g., albuterol). Aspirin, Benadryl, and atropine may be administered by only advanced EMS providers.

2. c. Benadryl is an over-the-counter medication.

3. b. EMT-Bs may assist a patient to take the patient's own nitroglycerin, under orders from medical control.

4. d. Activated charcoal is available under many trade names.

5. c. The official name is the same as the generic name and is followed by the initials USP (United States Pharmacopeia) or NF (National Formulary), denoting its listing in one of these official publications.

6. a. The EMS provider is primarily responsible for knowing the generic and brand names of a drug.

7. a. Seizures can cause hypoxia due to brief periods of apnea. The patient needs oxygen first. Further assessment must be completed before determining the need for any additional pharmacological treatment (e.g., glucose for low blood sugar).

8. a. With a history of asthma, a chief complaint of difficulty breathing, and assessment findings of wheezing, anxiety, and confusion, it is appropriate to assist the patient with her own albuterol. Chest tightness is a symptom frequently associated with dyspnea from asthma or an exacerbation of a respiratory condition, and is different from cardiac chest pain.

9. d. The signs and symptoms described indicate anaphylactic shock. The airway swelling is of primary concern, making epinephrine the treatment of choice.

10. a. Glutose is a brand or trade name for oral glucose.

11. a. The brand or trade name is a name assigned by the manufacturer, which usually registers the name as a trademark to protect it. One drug may have several trade names. A registered trade name begins with a capital letter and may be followed by the symbol ®.

12. b. Albuterol is the generic name. Ventolin, Proventil, and Combivent are trade names.

13. a. Solutions are liquids that contain dissolved drugs (e.g., eyedrops).

14. a. A tablet is a single dose that is shaped like a disc and can be chewed or swallowed whole (e.g., baby aspirin).

15. d. Suspensions are liquids with solid particles mixed in but not dissolved (e.g., activated charcoal).

16. a. Any patient with respiratory distress should receive oxygen first. For the patient with an asthma history and signs and symptoms consistent with an asthma attack, assisting the patient with her own inhaler is appropriate if medical control allows it.

17. d. In anaphylaxis, epinephrine is the main treatment. It works as a bronchodilator and it decreases vascular permeability.

18. c. Activated charcoal is used to absorb ingested poisons to prevent absorption into the body.

19. a. Epinephrine decreases vascular permeability by constricting blood vessels; this helps to increase the blood pressure. Epinephrine is also a bronchodilator.

20. d. The six "rights" of medication administration are: right patient, right drug, right dose, right route, right time, and right documentation.

21. c. The *classification* of a drug is a categorization based on how the drug works or what it is made of.

22. d. A *contraindication* is something that makes a particular treatment or procedure inadvisable (e.g., giving nitroglycerin to someone who is hypotensive).

23. d. Drugs and drug products are derived from several sources. Epinephrine and insulin are derived from both animals and humans.

24. c. Immunization is the creation of immunity against a particular disease.

25. c. Sublingual drugs are dissolved under the tongue and absorbed across the mucous membrane of the mouth.

26. b. A side effect may be considered desirable or undesirable, depending on the effect it produces. Some of the most common undesirable side effects include headache, nausea, and dizziness.

27. b. Epinephrine increases the heart rate and increases the work load on the heart. In a patient with a pre-existing heart condition or an acute condition such an MI, this side effect is significant.

28. b. Nitroglycerin dilates coronary vessels. This increases the blood supply to the heart, thus improving oxygenation to the heart and reducing pain.

29. a. Bronchodilators (e.g., albuterol and epinephrine) increase the heart rate.

30. a. Activated charcoal is used to absorb ingested poisons to prevent absorption into the body.

31. b. A known allergy to bee stings, signs and symptoms of allergic reaction, and hypotension indicate anaphylactic shock.

32. b. Anaphylactic shock is progressing in this patient. Perhaps the auto-injector was not administered correctly or the reaction is severe. Airway management and additional epinephrine are the treatment needed that the EMT-B can provide.

33. c. Tremors are a side effect of the medication. It is not uncommon for the MDI to be abused and used too much when someone is in distress. When obtaining a focused history, remember to ask how many times the inhaler was used before EMS arrived.

34. b. When a patient experiences an adverse reaction or an undesired side effect, the first thing to do is stop the medication and then provide supportive care for the symptoms. In this case, assist ventilations. Calling for ALS is also appropriate.

35. b. Reassessing a COPD patient who is on high-flow oxygen includes observing for a decreased respiratory drive. In COPD patients, the stimulus to breathe is abnormal and is driven by low oxygen levels. Prolonged administration of high-flow oxygen may cause the patient's respiratory drive to slow down, so the patient must be coached to increase the breathing rate.

Chapter 17: Respiratory Emergencies

1. d. The diaphragm is the major muscle of breathing. It is dome-shaped and separates the chest and abdominal cavities.

2. b. The trachea extends from the larynx to the bronchi.

3. c. Smooth muscle or involuntary muscle is located in the respiratory tract, blood vessels, and most of the intestines and urinary system.

4. a. With a history of asthma, a chief complaint of difficulty breathing and dizziness, and assessment findings of wheezing, it is appropriate to assist the patient with her own albuterol. Chest tightness is a symptom frequently associated with dyspnea from asthma or an exacerbation of a respiratory condition, and is different from cardiac chest pain. The tingling in the hands is likely due to hyperventilating and will subside when the patient can get her breathing rate back to normal.

5. d. A *symptom* is something the patient describes and a *sign* is something you can observe. You cannot always observe when it is difficult for a patient to take a deep breath.

6. b. Give the patient the benefit of the doubt and treat her symptom. Provide high-flow oxygen and reassess. To do otherwise could be disastrous.

7. b. The patient may have fallen asleep. Check for responsiveness first and then assess the ABCs.

8. d. The NRB is the oxygen delivery device of choice for any patient with respiratory distress who can tolerate a mask and has a good respiratory effort.

9. a. A *contraindication* is something that makes a particular treatment or procedure inadvisable. A nasal cannula on a mouth breather would not deliver the oxygen the patient needs.

10. a. The 14-year-old asthma patient needs a dose of her inhaler; medical direction must approve your assisting her with this medication.

11. b. It is appropriate to place the patient on high-flow oxygen by your NRB, not her home oxygen delivery (which is most likely a cannula) and then consider assisting her with her MDI.

12. d. The patient has signs and symptoms of allergic reaction, with respiratory symptoms indicating a progression to anaphylaxis. The administration of epinephrine is indicated.

13. a. The initial management of this patient includes providing a higher concentration of oxygen with your NRB, and supportive care such as position of comfort and warmth. Upon further assessment, additional treatment may be found appropriate. Aggressive airway management (e.g., BVM ventilations) at this point may worsen his condition, and a liter flow of 8 lpm through a cannula is not appropriate.

14. c. The NPA is a great airway adjunct for anyone with a gag reflex, and ventilating at a rate of once every 5 seconds is the recommended standard for an adult in need of ventilation assistance.

15. a. The goal is to get the medication into the lungs, but coordinating this skill can be easier said than done. Very often the patient's breathing is fast and labored. Coach the patient to exhale, then suck in the medication while inhaling and hold the breath.

16. a. Chest rise and fall, especially in children, is one indication that the ventilations being delivered are effective. Oximetry readings are not completely reliable. Compliance of the bag while you are squeezing is helpful but not completely reliable.

Fighting can mean either that the patient is getting better, or that he is hypoxic or has a head injury, so that is not reliable either.

17. d. Each of the answers provided suggests a decline in the patient's condition, thereby indicating the need for ventilatory assistance.

18. c. Seizure patients are great candidates for NPA use, because they often become apneic for a brief time, have clenched teeth, and usually have a gag reflex. The NPA is a safe and easy method of opening the airway with little effort.

19. a. When you are approaching a patient and forming a general impression, the patient's skin color is one of the first indications of how well the patient is perfusing.

20. a. Making sure the mask is tight on the face and making a good seal is the first step in assuring adequate ventilations using a BVM.

21. b. Inability to speak, unilateral breath sounds, and unequal chest rise are more often signs of inadequate rather than adequate air exchange.

22. b. The six rights of medication administration are: right patient, right drug, right dose, right route, right time, and right documentation.

23. c. Before assisting with the administration of any medication, vital signs and part or all of the focused history must be obtained. The EMT-B needs a baseline assessment to determine if the patient is getting better, worse, or not changing.

24. b. Albuterol is a bronchodilator, which means it reduces airway constriction.

25. a. Ventilating at a rate of once every 3 seconds is the recommended standard for a child who is in need of ventilation assistance.

26. a. Keeping the child calm is key. Providing high-flow oxygen by mask (or blow-by oxygen if the child does not tolerate the mask) is the crucial treatment for a sick child in respiratory distress.

27. c. This is the correct sequence for an FBAO in an infant.

28. b. Difficulty swallowing and drooling, together with difficulty breathing, are the classic signs of epiglottitis.

29. a. A recent infection and the distinctive seal-like barking cough are classic signs of croup.

30. c. Bronchiolitis affects the lower airways. Croup and epiglottitis affect the upper airway, and emphysema does not appear in children less than 2 years old.

31. a. Gas exchange occurs in the alveoli and pulmonary capillaries that surround them.

32. d. The epiglottis is a flap of cartilage that closes over the trachea during swallowing to prevent aspiration into the lungs.

33. a. The primary respiratory center controlling the stimulus to breathe is located in the medulla oblongata in the brain stem.

34. b. The body eliminates carbon dioxide during exhalation.

35. d. *Hypoxia* is the absence or shortage of oxygen in the tissues (cells) of the body.

36. d. Wheezing is caused by constriction of the lower airways, and may be heard on both inspiration and exhalation.

37. c. The tripod position is sitting up, leaning forward with both arms extended, with hands on the thighs or sitting surface. This position allows expansion of the rib cage and lungs.

38. b. Grunting is typically associated with respiratory distress in infants and children.

39. c. Kussmaul's respirations are deep and rapid respirations associated with conditions that create acidosis in the body, such as diabetic ketoacidosis.

40. b. Colorful sputum tells a lot. Green or yellow signals infection, and pink, red, or black sputum contains blood.

41. d. Smoking or proximity to second-hand smoke kills 1,200 people per day in the United States; it can cause any of the conditions listed.

42. a. Sounds heard through the posterior (back) of a patient are clearer than the front in most cases. This is because there is little or no fat on the back to diminish sounds.

43. d. The oxygen tubing connects to the regulator at one end and to the reservoir bag at the other end.

44. d. The pulse oximeter is a device that measures the saturation of hemoglobin with oxygen; it provides a percentage reading.

45. c. *Pneumothorax* means air in the chest. This is an abnormal condition that can progress to a life-threatening condition called *tension pneumothorax,* with a collapse of one or both lungs.

46. a. It takes years to develop chronic obstructive pulmonary disease (COPD); hence, it is a condition of the elderly.

47. b. An asthma attack is bronchospasm and/or bronchoconstriction combined with increased production of mucus, airway swelling, and inflammation.

48. b. Prolonged hyperventilation causes too much carbon dioxide to be blown off. When this happens, the patient begins to experience symptoms of anxiety, dizziness, rapid heart rate, and numbness or tingling in the mouth, hands, and feet.

49. d. Any of the traumatic injuries listed can cause difficulty breathing and respiratory distress.

50. c. *Retractions* is a term for the excessive use of respiratory muscles of the neck and chest.

Chapter 18: Cardiovascular Emergencies

1. a. The aorta is the largest artery in the body.
2. b. The right ventricle pumps blood from the heart to the lungs and the left ventricle pumps blood from the heart out to the body.
3. d. The atrioventricular (tricuspid and mitral) and semilunar (pulmonic and aortic) valves of the heart open and close alternately to promote forward flow of the blood through the heart; this valve action creates the classic heart sounds (lub-dub).
4. a. Unless the patient is hypotensive, let the patient assume a position of comfort.
5. d. Until a cardiac problem can be ruled out, consider chest pain to be a life-threatening event and give the patient high priority.
6. d. The goal when treating a patient who has cardiac chest pain is to reduce the pain and provide rapid transport to the appropriate hospital. The EMT-B's role is to provide high-flow oxygen; keep the patient calm, thereby preventing any further stress to the heart; assist with nitroglycerin when appropriate; and get the patient ALS.
7. a. The current guidelines are to attach the AED electrodes to patients who are unresponsive, apneic, and pulseless.
8. a. Use of an AED is indicated for a patient who is unresponsive and has no signs of circulation (e.g., apneic and pulseless).
9. a. Use of an AED is indicated for a patient who is unresponsive and has no signs of circulation (e.g., apneic and pulseless).
10. b. A patient with a pulse is a contraindication for using an AED, as is a malfunctioning AED.
11. a. The patient has all the indications for attaching and turning on an AED: unresponsive, apneic, and pulseless.
12. c. The role of the EMT-B in the chain of survival is to provide basic life support in the first few minutes of a life-threatening emergency.
13. d. Currently the standard is to use the same energy settings for defibrillation on all adults.
14. d. An AED with pediatric pads (electrodes) delivers a reduced energy level appropriate for the child who is under the age of 8 or weighs less than 25 kg (55 lbs).
15. a. Fowler's position is the patient lying down, with the upper body elevated at 45° to 60° angle; in high Fowler's, the upper body is upright, near 90°; in semi-Fowler's position, the patient's upper body is at an angle less than 45°. As this patient has no dyspnea, but does have weakness and dizziness when he mildly exerts himself, his BP may be low, so semi-Fowler's is likely to be the most comfortable position.
16. b. Crackles indicate that fluid is present in the lungs. Fluid responds to gravity, so when you lay a patient down the fluid in the lungs covers more surface area, making oxygen exchange very poor. Sitting upright will be the most comfortable position for the patient and is appropriate unless the BP is very low.
17. d. A decrease in mental status is a sign that the patient is not perfusing adequately. Provide high-flow oxygen and reassess the patient while she is lying down.
18. d. The primary goal in airway management is to make sure that the airway is open, that it stays open, and that the patient is adequately ventilated.
19. b. BLS in a cardiac-arrest scenario begins with assessing for airway, breathing, and pulse; if no breathing or pulse is detected, begin CPR.
20. b. A postarrest patient is unstable even after a successful conversion, and requires ALS. Such patients must be closely monitored for the possibility of deteriorating into cardiac arrest again.
21. d. The best chance of survival following a cardiac arrest from V-fib is when defibrillation is delivered within 4 to 6 minutes. The best chance of this happening in most cases is with public access defibrillation (PAD).
22. c. V-fib is disorganized electrical conduction that does not allow the heart to produce effective contractions. AEDs are programmed to recognize this rhythm and to indicate "Shock advised."
23. d. The chest pain the patient is describing (pain with breathing in the lower left chest) is not typical cardiac pain. It is muscular pain associated with respiratory infection and coughing. Provide oxygen and supportive care.
24. d. The patient should be transported for evaluation even though his chest pain was resolved with nitroglycerin. He may attempt further exertional activity, reproducing the pain or inducing an MI. Oxygen and supportive care en route are appropriate.
25. d. Advanced airway skills and pharmacologic therapy may improve patient outcome in the patient with a cardiac emergency, but they are not a substitute for early defibrillation in a V-fib cardiac arrest.
26. d. The best chance of survival for the patient with cardiac arrest is when advanced airway skills and pharmacologic therapy are available rapidly following cardiac arrest.
27. c. A patient with severe chest pain and hypotension is a critical patient who requires rapid transport and ALS. This patient will not get nitroglycerin even from advanced providers until her BP is higher, but there are other treatments ALS can provide, so begin rapid transport and request ALS en route.
28. a. This patient is unstable and needs rapid transport and ALS. The closest ALS is at the hospital, so begin transport immediately.

29. c. The monophasic defibrillator with escalating doses will provide approximately 200 joules for the first dose. The biphasic defibrillator provides nonescalating defibrillation energy doses of 150 joules. Implanted defibrillators deliver very low energy doses.

30. c. The biphasic defibrillator provides nonescalating defibrillation energy doses of 150 joules.

31. d. A fully automated defibrillator delivers the shock and a semi-automated defibrillator indicates to the user when to provide a shock.

32. d. Fully automated defibrillators have been prescribed for postdischarge cardiac patients for many years. The idea is for a family member to be able to attach the device and turn it on in the event of a cardiac arrest at home.

33. d. Even when the victim of a cardiac arrest has an implanted defibrillator that is firing, the AED defibrillation sequence should not be stopped or delayed.

34. d. Do not delay early defibrillation. The safest and quickest way to do this is to quickly dry off the patient's chest, attach the electrodes, and begin analyzing.

35. d. Always assess and treat the ABCs in order. Airway—open the airway and insert an adjunct. Breathing—begin ventilations. Circulation—begin CPR if pulseless.

36. d. Every answer provided is a good reason not to attach an AED to a patient who is breathing and/or has a pulse.

37. b. To prevent accidental or inappropriate defibrillation, do not attach an AED to a patient with a pulse or who is breathing.

38. b. The technology used in AEDs today is very good, so it is rare for an AED to give the prompt to shock when the patient does not exhibit a shockable rhythm.

39. a. The current recommendation is to reanalyze every 5 minutes en route to the hospital.

40. a. Do not delay defibrillation.

41. b. The recording technology is an advantage of the AED. With this information, the medical director or her designee can review each call for quality assurance.

42. a. There are very few disadvantages to AEDs; the need for ongoing training is the greatest.

43. b. Learning to use an AED is easy for laypersons and health care professionals alike.

44. c. The current recommendations are for the EMT-B to be able to deliver three successive shocks within 90 seconds after reaching the patient's side.

45. b. This technology is referred to as "hands-off" defibrillation because the rescuer presses the "Shock" button without touching the patient.

46. c. Remote or hands-off defibrillation is exceptionally safe for the rescuer.

47. d. Unless there is an acceptable reason to terminate resuscitation, the AED should remain attached and turned on.

48. d. AEDs can be set to recognize ventricular tachycardia (V-tach) as a shockable rhythm. The problem is that this rhythm can produce a pulse for a short time before the patient deteriorates. Technically, this rhythm is shockable when the patient is unstable; however, only advanced EMTs are trained to treat pulsed V-tach this way. This is another reason for not attaching an AED to a patient who has a pulse.

49. d. Finding that the batteries are dead when you need them the most, because you failed to check the AED at the beginning of your shift, is unprofessional and unnecessary.

50. d. This sequence allows the fastest possible delivery of a shock for a victim of cardiac arrest.

51. c. In this scenario, the patient should be shocked when the AED advises.

52. d. Transport should begin as soon as possible, so continue CPR and prepare the patient for transport by placing him on a long backboard. Reanalyze every few minutes.

53. a. In this scenario, the patient should be shocked when the AED advises.

54. c. Refractory V-fib is not uncommon in a cardiac arrest, and requires rapid reanalysis and defibrillation as needed.

55. b. Do not delay early defibrillation.

56. a. This sequence allows the fastest possible delivery of a shock for a victim of cardiac arrest.

57. d. The next pulse check should occur after a set of three shocks, or if the AED reads "No shock advised" before the set of three shocks is delivered.

58. b. Assessing for a pulse during the set of three shocks can significantly delay delivery of the shocks, and thus is not recommended.

59. c. The EMT-B's role is to provide basic life support.

60. d. Each chain is only as strong as its weakest link, so each link must have functional and practiced coordination with the next link.

61. c. After a return of pulses, the airway and breathing should be reassessed and assisted if necessary. Following an electrocution, it is common for the patient to remain apneic, because the electrical shock often temporarily paralyzes the breathing muscles.

62. a. Refractory V-fib is not uncommon in a cardiac arrest, and requires rapid reanalysis and defibrillation as needed. Until the patient is placed on an ECG monitor and ALS begun, the patient should remained attached to the AED with the unit turned on.

63. c. Always revert to the ABCs. Assure an open and patent airway and assist ventilations if needed.

64. d. Hypoxia, hypothermia, and vomiting are associated with near-drowning.

65. a. Giving a patient's family false hope is never appropriate.

66. c. Every victim of cardiac arrest will need some form of ALS support and follow-up.
67. d. Hands-on practice with a coach yields the best results when training to use an AED.
68. a. Frequent hands-on practice with a coach yields the best results for staying proficient in the use of AEDs.
69. d. Any EMS provider who carries an AED should check it regularly, preferably at the beginning of each shift.
70. a. Dead batteries is the primary reason for AED failure when it is needed to treat a cardiac arrest.
71. d. For citizens in a community to have the best chance of surviving a cardiac event, each of the listed elements has to be present.
72. b. The links in the AHA "Chain of Survival" are early access, early CPR, early defibrillation, and early ACLS.
73. d. An agency's medical director is the only one who can authorize agency use of the device. Any member of the agency who will use the device must meet the training requirements of the medical director.
74. d. This is the role of the medical director; if she wishes to be more directly involved, that is her option.
75. c. Reviewing each AED case for quality assurance is a great tool for improving future training and patient care.
76. d. Talking with the supervisor is a good and often quick way of getting reassurance about your performance on a call, based on the patient care report. However, discussing the call with the medical director following a full case review can give you more specific feedback and thus help you improve your performance on the next call.
77. d. This is a point of discussion for an advanced provider with knowledge of ECGs and how they correlate to specific pathophysiologic findings.
78. d. Any of these examples, and more, could be discussed with your medical director during review of a cardiac arrest call.
79. a. This is an example of what can be assessed and/or improved as a result of a quality improvement review.
80. c. The goal of the quality improvement team is to identify aspects of the system that can be improved, and to develop and implement plans to resolve any weaknesses.
81. b. When an irregular pulse is detected, the EMT-B should count the pulse for a full minute to obtain an accurate rate.
82. a. Not every patient who gets an implanted defibrillator has had a heart attack in the past, and in many the heart's natural pacemaker still works. The problem is that the sick heart has tendency to fire irregularly and can change the rhythm to a lethal one.
83. d. Laying the patient down is the right treatment for a drop in blood pressure. The patient needs ALS, so rapid transport is also appropriate. If ALS cannot meet you en route, call medical control to discuss the patient's condition.
84. a. Always follow your local protocols.
85. d. The EMT-B follows local protocols and medical control, not the orders of the patient's physician.
86. a. These are classic signs of cardiac chest pain.
87. a. The patient's blood pressure is too low; this is a contraindication for the use of nitroglycerin in this patient.
88. d. A drop in blood pressure can cause the patient to feel dizzy or lightheaded. Placing him on the stretcher before administering nitroglycerin is an excellent idea.
89. d. Although there are many different brands, the operation of each AED is very similar.
90. d. Always follow the manufacturer's recommendations for use, care, and maintenance.

Chapter 19: Diabetes, Altered Mental Status, and Seizures

1. b. Type 2 patients are non-insulin-dependent. Though they may require insulin injections for optimal regulation of blood sugar levels and the prevention of complications, insulin injection is not routinely necessary.
2. b. Insulin requires refrigeration, so check the refrigerator quickly to confirm. Searching for needles or syringes could take a lot longer.
3. b. After forming a general impression, the next step is to complete an initial assessment.
4. b. Until a cervical injury can be ruled out, the EMT-B should take C-spine precautions, while assessing and managing the ABCs. This should be followed up with a rapid trauma exam and then a baseline set of vital signs. If a glucometer is available, get a blood sugar reading.
5. b. For the patient with AMS and a diabetic history, the safest approach is to assume that the blood sugar is too low and begin treatment. Hypoglycemia is the more serious condition and can quickly become life-threatening. Of course, calling for ALS, if it is available, is also appropriate.
6. d. Any of the answers are appropriate for this scenario.

7. a. With no further information about the patient's medical history, it is practical for the EMT-B to expect that the patient might vomit during transport, and to be alert for a potential airway problem.

8. b. Seizing patients tend to clench their teeth, drool, experience brief periods of apnea, and sometimes bite their tongues. The NPA is an excellent adjunct for maintaining the airway until the patient becomes alert enough to remove it on his own.

9. d. Many medications, when taken in excess, cause respiratory depression. This patient's rate is within the normal range (12 to 20 bpm); it is shallow, but in a regular pattern. The EMT-B should attempt to place an airway adjunct, provide high-flow oxygen by NRB, and be prepared to assist ventilations if the patient's condition worsens.

10. d. Obtaining this part of the SAMPLE history is typically done concurrently with the focused physical exam, and is completed before providing this type of treatment.

11. d. Each of these products contains a high concentration of glucose, and is commonly used to raise the blood sugar in diabetics.

12. d. The *buccal area* is the space between the cheek and gum. This area and the area under the tongue (sublingual) are highly vascular, which allows for rapid absorption.

13. a. If the patient is not fully alert at this point, transportation should be started. However, many diabetics will refuse transport and the EMT-B will need to stay on the scene and provide additional care until the patient is fully alert and able to sign a refusal form.

14. b. Always follow local protocols!

15. b. The unresponsive diabetic needs glucose fast. If available, request ALS to meet you en route, provide high-flow oxygen, and begin transport. If ALS is not available, call medical control while en route. Do not administer oral glucose to an unresponsive patient, as this may cause airway obstruction or aspiration.

16. d. The combination of too much insulin and not enough food can cause all of the effects listed.

17. a. Appropriate care for the hypoglycemic patient by the EMT-B includes the use of oral glucose under specific criteria and local protocols.

18. d. Left untreated, hypoglycemia can progress to unresponsiveness, seizures (damage to brain cells), coma, and death.

19. a. Insulin moves sugar molecules from the blood into the cells, where the sugar is stored.

20. d. Febrile seizures are very common in the toddler age group. At this age, the thermoregulatory system is still immature and unable to prevent a fever from rising too quickly. It is the rapid change or spike in temperature that causes the seizures.

21. a. The EMT-B should be alert for another seizure with a patient who has just experienced a seizure. This is true whether or not the patient has a history of seizures.

22. c. Seizures are a disruption in one or more neurons in the brain. Prolonged seizures can cause brain damage and must be stopped quickly.

23. b. Infection, dehydration, and new-onset diabetes can also cause AMS, but the history makes this patient a high risk for TIAs and stroke.

24. c. The patient has symptoms of stroke and a history that puts him at high risk for stroke. He needs high-flow oxygen, supportive care, and rapid transport to a stroke center.

25. a. The family has described the patient as having stroke symptoms. The fact that the symptoms are resolving quickly are an indication of mini-stroke (TIA).

26. a. When the body fights an infection, a lot of energy is expended. The diabetic patient can easily use up her glucose reserves when sick or fighting an infection.

27. b. A sudden sickness with fever and AMS suggests an infection. However, hypoglycemia should be ruled out in any patient with AMS.

28. d. The first two conditions to rule out in any patient with an AMS are hypoxia and hypoglycemia.

29. a. This patient has taken an overdose of acetaminophen, which is affecting her liver. Calling medical control to discuss the treatment for an accidental overdose is prudent.

30. a. Perform an initial assessment while managing the ABCs as needed; these are the first steps in caring for any patient.

31. b. The fainting (syncope) and loss of speech are stroke symptoms. Continue the focused physical exam and include a stroke score.

32. a. Serial vital signs and neurological assessments (e.g., stroke score) are especially important in making a diagnosis with any neurological event.

33. c. The history, together with the patient's presentation, suggests that the patient may be hypoglycemic. Oral glucose is indicated; however, it is appropriate to administer oxygen and move the patient off the cold floor, providing warmth, and to obtain vital signs first. By the time these actions are completed, ALS will have arrived.

34. a. The patient is presenting with stroke symptoms even though she appears to be young and healthy. Stroke can occur at any age for a variety of reasons.

35. a. The stroke score assesses for facial symmetry, arm (pronator) drift, and abnormal speech.

Chapter 20: Allergies

1. a. Stridor is associated with the upper airway; wheezing, bronchospasm, and pulmonary edema are associated with the lower airways.

2. c. Signs and symptoms indicating that an allergic reaction *is* progressing to anaphylaxis include respiratory problems, shock, and AMS.

3. d. Jaundice (yellowing) is associated with liver dysfunction, and blisters are not typically associated with an allergic reaction.

4. b. Gloves with powder contain the proteins responsible for latex allergies. Studies indicate that 8 to 12 percent of health care workers who are regularly exposed to latex become sensitized and experience a reaction, such as a rash, to the latex.

5. a. Swelling of the lips can progress to swelling of the airway and should be watched carefully.

6. b. The initial assessment and baseline vital signs indicate that the patient is stable. However, the patient is stating that she is having some type of reaction. Provide supportive care and transport her for further evaluation.

7. a. The patient's airway is open and patent, so begin with the basics. Administer high-flow oxygen by NRB and monitor the airway carefully.

8. d. This patient has serious signs indicating that her allergic reaction is progressing to anaphylaxis. It is important to keep her calm and in a position of comfort while you administer high-flow oxygen. This patient is going to need epinephrine and may deteriorate to a state that requires ventilatory assistance. The EMT-B must anticipate and be prepared for this.

9. a. An unresponsive patient with inadequate respirations and cyanosis is in need of aggressive airway management. Begin by opening the airway; insert an airway adjunct to make sure it stays open, and assist ventilations with a BVM.

10. d. Epi Pen Jr. is the trade name of a pediatric-dose epinephrine auto-injector.

11. c. The generic name is often an abbreviated form of the drug's chemical name.

12. c. Epinephrine is the main treatment in the management of anaphylaxis, because it acts as a bronchodilator.

13. a. The epinephrine auto-injector has a safety cap over a recessed needle, so the cap must be removed first. The device is placed against the patient's thigh muscle (preferable with clothing removed). When the device is pressed against the thigh, a spring-activated plunger pushes the needle into the thigh and injects a dose of the drug. It takes a few seconds to empty the container. Record the time of administration and dispose of the injector in a sharps container.

14. b. The form of epinephrine used for injection is a liquid.

15. c. Signs and symptoms of shock and/or respiratory compromise are indications for calling medical control as soon as possible.

16. a. A history of allergies alone is not an indication for the use of epinephrine as a treatment for allergy. The patient must exhibit signs and symptoms of a severe allergic reaction, such as shock and/or respiratory compromise.

17. a. When the patient is exhibiting any sign or symptom of an allergic reaction that is progressing to anaphylaxis, the EMT-B should call medical control as soon as possible. Do not hesitate to call right away, as anaphylaxis can develop quickly, within minutes.

18. d. Latex is in nearly every medical product we use (e.g., stethoscopes, gloves, tourniquets, bandages, tape); latex is also associated with allergies to foods such as potatoes, bananas, tomatoes, kiwi fruit, papayas, chestnuts, and apricots. The symptoms of a latex reaction include a skin rash and inflammation, respiratory irritation, asthma, and in rare cases, anaphylaxis.

19. d. Many cases of anaphylaxis progress rapidly—within 20 to 30 minutes—from the time of exposure. However, the reaction time can vary from moments to hours.

20. b. The patient is exhibiting local signs of an allergic reaction; this requires continued observation and follow-up with a physician. Transportation to the ED should be strongly recommended in case the condition worsens.

21. c. Any patient with any type of acute anaphylactic reaction needs to be treated with epinephrine. Epinephrine is the main treatment because it acts as a bronchodilator and decreases vascular permeability.

22. d. Because it is a vasoconstrictor, epinephrine decreases the vascular permeability associated with vascular dilation from anaphylaxis.

23. d. The BLS management of anaphylaxis begins with airway maintenance, position of comfort, oxygen administration, and assistance with the administration of an epinephrine self-injector (if the patient has one). Treat for shock and then transport to the nearest hospital.

24. d. An allergic reaction may quickly progress to acute respiratory obstruction and circulatory collapse or anaphylactic shock. The goal in the treatment of anaphylaxis is to rapidly restore respiratory and cardiac efficiency to prevent death.

25. b. Nausea, vomiting, headache, dizziness, seizure, and tachycardia are signs and symptoms of allergic reaction and anaphylaxis. Epinephrine is a very

potent drug and a common side effect associated with it is tachycardia.

26. d. Epinephrine works quickly to relieve bronchoconstriction and improve blood pressure. However, side effects include tachycardia and palpitations.

27. c. Epinephrine is to be used with caution in patients who are more than 50 years old and have preexisting dysrhythmias. However, in a life-threatening situation, there is no real contraindication because the medication could be life-saving.

28. a. The adult auto-injection contains 0.3 mg and the pediatric auto-injector contains 0.15 mg.

29. c. Epinephrine is a very potent drug that increases the workload on the heart. Tachycardia is common in patients of any age following the administration of epinephrine; those who are over 50 years of age and who have preexisting heart conditions may experience life-threatening dysrhythmias, including ventricular fibrillation.

30. c. Epinephrine is fast-acting, taking effect within seconds, but the effects are short-lasting (about 10 to 20 minutes).

Chapter 21: Poisoning/Overdose

1. b. Pediatric ingestions of toxic substances account for a significant percentage of the total number of toxic emergencies in the United States. Unattended children and failure to "childproof" homes are the major reasons that children are at high risk for toxic exposures, especially ingestion.

2. c. Carbon monoxide is a colorless and odorless gas that may be inhaled.

3. b. Pesticides may be ingested by eating unwashed fruits or vegetables, or may be inhaled during application. However, by and large pesticides get into the body by absorption through the skin. Lead paint and mushrooms are ingested and CO is inhaled.

4. b. Just about any body system may be affected by a toxic emergency. The most dangerous toxic substances affect the nervous system, respiratory system, and the endocrine or metabolic systems. The most significant problems occur when substances cause abnormalities in airway, breathing, circulation, or level of consciousness. The type and amount of toxic substance, as well as length of exposure, will have an effect on the severity of the toxic emergency.

5. d. The most dangerous toxic substances affect the nervous system, the respiratory system, and the endocrine or metabolic systems.

6. d. The most significant problems associated with poisoning are those that affect the ABCs.

7. d. The EMT-B must consider other causes of altered mental status that can resemble intoxication (e.g., hypoxia, hypoglycemia, or trauma) and attempt to rule them out.

8. c. The ABCs are stable, so a focused history and physical exam are appropriate at this point in the scenario.

9. c. The care of a child often includes supportive care for an adult or caregiver of the child. That person is often upset or frightened; may have feelings of mis-

giving, fault, guilt, or remorse; and may need reassurance and understanding.

10. d. Without contaminating yourself or crew, the patients should be removed from the possible source of the chemical that potentially caused the symptoms. Administer oxygen while obtaining a focused history. If the patients have any chemicals on their clothing, have them remove the contaminated items. Obtain an MSDS and proceed to treat as recommended there.

11. c. This question would be more appropriate for a patient with an allergy than for a possible poisoning.

12. c. Do not wait for EMS. Pediatric ingestions of toxic substances account for a significant percentage of the total number of toxic emergencies.

13. c. As always, begin with the ABCs. Insert an airway adjunct and assist with ventilations, as this patient's respiratory rate and effort are too low.

14. d. The initial assessment of this patient shows an unresponsive patient with snoring respirations and good circulation. Consider taking C-spine precautions until more information is obtained. Unless the patient is deeply unresponsive with no gag reflex, an NPA is the best adjunct.

15. c. Any chemical exposure in the eyes requires quick treatment, with continuous irrigation right through to arrival at the ED. Remove the patient's shirt and any other clothing that may have chemical product on it.

16. d. Activated charcoal in its slurry form is black. It looks and tastes unpleasant. A common method for getting a patient to drink the slurry is to place it in a foam cup with a lid on it and have the patient sip it through a straw.

17. d. The generic name of a drug is often an abbreviated form of the drug's chemical name.

18. a. Activated charcoal is administered in a liquid slurry (syrup) form.

19. c. At this point you are out-resourced, with five patients and one ambulance. Declare an MCI, triage

the patients, request the appropriate resources, and then begin treatment and transport.

20. a. Call for medical direction whenever you have a concern about a specific treatment. If you know what the product is, calling poison control is another option.

21. c. Calling medical direction for advice is appropriate, but not before managing the ABCs. Consider the use of an NPA for a seizing patient; administer high-flow oxygen and be prepared to suction and ventilate as needed.

22. c. Activated charcoal is a treatment option for aspirin overdose, with orders from medical direction. The patient must be alert and able to swallow to administer activated charcoal.

23. b. Without a blood test, it is not possible to know how much of the toxin was eliminated from the body. Activated charcoal is indicated in this case, with orders from medical direction.

24. d. To administer activated charcoal, the patient must be alert and able to swallow. The concern is for possible aspiration.

25. c. Medical control may have more specific treatment options for the patient.

26. d. Do not hesitate to call for medical direction whenever you have a concern about a specific treatment.

27. c. Activated charcoal binds immediately to a variety of substances, inhibiting GI absorption thereof.

28. d. Activated charcoal does not cause decreased mental status. However, the ingested poison or overdose may cause AMS.

29. a. The dose of activated charcoal is 1 gram per kilogram of body weight in an adult.

30. b. After the initial assessment, it is appropriate to obtain vital signs while you obtain a focused history and proceed with a focused physical exam.

Chapter 22: Environmental Emergencies

1. d. *Evaporation* is loss of heat at the surface from vaporization of liquid (e.g., sweating).

2. c. *Convection* is the transfer of heat by the circulation of heated particles (e.g., cooling soup by blowing on it).

3. b. *Conduction* is the transmission of heat from a warmer object to cooler objects in direct contact (e.g., lying on a cold surface).

4. a. Deeply frostbitten skin has a white, waxy appearance. It feels hard, as if frozen. Generally there is a complete loss of sensation that does not recover within a short time.

5. a. Diminished coordination and psychomotor function set in quickly and progress rapidly after a sudden and extreme exposure, such as falling into freezing water.

6. c. Decreasing mental status is the most significant indication that a patient's condition is becoming critical, in either a hot or a cold exposure.

7. b. Manage the ABCs first as needed. Then quickly splint the extremity to prevent further damage, gently move the patient out of the cold, remove any wet clothing to prevent further heat loss, and begin to warm the patient.

8. a. The priority is to prevent any further heat loss. Move the patient into a warm environment, remove any wet clothing, and begin to warm the patient.

9. b. The patient should not bear any weight on the extremity, and the EMT-B should carefully splint it. Presuming that transportation will not take too long, it is appropriate to just keep the extremity from rewarming and let the ED provide additional care for the injury. Follow local protocol!

10. d. The loss of fluid and electrolytes is a significant factor in the development of heat illness. Signs and symptoms of dehydration associated with prolonged heat exposure may include any of those seen with heat illness and a rapid weight loss (typically more than 7 percent of body weight).

11. d. Weak pulse, shock, and AMS are later signs of more severe heat illness.

12. b. The most significant signs or symptoms are those that affect the ABCs.

13. a. The scenario describes a febrile seizure. The proper steps to take are to remove warm clothing and allow the child to cool off. Provide oxygen to the patient and supportive care to the parents and transport the patient in his car seat for evaluation.

14. d. Each of the steps described is appropriate treatment. The ABCs must be managed first and the patient must be cooled.

15. d. As the body temperature climbs rapidly, to 104°F to 106°F, a life-threatening emergency develops. Treatment must be rapid or the patient will progress from AMS, to convulsions, brain damage or renal failure, and death.

16. d. The MOI, together with the loss of consciousness, indicates the potential for a head or spinal injury. Cervical precautions must be taken immediately and continued until head and spinal injuries can be ruled out.

17. c. A prolonged exposure in any body of water will cause heat loss leading to hypothermia.

18. b. The patient has symptoms of decompression sickness. The history is key here. Anyone who has breathed compressed air underwater is at risk for

decompression illness. Any patient with a complaint of joint soreness 24 to 48 hours after a dive should be considered for decompression therapy.

19. b. Hypoxia can result from aspiration of any type of fluid, not just during a near-drowning.

20. b. When examining victims of near-drowning, it is important to note that they may initially appear normal, but typically will develop symptoms that affect breathing and respiration (e.g., progressive dyspnea, wheezing, and cyanosis).

21. b. Factors typically associated with drowning include: use of alcohol, teenage male in his 20s, spinal injury, and hypothermia. Frostbite is seldom a factor.

22. d. Regardless of the patient's age, a human bite that breaks the skin should be evaluated. The patient's tetanus vaccination must be verified or brought up to date, and the wound must be cleaned and dressed to prevent infection.

23. d. When it is not known what type of snake made the bite, the general wound care for this type of injury includes managing the ABCs, splinting the extremity, keeping the patient still, and transporting the patient to the ED.

24. a. Assessment and care are the same for every patient. Assess and manage the ABCs, then proceed with the focused history and physical exam, treating as you go.

25. b. *SCUBA* stands for self-contained underwater breathing apparatus.

26. a. Decompression illness or the bends is a sickness occurring during or after ascent secondary to a rapid release of nitrogen bubbles from the blood.

27. b. Anyone who has breathed compressed air underwater is at risk for decompression illness. Snorkeling does not involve breathing compressed air.

28. b. *Frostbite* is the formation of ice crystals within the tissues. These crystals damage the blood vessels and other tissues.

29. c. The young, the elderly, and intoxicated individuals are at a higher risk for developing hypothermia.

The young and elderly have immature or failing thermoregulatory systems and intoxicated persons have impaired judgment; these factors predispose these groups to develop hypothermia.

30. a. Small marine animal stings (e.g., Portuguese man-of-war, lionfish, jellyfish, sea urchins) are very painful. Heat is typically more effective than ice in destroying the venom of marine organisms. Generally, unless anaphylaxis is present, no medication is warranted.

31. a. Because the patient has no history of seizures, and this episode occurred in the pool, the EMT-B must consider a possible traumatic injury as the MOI for the seizure. Attempt to get more information about the possible MOI as you begin a rapid trauma assessment.

32. c. A submersion or near-drowning occurs when the process of drowning is interrupted or reversed. The victim of near-drowning may appear normal initially, with symptoms (e.g., difficulty breathing, wheezing, tachycardia, or cyanosis) developing over the next few hours. The patient was also witnessed having seizure activity, though she had no prior history of seizures, and this must be followed up.

33. c. Symptoms of a black widow spider bite include feeling a small sting at the site followed by a dull ache. The patient will develop severe muscle spasms, especially in the abdomen, chest, back, and shoulders. The bite from a tick or brown recluse spider is typically not felt and may go unnoticed for hours. The bite of a fire ant is very painful. The area becomes red, swollen, and the bites produce vesicles that are filled with fluid.

34. a. Abdominal rigidity is another indication of a black widow spider bite. Management of this patient includes wound care, supportive care for shock, and transport.

35. a. Shivering is the body's heat-producing mechanism; it begins when the core body temperature (CBT) is around 95°F and may continue for a few hours until the body's energy reserves are depleted.

Chapter 23: Behavioral Emergencies

1. a. Fasting (purposely abstaining from eating for a specified period) is an accepted practice for many reasons, including religious observance. However, if fasting is prolonged, it may lead to physical and psychological emergencies.

2. d. A *behavioral emergency* is a display of abnormal behavior, which typically results from a perceived crisis in a person's life.

3. a. An *emotion* is a psychological and physical reaction that is subjectively experienced as a strong feeling.

4. b. The EMT-B must rule out hypoxia first (administer oxygen) and hypoglycemia next for any patient exhibiting altered mental status.

5. d. There are many causes of abnormal or unusual changes in a person's behavior.

6. a. This statement is a classic example of something a person experiencing a behavioral emergency might say or agree to if asked. The remaining selections involve the patient's history, and a history alone does not indicate that the patient is currently experiencing a behavioral emergency.

7. d. Any major stress or accumulation of minor stresses can lead to psychological crisis (e.g., behavioral emergency).

8. a. A *crisis* is an emotionally significant event or radical change of status in a person's life.

9. b. Any injury or illness creates some form of psychological stress for the patient. How well the patient manages that stress is based on many factors, including past experiences and level of distress. The remaining statements are inaccurate.

10. a. Paranoia is a personality disorder in which the affected individual tends toward excessive or irrational suspicion and distrustfulness of others.

11. d. Any patients who have indicated that they want to harm themselves or have attempted to harm themselves must be transported for evaluation.

12. c. Depression is a dejected state of mind accompanied by feelings of sadness, discouragement, and hopelessness. Patients often exhibit reduced activity levels, an inability to function, and sleep disturbances. Depending on the patient, severe depression may also be accompanied by lack of self-care. This, by itself, could worsen any underlying medical condition. Studies have also shown that depressed people have a higher incidence of cardiovascular disease.

13. c. Numerous cases in the medicolegal literature report serious patient injury from inappropriate restraint techniques. Face-down restraint carries a high risk of patient suffocation, especially if the patient is violent.

14. d. Always follow the directions of medical control, as well as your local protocols.

15. a. Personal safety and the safety of the crew is always the first priority. Protecting the patient and bystanders comes next.

16. a. Rapid intervention is necessary for a behavioral emergency, but intervention does not always mean rapid transport. Unless the patient is also experiencing a medical emergency that requires rapid transport, the EMT-B should be prepared to spend extra time with the patient to avoid further agitating the patient.

17. d. Organic problems can cause or worsen an emotional illness. Be alert for organic or emotional causes (e.g., drug-induced sedation or psychosis).

18. d. Any injury or illness creates some form of psychological stress for the patient. The stress may cause minor behavioral changes or total crisis following a trauma or illness, so the EMT-B must assess the patient thoroughly to rule out a physical cause.

19. d. The EMT-B may provoke a violent action by the way she is dressed (e.g., uniform similar to that of a police officer) or behaves (e.g., rushed or aggressive.)

20. b. Behavioral clues indicating that a patient could become violent include yelling, cursing, clenched fists, nervous pacing, or verbal or physical threats.

21. d. Aggressive or violent behavior by a patient is classically an attempt to gain control of the situation.

22. a. Physical and chemical restraints are dangerous for the patient and a high risk for the person restraining the patient. Numerous cases in the medicolegal literature report serious patient injury from inappropriate restraint techniques.

23. d. The EMT-B should attempt to calm the patient by establishing a rapport with the patient using therapeutic interviewing techniques. Despite the need for physical restraint, attempt to help the patient maintain his dignity, and ask for permission to assess him. Limit the physical assessment to vital signs and any other absolutely necessary evaluations.

24. d. During an anxiety or panic attack, the patient will feel as though she is overwhelmed and has lost control. The EMT-B must assure the patient that he is here to take care of her now and will help her to begin to regain control.

25. c. Restraint options vary from system to system. Always follow medical control and local protocols!

26. a. During a behavioral emergency, the patient may feel overwhelmed or that he has lost control. The EMT-B must demonstrate control in a calm, professional, and nonthreatening manner to help the patient begin to cope with the present situation.

27. d. The patient's appearance, hygiene, and dress can all provide clues to a possible behavioral or psychiatric disorder. Some people with behavioral problems (both organic and psychiatric) exhibit an abnormal lack of regard for their own personal hygiene.

28. c. Rapid intervention is necessary for a behavioral emergency, but intervention does not always mean rapid transport. Unless the patient is also experiencing a medical emergency that requires rapid transport, the EMT-B should be prepared to spend extra time with the patient to avoid further upsetting the patient.

29. a. Therapeutic interview techniques include engaging in active listening while limiting interruptions, being supportive and empathetic, and centering questions on the immediate problem.

30. a. Males tend to use more violent means of suicide, and that makes them more successful than females. For the same reason, females make more attempts at suicide than males.

Chapter 24: Obstetrics/Gynecology

1. c. The umbilical cord, which connects the fetus with the placenta, contains two umbilical arteries and one umbilical vein.

2. b. The placenta is often referred to as the *afterbirth* because it is delivered in the third stage of labor, after delivery of the baby.

3. c. The examiner can best feel contractions of the uterus by placing a hand on the top of the uterus (top of the abdomen). This muscle contraction is quite strong as it pushes the fetus down the birth canal.

4. a. The contents of an obstetric kit are sterile prior to opening of the kit.

5. a. If the patient delivers the placenta before arriving at the hospital, the EMT-B should save it for inspection. The placenta can be transported in a plastic bag from the obstetrical kit or in a large pan.

6. a. A commercially prepared obstetric kit includes: sterile surgical gloves, disposable sheets for draping the mother, 4 × 4 gauze pads, a small rubber-bulb syringe, cord clamps, surgical scissors or blade, infant swaddler, sanitary napkins, and a plastic bag for the placenta.

7. c. The first step to take when a patient suddenly becomes unresponsive is to assess for breathing and a pulse. A pregnant patient in her third trimester may lose consciousness when placed in a supine position. When the large fetus lies directly on the vena cava, as it does in the supine position, blood return to the heart can be severely restricted, causing a loss of consciousness. The remedy is easy: turn the patient on her side.

8. c. The signs and symptoms of abruptio placenta that distinguish this obstetrical emergency from others are the sudden onset of severe abdominal pain and blood loss that is not always apparent, because it may be trapped behind the placenta.

9. a. The sign and symptom of placenta previa that distinguishes this obstetrical emergency from others is blood loss that can be significant; however, the patient usually experiences no pain.

10. a. Crowning indicates that the baby is ready to be delivered. Stop the ambulance and assist with the delivery. Call for additional help if needed.

11. c. The feeling of having to move her bowels comes from the baby being in the birth canal and pressing on the rectum. This is a reliable sign that the baby is being delivered.

12. a. Contractions that are 5 minutes apart are an indication that there is enough time to begin transport to the hospital.

13. c. Braxton Hicks contractions, or false labor, are irregular and often painless. These contractions are practice contractions that prepare the uterus for the

real thing. They can begin as early as the first trimester, but more often occur in the third trimester.

14. a. Eclampsia is the most serious condition of hypertension during pregnancy, and usually occurs between 20 weeks and 1 week postpartum. Eclampsia is marked by convulsive seizures and coma and is a life-threatening condition for both mother and fetus.

15. a. Request ALS to meet you and provide care as for any other seizure patient. Manage the airway, provide high-flow oxygen, and assist ventilations if needed. Begin gentle but rapid transport.

16. a. Pregnant women are predisposed to nausea and vomiting because of the pressure of the fetus on the stomach. Always be alert for vomiting.

17. c. Allowing the spouse and/or friend to be present during the delivery is an accepted and appropriate practice. This may help to keep the patient relaxed and better able to concentrate on your instructions.

18. d. The patient should be lying back with her head elevated and knees flexed, preferably on your stretcher.

19. c. It is rare to be exposed to CSF during childbirth.

20. a. Childbirth is messy. Eye protection, or face mask, gloves, and a gown, are recommended for an EMT-B who is assisting with childbirth.

21. a. Childbirth is messy and risk of exposure to body fluids is high. The EMT-B who assists with childbirth should use a high level of protection.

22. d. The third stage of labor is the delivery of the placenta. During this time and after the delivery of the placenta, the patient should be monitored for excessive blood loss and signs of shock.

23. c. Nuchal cord (umbilical cord wrapped around the neck) is not uncommon during childbirth. Immediately after the head delivers, the EMT-B must look to see if this condition is present. If it is, the cord must be carefully lifted off the neck and over the head without tearing the cord.

24. d. As the head begins to emerge from the vaginal opening, the EMT-B must place a gloved hand gently over the head to prevent an explosive birth, which can rip and tear the mother's perineum.

25. a. After assessing the neck for a wrapped cord, the EMT-B can begin to suction the baby's mouth and nose while waiting for the next contraction.

26. d. Once the head is delivered, the EMT-B can begin to suction the baby's mouth and nose while waiting for the next contraction. The mouth is suctioned first, because the baby takes its first breath through the mouth.

27. b. The most common presentation of the baby through the vaginal opening is face down, although

face up is very common, too. From there the baby's head will turn to the side.

28. d. Almost any sterile cutting device may be used, although a sterile blade or scissors is preferable.

29. d. When a nuchal cord cannot be unwrapped from the baby's neck, the EMT-B must clamp and cut the cord to prevent the baby from rapidly deteriorating.

30. b. The bleeding must be controlled immediately, because even a little blood loss is a lot for a newborn. Keep the first clamp in place and use a second clamp proximal to the first; then reassess.

31. a. The placenta is a large organ, and it is easy to see when a piece is missing. Any portion of the placenta that is left undelivered can cause moderate to severe bleeding.

32. d. The contractions that expel the placenta may be as painful as the contractions experienced during delivery of the baby.

33. d. The placenta must be inspected for completeness, because any potion of the placenta that is left undelivered can cause serious hemorrhaging.

34. b. The care for this patient is the same as for any patient with hemorrhagic shock.

35. d. The *perineum* is the area between the anus and the vaginal opening. This area can tear during delivery (especially with the first baby), causing a wound that looks like a laceration.

36. d. For uncomplicated childbirth, postpartum care of the mother includes giving supportive care, making her comfortable, and reassessing her for signs of shock.

37. d. When drying, warming, and suctioning do not stimulate the baby to breathe normally immediately after birth, the EMT-B should administer oxygen. If oxygen does not improve respiratory effort, ventilations by BVM must be started.

38. d. Holding a baby upside down or by the feet is unsafe and not an acceptable practice.

39. d. A heart rate of less than 60 beats per minute at 1 minute after delivery is critically low and requires cardiopulmonary resuscitation.

40. d. The EMT-B should assist in the delivery of a breech presentation (buttocks first) by supporting the buttocks and legs as they deliver, to prevent pulling and tearing of the neck muscles as the baby's head delivers.

41. d. This condition is prolapsed cord and it is a true emergency. Begin safe but rapid transport.

42. c. A limb presentation is a complication of childbirth that the EMT-B should not attempt to deliver. This type of delivery may require cesarean section.

43. c. Identical twins develop from the same cell, are the same gender, and share the same placenta. Fraternal twins develop from two separate cells and each has its own placenta.

44. b. Twin babies are smaller than single babies at birth and often are premature.

45. d. Additional help will be needed to care for and transport twins, but assistance with the delivery is the same as for a single baby. The first baby is usually the biggest and delivers head first. The second baby is usually smaller and breech.

46. d. The aspiration of meconium is dangerous because it causes serious complications in the lungs, including respiratory infection and death.

47. a. The mouth and nose should be suctioned as soon as the head is delivered. If meconium is still present after delivery, do not stimulate the baby until additional suctioning to remove the meconium has been completed.

48. d. Meconium is the baby's first bowel movement, which may occur while in the uterus when the baby is under stress or is overdue for delivery.

49. d. Each of the answers provided is a reason that a premature infant is at high risk for losing body heat.

50. b. Premature infants are at higher risk than full-term babies for developing hypothermia because they have a very small amount of body fat and a larger body surface area in relation to their weight; also the temperature regulating system of a premature infant is too immature to be reliable.

51. a. A premature baby weighs less than 5.5 pounds or is born before 38 weeks gestation.

52. c. This patient complaining of abdominal pain has signs of internal bleeding (pale skin, persistent tachycardia); management includes high-flow oxygen and treatment for shock. Pale skin and tachycardia maybe associated with severe pain alone, but the EMT-B should consider the more serious condition of shock first and treat for that.

53. d. The combination of all these symptoms suggests an STD.

54. d. The EMT-B should consider any female of childbearing age who is complaining of abdominal pain to be experiencing an ectopic pregnancy (a life-threatening condition) until proven otherwise (e.g., a negative pregnancy test at the ED).

55. c. The consumption of vitamin A supplements during pregnancy has been shown to cause irregular fetal development.

56. c. The body's self-preservation mechanism shunts blood from all areas of the body, including the fetus, to the mother's vital organs (brain, heart, and lungs).

57. d. For the baby to survive, the mother must survive until reaching the ED/OR.

58. b. Full-term gestation is 38 to 42 weeks. Less than 38 weeks is premature and more than 42 weeks is overdue.

59. c. The amniotic sac is actually a thin fetal membrane that forms a closed sac around the fetus and contains serous fluid in which the fetus is immersed.

60. c. The *perineum* is the area between the anus and the vaginal opening.

Chapter 25: Bleeding and Shock

1. b. The primary function of the circulatory system is to provide a continuous source of nutrients and oxygen to the tissues.
2. b. The plasma portion of blood carries cells and nutrients to all body tissues.
3. d. The functions of blood include providing nutrients to tissues, sustaining fluid balance, and temperature regulation.
4. a. Venous bleeding is characterized by dark blood with a steady flow.
5. a. Arterial bleeding is characterized by bright red blood with a fast flow that may pulse with each heartbeat.
6. c. Skin abrasions are associated with capillary bleeding, which is characterized by dark blood with very slow bleeding.
7. c. Using gravity to help control bleeding works well. Raising the bleeding extremity above the level of the heart helps to slow bleeding.
8. d. The steps in controlling any external hemorrhage include applying direct pressure and elevating the injured area. When bleeding continues, apply a pressure dressing and use a pressure point.
9. d. The EMT-B should use a tourniquet to control bleeding only when all other methods have failed and the bleeding is life-threatening. Once a tourniquet is applied in the prehospital setting, it cannot be removed.
10. b. Handwashing is the single best method of preventing disease transmission.
11. b. Hepatitis is easily transmitted from persons who exhibit no signs or symptoms of the disease. Health care providers are at risk of exposure when PPE is not used with every single patient.
12. d. Even a large amount of blood poses no risk when there is no contact with it.
13. d. To avoid an airway problem from draining of a nosebleed, have the patient lean forward and instruct him to spit out the blood. Ingested blood causes nausea.
14. d. When a patient who is immobilized to a long board gives notice that she is going to vomit, release the stretcher straps, keep the patient secured to the long backboard, and turn the patient on the board.
15. b. A poor mask seal is the most obvious reason for an air leak.
16. d. Any of these forces, when sustained in a MVC, can cause internal injuries.
17. d. A head, ankle, or spinal injury does not produce enough blood loss to cause shock.
18. d. The diaphragm, liver, large intestine, and right lung are all within reach of a 3-inch knife blade in the URQ of the abdomen.
19. d. Early signs of shock caused by intraabdominal bleeding are persistent tachycardia with normal or low blood pressure. As shock progresses, the blood pressure will drop, and the patient will feel weak, dizzy, or lightheaded and may pass out.
20. b. In the prehospital setting, bowel sounds are not a reliable assessment finding. To properly assess bowel sounds, the evaluator must listen for at least a couple of minutes before the patient moves or any palpation of the abdomen is done. If there is time to listen, the one finding that is significant is complete absence of bowel sounds for at least 2 minutes.
21. c. When a patient is exhibiting signs and symptoms of shock with no apparent reason, the EMT-B should consider the patient to have intraabdominal bleeding, until it can be ruled out in the ED. Treat the patient for shock!
22. d. This patient is exhibiting signs of decompensating shock. He needs ALS en route to the hospital and will likely require emergency surgery.
23. c. The MOI indicates that the patient needs full spinal immobilization. Any drainage from the ears should not be occluded. If the drainage is cerebrospinal fluid, the ear should be covered lightly with a gauze dressing that allows nothing in yet permits continuous drainage.
24. a. The steps in controlling any external hemorrhage begin with applying direct pressure.
25. b. During hypoperfusion, the body shunts blood away from nonvital organs (e.g., skin and intestines) to vital organs (e.g., brain, heart, and lungs). This causes the skin to appear pale, moist, and cool, especially in the extremities and face.
26. c. With severe blood loss, the oxygen-carrying red blood cells are lost and the tissues suffer a decrease in their oxygen supply (hypoxia).
27. c. In an effort to compensate for a loss of blood volume, the body will increase the heart rate and effort and constrict blood vessels to maintain the blood pressure.
28. d. This patient is exhibiting signs of decompensating shock. He needs ALS en route to the hospital, if available.
29. b. The patient could not have lost enough blood from this injury to develop anything but psychogenic shock.
30. d. The blood loss from a single femur fracture over the first hour can be as much as one to two liters. Two femur fractures from a significant MOI like this can quickly produce a state of decompensating shock.
31. c. Studies have shown that patients have the best chance of survival from a significant traumatic

MOI if they can reach an OR in less than one hour. This is the "Golden Hour" concept. Barring extrication, EMS should take no longer than 10 minutes (the "Platinum Ten") on the scene with this type of patient.

32. d. A significant MOI alone makes a patient a high priority; however, in the less common case when signs of shock are also present, the decision to provide rapid transport is absolute.

33. a. Definitive care of the patient with internal bleeding is most often done in the OR.

34. d. The potential for abdominal trauma is often overlooked or unrecognized in early assessments. This leads to a high mortality for victims of abdominal trauma. The key to correcting this is for the EMS provider to quickly and properly associate certain injury patterns with specific MOIs and make a proper priority treatment decision for the patient. This is one area in which the EMT-B can make life-saving decisions.

35. c. The severity of a hemorrhage can best be determined when you can get an estimate of how much blood has been lost.

Chapter 26: Soft-Tissue Injuries

1. b. The major functions of the skin include temperature, water, and electrolyte regulation; protection from the environment; and sensing touch.

2. a. One of the major functions of the skin is to protect the body from the environment, by keeping bacteria and other sources of infection out.

3. d. One of the major functions of the skin is to help regulate water and electrolytes in the body. When a large body surface is affected by trauma, such as when it is burned, the patient loses a large amount of fluids; this condition can rapidly lead to hypovolemic shock if fluids are not adequately restored.

4. c. The order of the layers of the skin, from the surface to the underlying tissue or muscle, is the epidermis, dermis, and subcutaneous tissues.

5. d. The subcutaneous tissues are the layers of skin that lie below the dermis and attach the upper layers of skin to the underlying muscles and/or bones.

6. d. Subcutaneous tissue is comprised of fatty tissue and lies below the dermis.

7. a. The first responders have indicated that there is no external bleeding or open wounds. At a minimum, gloves are needed to further assess the patient.

8. a. Abrasions create capillary bleeding, a slow oozing of blood. At a minimum, gloves should be donned prior to examining and treating this patient.

9. c. Scalp wounds can bleed a lot, and any blood in the airway creates a high risk of exposure for the rescuer. Blood that is spit can spray into the rescuer's face. Gloves, eye protection, and a mask are recommended for managing these injuries.

10. a. A soft-tissue injury that involves bone with no broken skin is a closed injury.

11. b. Edema is an abnormal condition that results when fluid leaks into areas of soft tissue.

12. a. A *contusion* is an injury to the soft tissue with no broken skin.

13. a. Facial fractures must be considered. The EMT-B should palpate the facial bones for stability and crepitus.

14. d. In this case, blood in the eye (*hyphema*) requires no specific treatment by EMS. However, the eye should be examined by a physician to rule out any complications.

15. a. The treatment for soft-tissue injury with a possible fracture includes splinting, elevation, and applying cold for pain relief.

16. a. An occlusive dressing provides an airtight seal over a penetrating injury to the chest, back, or abdomen.

17. b. A pericardial tamponade is a condition in which fluid fills the sac around the heart. This sac does not expand, so the fluid keeps the heart from effectively filling during contractions. If this condition is not quickly recognized and managed, the patient will die.

18. a. A penetrating wound to the chest can create what is referred to as a sucking chest wound. Each time the patient inhales, air is drawn into the chest through the wound. The air does not reach the lungs, but instead fills the chest, creating a pneumothorax. An occlusive dressing should be applied quickly.

19. a. An occlusive dressing should be applied immediately to help prevent the development of a pneumothorax or tension pneumothorax.

20. a. The object should be immobilized in place with bulky dressings to prevent further movement of the object.

21. b. An injury in the area described should not have penetrated the chest cavity; therefore, direct pressure and bandaging should be appropriate. If you suspect that the chest cavity has been penetrated, then apply an occlusive dressing.

22. d. An extremity that is red and hot to the touch is a sign of severe infection that requires immediate evaluation and care at the ED.

23. c. Exposed bowels should be kept moist with a moist dressing and warmth. Never attempt to replace bowel in the abdomen in the prehospital setting.

24. d. In addition to a penetrating abdominal injury, a gunshot wound can also create any of these

associated injuries: chest trauma, rib or spinal fractures, and spinal cord injury. The EMT-B must be highly suspicious of and alert for these potential injuries.

25. a. An electrical burn can create significant internal tissue damage that is not readily apparent and may require the care of a burn specialty unit. The other burns described are minor ones that can be managed at any ED.

26. c. A partial-thickness burn covering the upper thigh (less than 9 percent BSA) is classified as a moderate burn.

27. a. The terms *superficial, partial thickness,* and *full thickness* all describe the depth of a burn.

28. b. With no blistering present, this can be called a superficial burn. The BSA involved is the face, at 4½ percent, and the front of both arms, at 4½ percent each, for a total of 13½ percent BSA.

29. a. With no blistering present, this can be called a superficial burn. Because the eyes are involved, however, this is a serious burn that requires the care of a burn specialty unit.

30. b. A superficial or first-degree burn is a mild burn characterized by pain, redness, and heat on the affected area with no blistering or charring.

31. d. The thighs have superficial burns from the splashing; the dermis of the lower legs has been affected, making the injury in that area a partial-thickness burn.

32. b. A second-degree or partial-thickness burn involves the epidermal and dermal layers of the skin.

33. d. The risk for infection comes with damage to layers of the skin below the epidermis.

34. c. The hands are considered a critical body area when affected by burns. The severity of the burn on the hands is also greater than the other areas affected.

35. a. The dermis contains many nerve endings, and a second-degree or partial-thickness burn will produce severe pain in the affected area.

36. d. This will vary depending on the specific body areas involved, but typically a partial-thickness or second-degree burn will not affect subcutaneous fat.

37. a. A full-thickness or third-degree burn involves all the layers of the skin in the affected area.

38. a. The immediate and potentially life-threatening injuries are the airway injuries that resulted from a blast in a confined area. The patient is exhibiting wheezing and may rapidly progress to severe respiratory distress or arrest.

39. c. A full-thickness or third-degree burn involves all layers of the skin in the affected area. The area may appear charred and feel rough. The area around a full-thickness burn may also be affected to a lesser degree and appear blistered and weeping, or may not be affected at all.

40. d. The injury described includes second- and third-degree burns.

41. d. A full-thickness or third-degree burn is characterized as a severe burn that affects all layers of the skin and may affect underlying muscle.

42. a. The description includes partial- and full-thickness burns that involve 12 percent BSA. The most critical factor with this patient is age. The young, the elderly, and patients with impaired immune systems do not recover well from burn injuries.

43. c. It is not appropriate to remove debris from a burn area, but it is appropriate to flush the area with cool water.

44. b. Determining the source of the burn is part of the scene size-up and identification of the MOI. This must be done before a full assessment can be made and proper treatment begun.

45. b. Management of a superficial burn may include flushing the area with cool water.

46. a. All clothing, including socks and shoes, must be removed, because they could contain some of the chemical and continue the burning process.

47. c. When such a large BSA is affected, a clean dry sheet can be used to cover and protect the patient during treatment and transport.

48. d. Quick removal of these items is appropriate because they can retain heat and continue to burn. The jewelry (especially rings) must be removed before tissue swelling from edema impairs circulation.

49. d. Each of these management steps is appropriate for this patient.

50. b. A circumferential burn on an extremity can constrict blood flow to the distal portion of the extremity, creating a limb-threatening condition.

51. c. Stop the burning process! Flush with water until the chemical is completely removed.

52. b. The use of sterile dressings will help to prevent any further contamination of an open wound.

53. c. Children (especially toddler to preschool age) often engage in magical thinking. Traumatic injuries with bleeding can be very frightening. Covering the wound quickly can help some children to keep from thinking they are going to die.

54. a. A bandage is used to keep a dressing in place.

55. a. Never rupture a blister that has developed from a burn. The risk of infection increases significantly when blisters are disturbed.

56. c. In addition to controlling a bleed, the use of a bandage will help reduce the risk of further contamination and possible infection.

57. a. The management of an abdominal evisceration includes the use of a large trauma dressing to cover the contents. The dressing should be moistened and kept warm to help preserve the bowel.

58. a. A blood pressure cuff inflated to occlude venous flow only (no greater than 70 mm Hg) may be used to help control bleeding from an extremity when other methods have not worked.

59. a. A pressure bandage is applied directly onto the open wound.

60. d. The steps for controlling continuous bleeding are: direct pressure, elevation, pressure bandage, and pressure on a pressure point.

61. d. The knife is long enough to reach each of the listed organs except the trachea.

62. d. Manage the ABCs, immobilize the patient, and begin rapid transport. Request ALS, if available, to meet you en route.

63. d. Wheezing is a sign of respiratory distress. In this case, the MOI is significant (working on a fire scene). Firefighters tend to initially downplay or ignore injury or illness while on the job, and this can cause both a delay in recognizing early signs and symptoms and a delay in treatment.

64. d. Increased tissue damage is a major complication commonly associated with improperly applied dressings. Loss of limb and death may occur, but are not common.

65. b. The use of a tourniquet is a method of last resort for controlling a severe arterial bleed. The tourniquet should be placed above the open wound. A strap or wide band of cloth can be used to occlude arterial blood flow. Do not use any smaller object, such as string, rope, or wire, as it can cause additional tissue damage at the site where it is applied. Once a tourniquet is applied, it cannot be removed in the prehospital setting; the ED should be notified immediately.

66. b. Keep the extremity elevated above the level of the heart and apply a pressure bandage.

67. c. Protect yourself first by applying the appropriate PPE for the situation.

68. a. Never remove an impaled object. Stabilize it in place.

69. d. Removing an impaled object from an extremity can cause further damage to blood vessels, nerves, and muscles.

70. d. Control the bleeding and, whenever possible, bring the amputated body part with the patient to the hospital for possible reattachment or reimplantation.

71. a. The use of dry ice on an amputated body part can cause irreversible tissue damage and failure of reattachment or reimplantation.

72. b. Lay the patient down before he falls down. The blood loss is not enough to cause hypovolemic shock, but the patient maybe experiencing psychogenic shock.

73. d. Wet or dry ice should never be placed directly on an amputated part. Freezing can occur and cause irreversible tissue damage, and the opportunity for reattachment or reimplantation may be lost.

74. b. The lenses must be removed as soon as possible. Leaving them in can hold chemical product or residue in and further injure the eye.

75. b. Pepper spray is an oily substance that can be difficult to remove. Do not allow the victim to rub it. Instruct the victim to spit if it is in the mouth, blow the nose, and reinforce the instruction of "no rubbing." Then blot the oil off and flush the area with water.

76. d. Alkalis are stronger than acids. Take the time to flush the patient adequately no matter what type of product is involved.

77. a. Manage the ABCs first! This type of injury can result in respiratory and/or cardiac arrest.

78. b. Do not put yourself in danger. High-voltage wires are commonly buried underground. Call for additional help.

79. a. Most likely, the patient was standing while working on the electrical box. Electricity looks for ground, so check the feet first. Also assess the patient from head to toe in the rapid trauma exam.

80. d. Arc and flash burns can cause external injuries and steam can reach the upper airways. Chemical burns can reach the lower airways.

81. c. Think of the eye as an eviscerated organ. Keep it covered with a moist sterile dressing and keep it warm.

82. c. A circumferential burn around the chest is a serious injury that can keep the chest wall from expanding properly during breathing.

83. b. The sources of electrical burns are flash, contact, and arcing.

84. a. Management of an avulsion injury includes placing the avulsed tissue back over the affected area and applying a dry sterile dressing and bandage.

85. b. The steps for controlling a continuous bleed are direct pressure, elevation, and pressure dressing. There is no pressure point to use for this type of bleeding.

Chapter 27: Musculoskeletal Care

1. a. The intercostal muscles (muscles between the ribs) are skeletal muscles.

2. d. The contraction of a muscle results in movement of a body part.

3. d. Muscles are named according to their size, shape, and/or location.

4. c. Cartilage, tendons, and ligaments are all types of connective tissue, and their function is to aid muscles in movement of the skeleton.

5. a. The majority of blood cells are formed in the bone marrow located within bones (e.g., ends of long

bones, flat bones of the head and pelvis, ribs, and vertebral bodies).

6. b. The skull, thorax, and spinal column protect the vital organs of the body (e.g., brain, heart, and lungs).

7. d. Metatarsals are bones in the foot.

8. c. Phalanges are finger bones.

9. b. The costal arch is a landmark on the anterior chest outlining the lower ribs.

10. a. The shoulder girdle is made up of the clavicle, humerus, and scapula.

11. a. Musculoskeletal injuries are classified as open or closed.

12. a. A soft-tissue injury with deformity and no opening in the skin is a closed injury.

13. a. A soft-tissue injury with deformity and no opening in the skin is a closed injury.

14. a. Long bones should be splinted in a straight or neutral position to prevent additional damage to bones, vessels, and muscle tissue.

15. d. Dislocations are typically splinted in the position they are found. The patient will be guarding in the best position of comfort for that patient and injury.

16. d. Long bones should be splinted in a straight or neutral position without causing further injury.

17. c. The goal in splinting a dislocation or fracture is to immobilize the bone ends and the joint both above and below the injury.

18. c. The ongoing assessment of an extremity fracture includes reassessing the splint to assure a proper fit and reassessing distal PMS.

19. b. DISTAL PMS is assessed before and after splinting and in the ongoing assessment.

20. b. When a patient experiences tingling and numbness after splinting, the most likely cause is that the splint was applied too tightly. Loosen the splint and reassess.

21. b. A splint that is applied incorrectly, either too tight or too loose, can cause further damage and increased pain and swelling.

22. d. Increased back pain or new back pain is a common complaint of patients who have been immobilized to a long backboard.

23. a. The patient is stable with an isolated extremity injury. This injury should be splinted on the scene.

24. d. At the very least, the patient is going to increase swelling and pain without the proper attention. If the injury is severe, bearing weight will increase the risk of bleeding and loss of function, either temporarily or permanently.

25. d. The injury is not life-threatening and should be assessed and managed accordingly on the scene. The patient needs some psychological support in addition to the care of the traumatic injury. Reassure the patient that you are taking the appropriate measures in the care of her injury.

26. d. A sling and swathe is very effective and commonly used to splint shoulder, humerus, elbow, and forearm musculoskeletal injuries.

27. d. Injuries to the elbow carry a high probability of blood vessel and nerve damage. The brachial artery is the largest blood vessel in the elbow joint.

28. b. The fact that splints can easily be made from many different materials is not an advantage of splinting.

29. b. Splinting and hemorrhage control can be done simultaneously with this type of injury.

30. a. The application of cold helps to reduce and minimize swelling, which helps to reduce pain.

31. b. The MOI and the patient's signs and symptoms suggest rib fractures. Use a sling and swathe to splint her left arm to the chest.

32. c. The carpals and metacarpals are the bones of the hands.

33. b. The pelvis is made up of two hip bones, the sacrum, and the coccyx.

34. b. A *pathological fracture* is a fracture of a bone weakened by disease such as osteoporosis.

35. d. *Crepitus* is the sound and feel of fractured bone ends grinding together.

Chapter 28: Injuries to the Head and Spine

1. d. The brain, brain stem, CSF, and spinal cord make up the central nervous system. The peripheral nervous system includes 31 pairs of spinal nerves.

2. a. The brain, brain stem, CSF, and spinal cord make up the central nervous system.

3. d. The autonomic nervous system is the part of the nervous system that controls involuntary muscles and glands.

4. d. One function of cerebrospinal fluid (CSF) is to act as a shock absorber to cushion and protect the brain and spinal cord within the skull and spinal canal.

5. c. The vision control areas are located in the occipital area of the brain.

6. b. The brain stem extends from the brain to the spinal cord.

7. b. The spinal nerves originate in pairs from the spinal cord and extend out to the extremities and trunk of the body.

8. a. The spinal canal is located in the openings of the spinal vertebrae.

9. b. The spinal cord originates at the brain stem and extends down the spinal canal.

10. b. A significant electrical shock can cause a victim to be thrown or knocked down. The MOI has the potential to cause a head, cervical, or spinal injury in addition the injury from the shock.

11. b. Altered mental status or a painful injury (broken bone) can initially distract a patient from sensing or realizing the potential for a spinal injury.

12. c. It is possible for a patient to have a significant injury (e.g., fractured cervical spine or spinal injury) without any immediately obvious physical or neurological deficits. Various MOIs are associated with certain injury patterns. The EMT-B must recognize the potential for these injuries and manage the patient with a high index of suspicion for these injuries based on the MOI.

13. c. Being placed on a long backboard, in most cases, is uncomfortable for the patient and may worsen pre-existing injuries. Filling the voids when splinting can help make the patient more comfortable during the time spent immobilized.

14. d. The inline neutral position allows the most space in the spinal canal for the spinal cord, thus making this position the safest for moving patients with suspected spinal injury.

15. b. Do no harm! The primary goal in caring for patients who have suspected spinal injury is to get them to the ED without compromising them further.

16. d. The potential for a spinal injury is the primary reason for immobilizing this patient to a long backboard. The other reasons are logical and practical too.

17. a. Pain or tenderness, especially upon palpation, is a clear indication for immobilizing a patient.

18. b. When you detect an abnormal finding in your assessment, remember to ask the patient whether this is normal for her or is new.

19. c. You may not detect tenderness unless you palpate for it. When an appropriate MOI is present, routinely examine the spine by palpating each vertebra for deformity, crepitus, pain, or tenderness.

20. b. The MOI is significant in this case, so the patient should be immobilized.

21. d. The MOI and the age of the patient are significant factors for deciding to immobilize. Remember, it is possible for a patient to have a significant injury (e.g., fractured cervical spine or spinal injury) without any immediately physical or neurological deficits.

22. d. Taking cervical precautions, begin with opening the airway.

23. c. A sudden loss of consciousness is an indication to quickly reassess the ABCs. If it becomes necessary to remove the helmet (e.g., to manage the airway), then take the necessary steps to do so safely.

24. c. This scenario can be challenging, especially when the patient is unconscious. A patient who requires suctioning and needs to be immobilized is going to need very close attention. Tilt the board and suction as often as needed.

25. b. After one unsuccessful attempt to place the patient's neck in a neutral position, it is then appro-priate to splint it in the position found. Never force the cervical spine into a splint!

26. d. Manual stabilization of the head and neck is maintained until the patient is properly secured to an immobilization device.

27. d. Instruct the patient not to move her head while manual stabilization is undertaken and a cervical collar is applied.

28. b. An isolated extremity injury alone does not indicate a need for cervical immobilization.

29. a. Because the patient is sitting in her vehicle when you reach her, it now becomes appropriate to have her remain still while manual stabilization of her cervical spine is held, a cervical collar is applied, and a short-board device is applied.

30. d. The decision to immobilize the cervical spine can be determined from the MOI and/or a patient's signs and symptoms.

31. c. Swelling or edema is associated with soft-tissue injuries.

32. c. Head injuries can cause a patient to become nauseated and vomit. When a patient has an altered mental status and vomiting, there is a high risk of aspiration. The EMT-B must be alert for this and be prepared to manage the airway.

33. a. Reassess the ABCs frequently for the unconscious patient, and pay a lot of attention to the airway and breathing. Head injuries can cause a patient to become nauseated and vomit. When a patient has an altered mental status and vomiting, there is a high risk of aspiration. The EMT-B must be alert for this and be prepared to manage the airway.

34. b. Cervical collars can be difficult to apply on babies and infants due to their short necks. A rolled towel is soft to the touch, easy to apply around the neck, and works effectively in place of a rigid cervical collar.

35. b. The more experience you have with immobilizing patients, the better you can estimate the size of a patient for fitting into various splinting devices. Until then, you should place the device next to the patient and size it for proper fit based on the patient's weight and height.

36. c. A pediatric equipment is typically selected based on the weight and height of the patient.

37. b. When immobilizing a patient with a suspected cervical or spinal injury, the rescuer holding stabilization of the head and neck makes the call to move the patient; she first checks with each rescuer to see that they are all ready, then all rescuers count and move the patient as a team.

38. d. Distal PMS is assessed before and after immobilizing the spine or an extremity.

39. b. When immobilizing the spine, remember the phrase "bone to board." Use the body's bones (shoulders,

thorax, hips, legs, and head last) to move and secure the body to the device.

40. a. When immobilizing the spine, use the body's bones (shoulders, thorax, hips, and legs) to move and secure the body to the device.

41. b. The body is secured before the head.

42. a. When immobilizing the spine, remember the phrase "bone to board." Use the body's bones (shoulders, thorax, hips, legs, and head last) to move and secure the body to the device.

43. d. Smoke or fire is an example of a hazard that would prompt a decision to rapidly extricate a patient.

44. c. A short spine board device would allow the least amount of movement for the patient and therefore create the least amount of pain. A rapid extrication onto a long backboard would not be inappropriate, but might cause more pain and injury for the patient.

45. c. The patient is stable following an MVC. The MOI is not described as being significant, so a short spine board is an appropriate device for this patient.

46. b. The short spine board device is used to move a patient from a location where a long backboard will not fit. The patient must be secured to a long backboard device prior to being transported.

47. d. Before placing the short spine board device behind the patient, the rescuers will move the patient forward to allow enough room for the device to fit.

48. b. Manual stabilization of the head and neck is maintained until both the torso and the head are secured to the immobilization device.

49. a. The patient is unstable and had a significant MOI, so rapid extrication is appropriate for this patient.

50. c. The indications for performing a rapid extrication include: unstable patient condition, a patient who is blocking access to an unstable patient, and unsafe scene.

51. a. The indications for performing a rapid extrication include: unstable patient condition, a patient who is blocking access to an unstable patient, and unsafe scene. Both patients in this vehicle meet the criteria for a rapid extrication.

52. d. A cervical collar is applied before the patient is moved.

53. b. Minimal cervical movement is the key to preventing any further injury to the patient with a suspected cervical spinal injury.

54. b. The EMT-B must have special training and practice to remain proficient in rapid extrication.

55. a. After one unsuccessful attempt to place the patient's neck in a neutral position, it is then appropriate to splint it in the position found. Never force the cervical spine into a splint!

56. a. The patient is conscious, alert, and stable and can be immobilized with the helmet on. Football players wear shoulder padding that elevates the back from the long backboard. If you need to remove the helmet and the shoulder pads are still in place, you will have to place a towel under the head to keep the spine in a neutral position.

57. d. Many types of helmets have face guards that can be removed to give access to the airway while the helmet is left on.

58. b. Bicycle, motorcycle, and auto racing helmets have the classic chin strap.

59. a. Helmets used in skiing or snowboarding and motorcycling are examples of the full-faced style. This type of helmet has a rigid chin guard that is continuous with the rest of the helmet.

60. d. Football players wear shoulder padding that elevates the back from the long backboard. If you need to remove the helmet and the shoulder pads are still in place, you will have to place a towel under the head to keep the spine in a neutral position.

61. b. When a helmet is fitted properly and has a snug fit around the head, the EMT-B can leave the helmet in place and immobilize the patient with it on.

62. d. When removing a full-face-style helmet, sometimes it is necessary to tilt the helmet slightly to avoid mashing the nose, but you must do so without moving the head or neck.

63. d. The rescuer holding stabilization will remove the helmet. The second rescuer supports the head by reaching under the patient's neck and into the helmet to support the back (occiput) of the patient's head.

64. b. When you need to access the airway or assist the patient's breathing, it is appropriate to remove the helmet immediately.

65. a. Each situation is a little different, but removing a helmet from a patient who is on his back allows the rescuers the easiest access to maintain cervical stabilization, see the airway, and support the head.

66. c. Manual stabilization of the head and neck is maintained until the patient is properly secured to an immobilization device.

67. c. The rescuer should ensure that the airway remains open by using a jaw-thrust maneuver.

68. c. When a face shield or guard is present on a helmet, the EMT-B should lift it up to gain access to the airway.

69. b. The patient who is immobilized with a helmet left on will not get a cervical collar.

70. d. Each of the answers listed is a valid reason for using a long backboard to immobilize a patient who has a suspected cervical spine injury.

71. d. Each of the answers listed is a valid reason for using a long backboard to immobilize a patient who has a suspected cervical spine injury.

72. c. Only the stretcher straps holding the patient on the long backboard should be unfastened. Keep the patient secured to the long backboard and turn the patient on the board.

73. d. The patient is secured to the long backboard first. Then the stretcher straps are secured over the patient.

74. d. The short spine board device is used to keep the spine from moving when a long backboard cannot be used as the first immobilization device. Once the patient is moved out to an area where she can be moved onto a long backboard, the patient is secured with both devices.

75. c. The short spine board device is used to keep the spine from moving when a long backboard cannot be used as the first immobilization device (e.g., when the patient is seated in an automobile).

76. a. The indications for performing a rapid extrication include: unstable patient condition, a patient who is blocking access to an unstable patient, and unsafe scene.

77. b. The use of rapid extrication increases the risk of further spinal injury for any patient. That is why this technique is used only in urgent circumstances.

78. b. This is an example of when to use a standing takedown.

79. d. Indications for immobilizing a patient with a helmet on include: the patient is stable, the helmet fits well, and proper immobilization can be accomplished with the helmet on.

80. b. Indications for immobilizing a patient with a helmet on include: the patient is stable, the helmet fits well, and proper immobilization can be accomplished with the helmet on.

Chapter 29: Infants and Children

1. d. Adolescents have the same respiratory rate range as adults.

2. b. The basics of language are usually mastered by the age of 36 months.

3. a. The normal heart rate at birth is 100 to 160 beats per minutes. It gradually slows to an average of 120 beats per minute during the first year of life.

4. a. Adolescents have the same respiratory rate range as adults.

5. c. Primary teeth are lost, and replacement with permanent teeth begins, in the school-age group.

6. a. Infants have higher metabolic and oxygen consumption rates. Thus, they have higher respiratory rates that may lead to rapid heat and fluid loss through exhaling condensation and warm air.

7. a. During the first month of life, the infant grows by approximately 30 grams per day. As a result, the infant's weight should double by 4 to 6 months, and triple by 9 to 12 months.

8. c. An infant's respiratory muscles are immature and fatigue faster than those of an adult.

9. a. *Grunting* is an abnormal respiratory sound produced by a partially closed glottis. Grunting is a characteristic of respiratory distress in children.

10. d. A slow respiratory rate in a child who is in respiratory distress indicates that the child is tiring; this is an ominous sign.

11. d. As the child become more hypoxic from inadequate oxygenation, the mental status will decrease. This is the most significant indication that the child is in failure and progressing to respiratory and cardiopulmonary arrest.

12. d. Secretions, positioning, and foreign bodies are all causes of airway obstruction in pediatric patients.

13. d. When the onset of respiratory distress is sudden, the EMT-B should suspect and assess for a foreign body, especially when stridor or wheezing is noted.

14. b. Respiratory distress from asthma is characterized by difficulty exhaling and a prolonged expiratory phase.

15. d. The method for opening the airway in any unconscious patient with no suspected injuries is the head-tilt chin-lift maneuver.

16. c. To properly assess an unresponsive patient who may have choked, you should place the patient supine on a flat surface. This position will also help to prevent any further injury from a possible fall.

17. a. The obstruction must be relieved (A = Airway) before proceeding with breathing and circulation.

18. c. The steps in the management of a FBAO in an unresponsive infant are: open the airway, attempt ventilation, deliver five back blows and five chest thrusts, and then perform a jaw-thrust maneuver and look for the FBAO. Never perform a blind finger sweep on an infant.

19. b. The patient is in need of a bronchodilator. The EMT-B can assist with an MDI under direct or indirect medical control. Always follow local protocols!

20. a. Mucus and nasal secretions are a real problem for small infants, because they breathe primarily through the nose. The obstruction can be easily relieved with a bulb syringe.

21. a. Further upsetting or agitating the child can cause a rapid deterioration in his condition. The EMT-B's general approach must be calm and reassuring during the management of such a patient.

22. d. Tachypnea (fast respiratory rate) and delayed capillary refill (poor circulation) in a sick child are signs of decompensated shock.

23. a. The patient's labored effort to breathe suggests distress, but the cyanosis indicates respiratory failure.

24. b. The child appears to have had a febrile seizure. Skin signs indicate that circulation is adequate.

25. a. Mental status, capillary refill, and pulses are direct measures of end-organ perfusion.

26. b. Urine output is an indirect but valid measure of end-organ perfusion in a sick child.

27. d. Cool extremities and a loss of distal pulses in warm ambient temperatures are signs of inadequate perfusion in a sick child.

28. b. Unlike adults, respiratory distress and failure are the primary causes of cardiac arrest in children. When the EMT-B can recognize respiratory distress and failure, she can act quickly to prevent the child from deteriorating to cardiac arrest.

29. d. Unlike adults, respiratory distress and failure are the primary causes of cardiac arrest in children.

30. a. Febrile seizures are caused when a child's body temperature rises too quickly. Management includes attention to the ABCs; gentle cooling of the child, such as removing layers of clothing; and then transporting for evaluation.

31. c. Febrile seizures are caused when a child's body temperature rises too quickly, which can occur when a child is sick with an infection.

32. a. Traumatic brain injury is a common pathology in children of all age groups.

33. b. BLS care for this patient includes managing the ABCs (e.g., oxygen, suctioning, and transport), and calling for ALS to meet you en route, if possible.

34. a. The patient has a history of seizures and may have another while in your care. The BLS care of this patient includes attention to the ABCs and transport for evaluation. If another seizure occurs, request ALS to meet you en route to the ED.

35. c. Brief periods of apnea are not uncommon with seizures. The EMT-B should administer high-flow oxygen during the postictal period of a seizure and longer if needed.

36. c. The heads of children are disproportionately large in relation to their bodies. This leads to more injuries to the head, face, and neck because children tend to land head first.

37. a. The heads of children are disproportionately large in relation to their bodies. This leads to more injuries to the head, face, and neck because children tend to land head first.

38. c. The growing bones in children are not as calcified and strong as those in an adult.

39. c. The use of an OPA is appropriate in any unconscious patient without a gag reflex.

40. a. The patient is unconscious with labored breathing following a traumatic MOI. Manage the ABCs. Ensure that the airway is open and assist with ventilations.

41. a. The patient appears to be stable, so it is both appropriate and safest to immobilize and transport the child in the car seat. Children tend to be less frightened and easier to manage when transported in their own car seats, because the seats are familiar to them.

42. a. Difficulty walking or sitting, anxiety, avoidance of eye contact, and uncooperativeness with certain aspects of assessment, together with other suspicious findings at the scene, may indicate that the child is a victim of sexual abuse.

43. c. Mouth and gum lacerations in a baby are a sign often associated with "baby bottle syndrome." The parent or caregiver repeatedly forces the bottle into the infant's mouth in an effort to stop it from crying.

44. b. Document only your specific findings and facts regarding the call. Opinions are not regarded as professional or reliable.

45. a. Suspected child abuse or neglect reporting is mandatory in every state. The specific method of reporting varies from state to state. However, the next health care provider (e.g., ED staff) to take care of the patient should be informed of your suspicions.

46. d. The EMT-B has the advantage of observing each of the facts regarding the call, and she should document the specific findings appropriately, without rendering opinions or judgments.

47. a. Child abuse is a crime; reporting of suspected child abuse or neglect is mandatory in every state. The specific method of reporting varies from state to state.

48. b. EMS calls involving children can be challenging for any EMS provider. Each person manages stress differently, so you should talk to your partner first and assess his reaction. He may need to take the rest of the shift off, or he may want (and be perfectly able) to return to service.

49. d. Each person manages stress differently. Any of the suggestions listed may be appropriate and helpful.

50. a. Talking about the call with your crew is very helpful in working through the stress of a call like this. However, it may not be enough for everyone. Consider utilizing critical incident stress management (CISM) and other techniques for those who need additional support.

51. d. No one is expected to remember all the ranges of vital signs for each age group. What is expected is that the EMT-B knows where to find a pediatric reference and how to read it.

52. c. The priority of the ABCs never changes, but the method of assessment should be modified according to the age of the patient. For example, with toddlers and preschool-age children, the toe-to-head direction of physical exam may be less threatening and upsetting than the head-to-toe method.

53. c. Children of grade-school age are typically reliable with information regarding their past medical history.

54. b. Studies have shown that families who are included in the initial and emergency care of a child in

cardiac arrest do better in the grieving process. Let the parents or caregivers know that the child is your first priority. Designate a crewmember to explain the treatment being provided and answer questions.

55. b. Parents of injured and sick children can experience a wide range of emotions. Often they may feel that the child's pain is somehow their fault. Maintain a professional demeanor, honestly explain any procedures, and keep him informed.

56. d. Parents of injured and sick children can experience a wide range of emotions. Often they may feel that the child's pain is somehow their fault. Reassure her that the bleeding is controlled and permit her to observe.

57. c. EMS calls involving children can be challenging for any EMS provider, and it is common for EMT-Bs who are parents to internalize the stress somewhat more than those who are not parents.

58. b. The experienced and professional EMT-B knows that a calm and reassuring disposition goes a long way toward establishing trust with patients and parents of patients.

59. c. Utilizing a parent in the management of a pediatric patient is a good practice, but is not always necessary nor appropriate for every call.

60. a. Do not risk losing the patient's confidence by getting involved in disputes or taking sides.

61. d. Cardiac arrests due to MI are more prevalent in adults than in children.

62. d. Further upsetting or agitating such a patient can cause a rapid deterioration in his condition. The EMT-B's general approach must be calm and reassuring during the management of this child. Let the patient stay in a position of comfort with minimal disturbance.

63. a. Croup is caused by viral or other infections (e.g., ear, throat) and is characterized by a two- or three-day onset of sickness progressing to respiratory distress. The patient may have a barking cough.

64. a. The poor skin signs, loss of distal pulses, and delayed capillary refill indicate hypoperfusion and inadequate circulation.

65. c. BLS management includes management of the ABCs, recognition of the need for ALS, and rapid transport.

Chapter 30: Ambulance Operations

1. b. A penlight is of little value in a cache of extrication equipment.

2. d. These items are a variety of miscellaneous patient care equipment.

3. d. A stretcher mount is not considered part of an emergency vehicle's mechanical system.

4. a. Unless there are special circumstances (e.g., prolonged scene time with extra personnel), on the scene of a call is not where the EMT-B would typically be checking the equipment or restocking the ambulance.

5. a. Permission to assess and treat a patient should be obtained before you touch the patient. In most cases, this will occur on the scene of a call.

6. a. The decision on which priority response to use is made at the time of dispatch in most cases.

7. c. State vehicle and traffic regulations do not typically approve the use of emergency lights and audible devices for drills, training, or returning from calls.

8. c. An ambulance is not exempt from the prohibition on leaving the scene of an accident, even when a patient is on board.

9. b. The driver of an emergency vehicle must drive with extreme care and due regard for other drivers. The proper action in this case is to wait for a safe location to pass the vehicle on the left.

10. d. The driver of an emergency vehicle is held to a higher standard than other drivers and must drive with extreme care and due regard for other drivers. If the driver of the ambulance continues with lights and sirens, the family member will most likely continue his unsafe driving. Ideally, the ambulance operator should stop and warn the family member to readjust how he is proceeding behind the ambulance.

11. a. Having completed an EVOC or ambulance accident prevention seminar (AAPS) driving course is an excellent method of obtaining training and practice in operating emergency vehicles. It does not, however, provide any immunity or confer special driving privileges.

12. d. The driver of an emergency vehicle is held to a higher standard than other drivers and must drive with extreme care and due regard for other drivers.

13. b. The actions to take in this case are the same as you would take with your personal vehicle.

14. a. The driver of an emergency vehicle is held to a higher standard than other drivers and must drive with extreme care and due regard for other drivers.

15. c. Drowsiness, smoking, talking on the phone, and obtaining dispatching information are all examples of driver distractions.

16. b. Use of escorts is dangerous and has caused many collisions. Whenever possible, avoid the vehicle escort scenario.

17. d. Use of escorts is dangerous and has caused many collisions. Whenever possible, avoid the vehicle escort scenario.

18. c. In this situation, each vehicle operator should use a different siren, to prevent confusion for other vehicle operators.

19. a. Courtesy to and safety of other drivers is the responsibility of the emergency vehicle operator.

20. c. It would be unusual for an investigation to consider whether the signaling equipment was routinely inspected, unless there was an indication that this caused the problem.

21. a. This is the definition of operating an emergency vehicle with "due regard."

22. a. Safety of other drivers is the primary responsibility of the emergency vehicle operator.

23. a. This information is not typically documented on the prehospital care report (PCR).

24. c. This situation describes a third-party caller.

25. d. Enhanced 9-1-1 has all of the features described.

26. a. A *repeater* is a device that receives transmissions from low-power sources and retransmits them at a higher power on anther frequency.

27. c. Currently, emergency calls made from cell phones can cause significant delays in emergency response. The situation is improving slowly with the use of GPS and stricter federal regulations.

28. c. If the patient is able to sit up, the stair chair is a valuable piece of equipment for spaces such as that described in the question.

29. b. At this point, the patient can be placed directly on a stretcher.

30. c. The long backboard is the ideal piece of equipment in this situation. It acts as a splint. and once the patient is secured and padded on the board, further patient movement is significantly reduced or eliminated.

31. a. The long backboard is the ideal piece of equipment in this situation. It acts as a splint. and once the patient is secured and padded on the board, further patient movement is significantly reduced or eliminated.

32. a. For the patient who is able to sit up, the stair chair is a valuable piece of equipment for moving through tight spaces. This patient should not walk or lie down, because of her condition.

33. b. Routinely documenting this information is a good practice. Some agencies routinely document the name of the nurse or physician to whom the patient was turned over.

34. c. The EMT-B who routinely completes patient care reports in a timely fashion, using accurate and complete information with no misspelled words, demonstrates professionalism.

35. a. The PCR contains administrative information, patient demographics, vital signs, patient narrative, and treatment.

36. d. The steps you take to prepare your ambulance for going into service will help to ensure the safety and health of you, your crew, and the patient.

37. b. The crew is responsible for cleaning and restocking as much of the ambulance as possible while at the hospital and before returning to service.

38. b. These are the OSHA-recommended steps for disinfecting an ambulance in such a situation.

39. b. Each of the other steps is necessary on every exposure call.

40. b. Verification of proper immunizations should be done well before you report to work.

41. c. These are the OSHA-recommended steps for disinfecting equipment in such a situation.

42. b. This product is designed for low-level disinfection.

43. b. *Sterilization* kills all forms of microbial life on medical instruments.

44. a. *Cleaning* is the process of removing dirt from the surface of an object with soap and water.

45. d. These are the OSHA-recommended steps for disinfecting an ambulance in such a situation.

46. c. A solution of bleach and water in a dilution of 1:100 is the OSHA-recommended concentration.

47. c. Yellow bags are used to transport reusable items, such as blankets or other equipment, back to the station for cleaning. The yellow indicates that the items are contaminated with possible infectious body fluids other than blood (e.g., urine, vomit, feces).

48. d. A complete verbal report is the standard for transferring patients from one health care provider to the next. A face-to-face report helps to minimize errors and missed information.

49. b. Verifying that the medication is prescribed for the patient is one of the six "rights" of medication administration, and is typically documented rather than verbally reported during patient transfer.

50. b. No emergency department appreciates the surprise of an emergency patient arriving without notice. Prearrival notice to the ED is standard practice and helps the staff to be prepared for the patient when that patient arrives.

51. d. This will vary from agency to agency. In many agencies, the EMT-Bs are responsible for checking fluid levels on a regular basis, but the agency's vehicle mechanic performs the maintenance.

52. a. Each of the answers is a valid reason for completing a daily ambulance checklist. However, the *primary* purpose is to have the vehicle prepared to respond to calls.

53. c. The patient with a head injury and AMS gets the air medical transport. Cardiac arrest victims are not flown, and the toddler and 10-year-old patient are stable and can go by ground transport.

54. d. 100×100 feet is the minimum required landing zone area for a small rotor aircraft.

55. b. $1,500 \times 1.56 = 2,340 \div 10 = 234$ minutes.

Chapter 31: Gaining Access

1. d. Extrication is not limited to motor vehicles; it can occur wherever a patient is trapped.

2. b. The purpose of an extrication is to free the patient and provide care on scene during the extraction.

3. c. This is the definition of *disentanglement*.

4. d. An EMT-B with the proper training and equipment may participate in any of the phases of a rescue for which he is qualified.

5. d. After sizing up the scene and managing hazards, the steps of a rescue include: gain access to the patient, assess and begin treatment, disentanglement, extrication, further assessment, treatment, and transport.

6. b. Each EMT-B is trained to the awareness level, which means they have the knowledge to recognize a hazardous scene, call for more help, and not enter unless they have a higher level of training and the proper equipment.

7. c. A personal flotation device (PFD) is the required minimum personal safety equipment for any rescuer working in or near water.

8. b. A helmet, turnout coat and pants, and hearing and eye protection are all items of the minimum-level protective equipment used at the scene of a rescue.

9. d. A helmet, turnout coat and pants, and hearing and eye protection are all items of the minimum-level protective equipment used at the scene of a rescue.

10. a. Estimating the severity of injuries and patient transport needs is part of the scene size-up, but the estimates may be modified at any point in the rescue.

11. a. Each EMT-B is trained to the hazmat awareness level, which means they have the knowledge to recognize a hazardous scene, call for more help, establish a safe perimeter, and not enter unless they have a higher level of training and the proper equipment.

12. c. After sizing up the scene and managing hazards, the steps of a rescue include: gain access to the patient, assess and begin treatment, disentanglement, extrication, further assessment, treatment, and transport.

13. c. There is not much you can do for these victims until they are extricated.

14. d. Short and long backboards are often used as additional protection for rescuers and patients during a rescue effort.

15. d. Any of these items will help to protect the patient from the breaking glass.

16. a. Hazardous terrain rescues are categorized as low angle, high angle, or flat with obstructions. A steep slope or "low-angle" terrain is capable of being walked up without using the hands. This terrain can become more dangerous because of difficult footing, especially when you are carrying a patient in a basket on snow, ice, rocks, or mud.

17. a. Sometimes the fastest and easiest method of gaining access is overlooked. Don't forget to check first for an unlocked door.

18. b. While wearing a PFD, you can attempt to throw a rope to the victim during the wait for the rescue team.

19. d. The window furthest from the patient should be the first one broken to gain access to the patient.

20. b. As the name indicates, this is a simple form of access requiring no tools or special equipment.

21. c. This term applies when tools or special equipment are used to gain access to a victim who is entrapped.

22. a. As the name indicates, this is a simple form of access requiring no tools or special equipment.

23. b. A personal flotation device (PFD) is the required minimum personal safety equipment for any rescuer working in or near water. An exposure suit is used when working in cold or icy water.

24. d. Ideally, each ambulance should be carrying one or more of these hazmat resource guides.

25. b. The amount of time it takes to gain access is the dynamic factor in rescue operations, and is very different from other types of EMS calls.

26. a. Traffic is the greatest hazard for emergency responders.

27. a. The A post supports the roof at the windshield; the B post is the support on the side of the vehicle behind the driver's door.

28. d. Of the choices listed, gamma radiation is the most dangerous form.

29. d. ID placards list the name of the chemical and the reactivity, flammability, and associated health hazards.

30. a. Confined spaces may contain very little oxygen or may contain dangerous gases. Rescues in confined spaces require continuous air monitoring during the rescue effort.

Chapter 32: Overviews

1. c. Each EMT-B is trained at least to the awareness level, which means they have the knowledge to recognize a hazardous scene, call for more help, and not enter unless they have a higher level of training and the proper equipment. The level of response and participation is predetermined in many communities.

2. b. The EMT-B must complete a scene size-up at each call, including potential hazmat incident scenes.

3. b. Each EMT-B is trained at least to the awareness level, which means they have the knowledge to recognize a hazardous scene, call for more help, and not enter unless they have a higher level of training and the proper equipment.

4. c. The incident commander has the primary responsibility of ensuring everyone's safety at the scene of an incident. He may designate an safety officer, especially at large incidents, to assist with this task.

5. b. Before work begins at an incident where a hazardous material is present, zones are established to prevent injury and unnecessary exposure to the substance.

6. a. Before work begins at an incident where a hazardous material is present, zones are established to prevent injury and unnecessary exposure to the substance.

7. a. Flammability hazards include: may cause fire or explosion; may ignite other combustible materials; and may be ignited by heat, sparks, or flames.

8. b. In such a case, the victims of a possible exposure should be removed right away. The longer the victims are exposed, the more serious their conditions may become.

9. c. The EMT-B is trained to recognize a hazardous scene, call for more help, and not enter unless she has a higher level of training and the proper equipment.

10. d. This is the recommendation for approaching and staging at the scene of a hazmat incident.

11. b. The EMT-B is trained to recognize a hazardous scene, call for more help, and not enter unless he has a higher level of training and the proper equipment.

12. b. Safety first for you and your crew!

13. b. The *cold zone* is the furthest outside the incident. It is the safe area for personnel trained to the awareness level or higher.

14. b. Gross decontamination should be completed by the patient if he or she is able.

15. b. One of the duties in a treatment sector (group) is to monitor the hazmat teams before and after entry into the hot zone.

16. d. Decon is the process of removing hazmats from exposed persons and equipment at a hazmat incident.

17. c. Victims who have been in a confined space where smoke and fire were present are at risk for carbon monoxide inhalation and should be evaluated for it.

18. d. Wind direction can change the dynamics of a hazmat incident very rapidly. Wind direction is routinely monitored during outside hazmat incidents for this reason.

19. d. This rescue is still an extrication for one patient, but now there is a second patient in need of evaluation.

20. c. At the onset, there is the potential for a number of patients here (more than you and your crew can effectively manage), so declaring an MCI is appropriate.

21. d. At the onset, there are a number of patients here (more than you and your crew can effectively manage), so declaring an MCI is appropriate.

22. d. The size and complexity of the incident, including the number of personnel on scene, are the primary factors that help determine how many sectors (groups) will be established at an incident.

23. d. The first unit to arrive should establish EMS command; notify dispatch of the first-in size-up report, and, when police and fire officers arrive on scene, work to establish a unified command.

24. a. This is the role of the treatment sector (group) officer.

25. a. To *triage* is to sort patients based on the severity of injury and the resources available.

26. a. The use of triage tags helps to reduce or eliminate the need to repeatedly count and get a baseline assessment of each patient.

27. c. This task can be done quickly and possibly help save a life without delaying the triage of other potential patients.

28. d. There are many causes of disasters other than natural forces.

29. b. During a disaster operation, the EMT-B provides medical and psychological support to those who need it.

30. a. Preplanning and training are the best way to prepare for disaster operations.

31. a. "Keep it simple and clear with plain English" is the concept used in such emergencies.

32. b. Each community needs to have an IMS that has been practiced and is understood by all of the providers in each of the agencies that may be asked to respond to any major incidents.

33. c. The four major components utilized during the management of a large MCI are operations, planning, logistics, and finance.

34. c. An ED with the resources will direct you to take your patient through a designated area in its facility for additional decon.

35. c. The cold zone is the furthest outside the incident. It is the safe area for personnel trained to the awareness level or higher.
36. a. The patient's clothing is removed early as part of the decon process.
37. d. The local fire departments should have all this information, as well as a preplan for possible incidents at the locations.
38. d. These are the common methods for learning more about local MCI preplanning and training in your community.
39. a. Weapons of mass destruction include explosives, chemicals, and biological and nuclear agents.
40. b. The role of the EMT-B in this type of incident is similar to that in other incidents. Upon arrival at the scene, report to command and then to any area designated by command.
41. d. This patient has minor injuries and none that affect the ABCs.
42. a. This patient is having a breathing problem, which makes her a high priority in need of immediate care.
43. b. Get the ball rolling and declare an MCI. Assess the amount and type of resources needed and request them.
44. c. This is the definition of a *multiple-casualty incident (MCI)*.
45. c. An EMT-B with the proper training and equipment may participate in any of the phases of a rescue that she is qualified for.

Chapter 33: Advanced Airway

1. b. The mediastinum contains the great vessels and is located in the center of the chest between the lungs.
2. a. The epiglottis is one of the anatomical structures visualized during endotracheal intubation.
3. b. The vocal cords are anatomically anterior to the false vocals.
4. d. The cricoid ring has the smallest circumference in the pediatric airway. The endotracheal tube used for infants, toddlers, and small children is uncuffed to fit through this small structure.
5. a. Until the age of approximately 8 years, the back of a child's head is proportionately larger. When the unconscious child is lying supine, the large occiput displaces the head in a flexed position and can close off the airway.
6. d. The trachea of an infant, toddler, or small child is more flexible than that of an adult.
7. b. Absence of a gag reflex is a reliable indication that the patient cannot protect her own airway.
8. a. An oral airway adjunct or OPA would be inserted at this point to keep the tongue from becoming an obstruction in the airway.
9. d. Any of the steps listed should be attempted as needed before attempting any advanced airway techniques. Do not forget the basic airway techniques!
10. b. The tissues of the infant airway are highly vascular and can bleed very easily.
11. b. BSI, including gloves, eye protection, and a face mask, must be utilized with either simple or advanced airway techniques, because the risk for exposure is very high.
12. d. The NPA is an excellent airway adjunct for seizing patients or any patient with clenched teeth and an AMS.
13. b. The AHA recommends at least 800 cc volume during ventilation without supplemental oxygen and a minimum of 600 cc volume with supplemental oxygen.
14. b. Positive pressure ventilation with a BVM is indicated when a patient's ventilations are inadequate.
15. d. Before attempting advanced airway procedures such as endotracheal intubation, the patient should be hyperoxygenated briefly.
16. a. Before inserting a gastric tube, the EMT-B must measure and mark the tube for proper placement.
17. b. The indication for inserting a nasogastric tube is an unconscious patient who is vomiting.
18. c. The primary indication for the EMT-B to insert a nasogastric tube is to relieve gastric distention following endotracheal intubation.
19. d. This step is required to confirm proper placement of the nasogastric tube.
20. c. Ideally, a third trained EMT-B helper would be the one to apply Sellick's maneuver to assist in the airway management of a patient.
21. b. When Sellick's maneuver is incorrectly applied, the airway can be occluded.
22. c. Making an adequate mask seal requires the rescuer to use both hands. This technique should be attempted first.
23. a. To insert an OPA, the patient must lack a gag reflex. An absent gag reflex is a reliable indication that the patient cannot protect his own airway and requires intubation.
24. c. The patient is being adequately ventilated and has good vital signs. With a short transport time, there is no immediate need to intubate this patient.
25. c. Endotracheal tube placement should be confirmed by a minimum of three methods. The EMT-B can use visualization of the tube going through the vocal cords, listening over the lung sounds and epigastrum, and the use of an esophageal intubation

detector (EID) or EtCO$_2$ device to confirm proper placement.

26. d. BSI, including gloves, eye protection, and a face mask, must be used with both simple and advanced airway techniques, because the risk of exposure is very high.

27. c. A lubricant such a lidocaine gel or a water-soluble gel would be used for a *naso*tracheal intubation.

28. b. The laryngoscope handle and blade are similar to a flashlight; you must check it to see that the light is working and bright before attempting an intubation.

29. d. Either a straight or a curved blade can be used to lift the epiglottis for visualization of the vocal cords.

30. c. The curved blade is designed to be placed into the vallecula.

31. d. The straight blade is designed to be placed under the epiglottis and lift it so that the vocal cords can be visualized.

32. a. The straight blade is more accommodating than the curved blade for visualizing the shorter and more anterior airway of the pediatric patient.

33. b. The technique described is used with all types of blades.

34. a. The stylet must be removed so that the BVM can be attached.

35. a. The Murphy eye is used as the point of reference on an endotracheal tube past which the stylet should not pass. Passing the stylet further can cause the stylet to come out of the tube and perforate the throat or trachea.

36. b. The stylet is a rigid piece of coated wire that gives an endotracheal tube shape and stability during placement.

37. c. Ideally, it is best to have one size larger and one size smaller tube ready prior to intubating, especially if you anticipate a difficult airway.

38. b. The average male will take an 8.0 size; the average female takes a 7.0.

39. b. The average female takes a 7.0, so try that first, but have a couple of smaller-sized tubes ready, as they may be needed.

40. d. The 3.0-sized tubes are used to intubate and suction meconium from the airway of a newly born infant.

41. c. $4 + (2/4 = .5) = 4.5$.

42. d. Any of the methods listed will get you close to or exactly at the proper size tube.

43. b. The tube slipping out of the trachea is a major complication associated with moving a patient. This is one reason why tube placement must be verified repeatedly throughout the care and transport of the intubated patient.

44. b. Reinflate the pilot balloon and verify tube placement by auscultation of lung sounds and negative epigastric sounds.

45. b. Placing objects into the throat stimulates the vasovagal response and slows the heart rate.

46. b. The right mainstem bronchi is wider and straighter than the left and is commonly intubated. The complication of not recognizing this is that only the right lung gets ventilated.

47. d. You are looking for equal chest rise and fall in addition to equal breath sounds. Many pediatric tubes have a black marking on the distal end of the tube that is used to assist in placing the tube to the proper depth.

48. d. The cricoid ring has the smallest circumference in the pediatric airway. The endotracheal tube used in infants, toddlers, and small children (less than 8 years old) is uncuffed so that it will fit through this small structure.

49. c. Start with a 2.5 and have one size smaller and one size larger ready for use if needed.

50. a. The laryngoscope handle is held in the left hand by both right- and left-handed EMT-Bs.

51. b. The sniffing position is the optimal position for visualizing the vocal cords.

52. b. AHA recommends stopping ventilations no longer than 30 seconds during an intubation attempt.

53. d. The straight blade is more accommodating than the curved blade when the EMT-B is attempting to visualize the shorter and more anterior airway of the pediatric patient.

54. a. A major difference is the size of equipment. The experience of the person performing the intubation can also make a significant difference.

55. b. Until the age of approximately 8 years, the back of a child's head is proportionately larger. When the unconscious child is lying supine, the large occiput displaces the head in a flexed position and can close off the airway. A mild extension is preferred over the sniffing position in infants during an intubation attempt.

56. b. The most likely cause of the rapid deterioration is a dislodged tube. First assess placement of the tube; if it is dislodged, extubate, ventilate, and reinsert a clean tube.

57. d. Ideally, the tube should be visualized going through the vocal cords, rather than blindly inserting the tube.

58. b. When the endotracheal tube is misplaced in the esophagus, the BVM will become more and more difficult to squeeze with each ventilation. The abdomen will quickly become distended and the patient will be at great risk for vomiting.

59. a. A tube misplaced into the esophagus will ventilate the stomach, not the lungs. The patient will deteriorate quickly and die if this condition is not rapidly recognized and corrected.

60. d. When an esophageal intubation or displaced tube is suspected, the EMT-B should first assess placement of the tube; if it is dislodged, he should extubate, ventilate, and reinsert a clean tube.

61. a. Immobilizing the head is an excellent way to help minimize the risk of tube displacement.

62. c. The size, not the length, of a tube is documented, as well as the centimeter mark at the level of the patient's teeth or lips.

63. b. One-inch tape and an OPA for a bite block were used for years before commercial restraining devices became available.

64. d. Each of these is an appropriate action in this scenario.

65. b. It is appropriate and necessary to explain the steps you are taking to resuscitate the family member. If you cannot do this because you are engaged in care, a designated crew member or supervisor should do this for you.

66. b. Endotracheal intubation is the gold standard for airway maintenance, as it provides the best control of the airway, especially for prolonged periods of time.

67. a. Endotracheal intubation is not typically considered an easy skill to learn or maintain proficiency with.

68. c. One advantage of the Combitube is that it can be inserted blindly and does not require visualization of the vocal cords.

69. d. An EMS agency's medical director is the person who can approve an EMT-B to perform advanced airway procedures.

70. d. These are all valid reasons for trained EMT-Bs to gain approval to perform advanced airway procedures.

71. c. Stylets are not routinely used to intubate newly-borns. The rigid stylet can cause injury to the small, delicate airways.

72. a. The stylet is a rigid piece of coated wire that gives an endotracheal tube shape and stability during placement.

73. a. Extubation often provokes vomiting, so suction must be turned on and ready for use during removal of the tube.

74. c. The soft tissues in the airway are highly vascular and bleed easily. Rough handling of the laryngoscope blade can cause soft-tissue injury with concomitant bleeding and swelling.

75. d. The right mainstem bronchi is wider and straighter than the left and is commonly intubated. The complication of not recognizing this is that only the right lung gets ventilated.

76. d. A tube misplaced in the esophagus will ventilate the stomach, not the lungs. The patient will deteriorate quickly and die if this condition is not rapidly recognized and corrected.

77. d. The stethoscope is placed over the stomach for the first ventilation and then over the left and right lungs to verify proper placement.

78. d. The centimeter markings on an endotracheal tube are used to mark the placement and identify any movement thereafter.

79. a. A displaced tube is the primary concern with patients who are intubated. This is why the EMT-B must frequently reassess placement during the care and transport of an intubated patient.

80. a. In the absence of a commercial restraining device, an OPA is used as a bite block to prevent the patient from biting the endotracheal tube; one-inch tape is used to secure the tube.

Appendix B: Tips for Preparing for a Practical Skills Examination

EMT-B courses are designed to cover the specific objectives outlined in the DOT National Standard Curriculum. The curriculum also suggests that EMS educators take the option of enriching these courses with more material if they or their medical directors so choose. What prohibits many educators from enriching their courses is limited time and resources.

During an EMT-B course, many educators teach the core curriculum and provide enrichment material as time, resources, and experience permit. Near the end of an EMT-B course, it is typical for educators to change their style of teaching and begin preparation for the exam. That is, they will provide examples of the material to be tested on state and national exams, and give tips on how to take the written exams. The educator may hold one or more practice skills sessions and a mock practical exam to help students prepare. Limited time and resources often do not allow for as much skills practice time as some students would like. Thus, I have included some tips to help you get ready for the practical skills exam.

If you have not done so already, obtain a copy of the skills testing sheets to be used for *your* practical skills exam, and carefully read the instructions well before the day of the exam itself. Note that each exam skill sheet has items that are identified as critical pass-or-fail items. These items, which are usually bolded for easy identification, include taking or verbalizing BSI or scene safety, as well as other critical tasks. National Registry skills sheets also list "Critical Criteria" at the bottom of each sheet. This is a list of items that were not performed and should have been. When an evaluator checks one of these items, the candidate will fail the station.

Often the course instructor will hand out a set of the skills testing sheets to be used for the state and/or registry exam during or near the end of the course, and you

will be given an opportunity to practice the skills in lab using the testing sheets. I strongly recommend that you take every opportunity provided during the course to do this. In addition, find one or more students or experienced EMT-Bs to practice skills with. While you demonstrate the skill, have another person use the testing sheet to evaluate your performance. Be tough on each other in a friendly way! Pay close attention to the critical failure items and then focus on obtaining every point available.

Before the day of the practical skills exam, make certain you are familiar with the location where the exam is being given. Arrive 15 minutes early on the day of the exam. Bring a copy of the skills sheets with you to review while you are waiting. On the testing day, be patient and prepared to be at the testing site for most of the day. Practical skills testing typically takes a lot of time. In addition to bringing the skills sheets to review, bring a book, a drink, lunch, and plenty of patience.

On the day of the practical exam, if you have the option of choosing the order of the testing stations, I recommend using one of two methods. The first one is this: If you are a little nervous and you want to build your confidence, start with a short skill station like AED. This is a skill you will have successfully completed in a CPR class. From there, continue to build your confidence by selecting the stations that you feel you can complete without difficulty.

The second method I recommend is selecting the most difficult stations and completing those first. For most people, the assessment stations seem the most difficult because they have the most steps and take the longest to complete. Once these stations are complete, you can breathe a little easier while completing the remaining stations.

If you do not have the option of choosing the order of skills to be tested, do not worry at this point; you have prepared and are ready for each skill station. During the exam, the evaluators are instructed not to tell you if you have passed or failed a skill station until you have finished testing at all of the stations, so do not expect or ask them to. (The reasoning behind this is that if you fail a station early in the testing, you may become distracted and fail another.)

Once in the station, you will be read a set of instructions and given the opportunity to ask questions for clarification and to check the equipment provided. I recommend that you do this, especially if you are the first candidate of the day coming into a station. The evaluator has been instructed to make sure that the equipment is functioning properly and that there will be no distractions for the candidates. They are not there to trip you up, but occasionally something goes amiss, such as a blood pressure cuff that is broken and is not detected before the exam starts.

In the patient assessment station, I recommend that you ask if the injuries or significant signs that you are supposed to detect are going to be visible with moulage or by another method. This is a common area where problems can develop. Verbalize the steps and tasks you complete as if you were talking to a new partner. After a long day of testing, evaluators become fatigued just like you. If an evaluator happened to have her head turned while you were performing a critical step, she will hear you verbalizing it.

If you should have to repeat a station, know the retest policy and do not overreact. You have spent a lot of time training and should persevere rather than throwing it in over one bad day! Remember, we humans do make mistakes occasionally. The key is how you learn from your mistakes, correct them, and move forward.

Lastly, get some sleep before the examination. Try to get a good night's rest two nights before in addition to the night before. Many people are very nervous about test taking and do not sleep well the night before no matter what. Getting a good sleep two nights before does help.

Best of luck and be prepared!

—Kirt

Appendix C:
National Registry Practical Examination Sheets

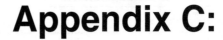

Patient Assessment/Management - Trauma

Start Time: _____

Stop Time: _____   Date: _____

Candidate's Name: _____

Evaluator's Name: _____

		Points Possible	Points Awarded
Takes, or verbalizes, body substance isolation precautions		1	
SCENE SIZE-UP			
Determines the scene is safe		1	
Determines the mechanism of injury		1	
Determines the number of patients		1	
Requests additional help if necessary		1	
Considers stabilization of spine		1	
INITIAL ASSESSMENT			
Verbalizes general impression of the patient		1	
Determines responsiveness/level of consciousness		1	
Determines chief complaint/apparent life threats		1	
Assesses airway and breathing	Assessment	1	
	Initiates appropriate oxygen therapy	1	
	Assures adequate ventilation	1	
	Injury management	1	
Assesses circulation	Assesses/controls major bleeding	1	
	Assesses pulse	1	
	Assesses skin (color, temperature and condition)	1	
Identifies priority patients/makes transport decision		1	
FOCUSED HISTORY AND PHYSICAL EXAMINATION/RAPID TRAUMA ASSESSMENT			
Selects appropriate assessment *(focused or rapid assessment)*		1	
Obtains, or directs assistance to obtain, baseline vital signs		1	
Obtains S.A.M.P.L.E. history		1	
DETAILED PHYSICAL EXAMINATION			
Assesses the head	Inspects and palpates the scalp and ears	1	
	Assesses the eyes	1	
	Assesses the facial areas including oral and nasal areas	1	
Assesses the neck	Inspects and palpates the neck	1	
	Assesses for JVD	1	
	Assesses for trachael deviation	1	
Assesses the chest	Inspects	1	
	Palpates	1	
	Auscultates	1	
Assesses the abdomen/pelvis	Assesses the abdomen	1	
	Assesses the pelvis	1	
	Verbalizes assessment of genitalia/perineum as needed	1	
Assesses the extremities	1 point for each extremity includes inspection, palpation, and assessment of motor, sensory and circulatory function	4	
Assesses the posterior	Assesses thorax	1	
	Assesses lumbar	1	
Manages secondary injuries and wounds appropriately 1 point for appropriate management of the secondary injury/wound		1	
Verbalizes re-assessment of the vital signs		1	

Critical Criteria   **Total:** 40

_____ Did not take, or verbalize, body substance isolation precautions
_____ Did not determine scene safety
_____ Did not assess for spinal protection
_____ Did not provide for spinal protection when indicated
_____ Did not provide high concentration of oxygen
_____ Did not find, or manage, problems associated with airway, breathing, hemorrhage or shock (hypoperfusion)
_____ Did not differentiate patient's need for transportation versus continued assessment at the scene
_____ Did other detailed physical examination before assessing the airway, breathing and circulation
_____ Did not transport patient within (10) minute time limit

(Reprinted with permission of the National Registry of Emergency Medical Technicians.)

Patient Assessment/Management - Medical

Start Time: _____

Stop Time: _____   Date: _____

Candidate's Name: _____

Evaluator's Name: _____

	Points Possible	Points Awarded
Takes, or verbalizes, body substance isolation precautions	1	
SCENE SIZE-UP		
Determines the scene is safe	1	
Determines the mechanism of injury/nature of illness	1	
Determines the number of patients	1	
Requests additional help if necessary	1	
Considers stabilization of spine	1	
INITIAL ASSESSMENT		
Verbalizes general impression of the patient	1	
Determines responsiveness/level of consciousness	1	
Determines chief complaint/apparent life threats	1	
Assesses airway and breathing — Assessment	1	
Initiates appropriate oxygen therapy	1	
Assures adequate ventilation	1	
Assesses circulation — Assesses/controls major bleeding	1	
Assesses pulse	1	
Assesses skin (color, temperature and condition)	1	
Identifies priority patients/makes transport decision	1	
FOCUSED HISTORY AND PHYSICAL EXAMINATION/RAPID ASSESSMENT		
Signs and symptoms (*Assess history of present illness*)	1	

Respiratory	Cardiac	Altered Mental Status	Allergic Reaction	Poisoning/ Overdose	Environmental Emergency	Obstetrics	Behavioral
*Onset? *Provokes? *Quality? *Radiates? *Severity? *Time? *Interventions?	*Onset? *Provokes? *Quality? *Radiates? *Severity? *Time? *Interventions?	*Description of the episode. *Onset? *Duration? *Associated Symptoms? *Evidence of Trauma? *Interventions? *Seizures? *Fever	*History of allergies? *What were you exposed to? *How were you exposed? *Effects? *Progression? *Interventions?	*Substance? *When did you ingest/become exposed? *How much did you ingest? *Over what time period? *Interventions? *Estimated weight?	*Source? *Environment? *Duration? *Loss of consciousness? *Effects - general or local?	*Are you pregnant? *How long have you been pregnant? *Pain or contractions? *Bleeding or discharge? *Do you feel the need to push? *Last menstrual period?	*How do you feel? *Determine suicidal tendencies. *Is the patient a threat to self or others? *Is there a medical problem? *Interventions?

	Points Possible	Points Awarded
Allergies	1	
Medications	1	
Past pertinent history	1	
Last oral intake	1	
Event leading to present illness (rule out trauma)	1	
Performs focused physical examination (*assesses affected body part/system or, if indicated, completes rapid assessment*)	1	
Vitals (*obtains baseline vital signs*)	1	
Interventions (*obtains medical direction or verbalizes standing order for medication interventions and verbalizes proper additional intervention/treatment*)	1	
Transport (re-evaluates the transport decision)	1	
Verbalizes the consideration for completing a detailed physical examination	1	
ONGOING ASSESSMENT (verbalized)		
Repeats initial assessment	1	
Repeats vital signs	1	
Repeats focused assessment regarding patient complaint or injuries	1	

Critical Criteria   Total: **30**

_____ Did not take, or verbalize, body substance isolation precautions when necessary
_____ Did not determine scene safety
_____ Did not obtain medical direction or verbalize standing orders for medical interventions
_____ Did not provide high concentration of oxygen
_____ Did not find or manage problems associated with airway, breathing, hemorrhage or shock (hypoperfusion)
_____ Did not differentiate patient's need for transportation versus continued assessment at the scene
_____ Did detailed or focused history/physical examination before assessing the airway, breathing and circulation
_____ Did not ask questions about the present illness
_____ Administered a dangerous or inappropriate intervention

(Reprinted with permission of the National Registry of Emergency Medical Technicians.)

Cardiac Arrest Management/AED

Start Time: _____

Stop Time: _____   Date: _____

Candidate's Name: _____

Evaluator's Name: _____

	Points Possible	Points Awarded
ASSESSMENT		
Takes, or verbalizes, body substance isolation precautions	1	
Briefly questions the rescuer about arrest events	1	
Directs rescuer to stop CPR	1	
Verifies absence of spontaneous pulse (skill station examiner states "no pulse")	1	
Directs resumption of CPR	1	
Turns on defibrillator power	1	
Attaches automated defibrillator to the patient	1	
Directs rescuer to stop CPR and ensures all individuals are clear of the patient	1	
Initiates analysis of the rhythm	1	
Delivers shock (up to three successive shocks)	1	
Verifies absence of spontaneous pulse (skill station examiner states "no pulse")	1	
TRANSITION		
Directs resumption of CPR	1	
Gathers additional information about arrest event	1	
Confirms effectiveness of CPR (ventilation and compressions)	1	
INTEGRATION		
Verbalizes or directs insertion of a simple airway adjunct (oral/nasal airway)	1	
Ventilates, or directs ventilation of, the patient	1	
Assures high concentration of oxygen is delivered to the patient	1	
Assures CPR continues without unnecessary/prolonged interruption	1	
Re-evaluates patient/CPR in approximately one minute	1	
Repeats defibrillator sequence	1	
TRANSPORTATION		
Verbalizes transportation of patient	1	
Total:	21	

Critical Criteria

_____ Did not take, or verbalize, body substance isolation precautions

_____ Did not evaluate the need for immediate use of the AED

_____ Did not direct initiation/resumption of ventilation/compressions at appropriate times.

_____ Did not assure all individuals were clear of patient before delivering each shock

_____ Did not operate the AED properly (inability to deliver shock)

_____ Prevented the defibrillator from delivering indicated stacked shocks

(Reprinted with permission of the National Registry of Emergency Medical Technicians.)

BAG-VALVE-MASK
APNEIC PATIENT

Start Time: _____

Stop Time: _____   Date: _____

Candidate's Name: _____

Evaluator's Name: _____

	Points Possible	Points Awarded
Takes, or verbalizes, body substance isolation precautions	1	
Voices opening the airway	1	
Voices inserting an airway adjunct	1	
Selects appropriately sized mask	1	
Creates a proper mask-to-face seal	1	
Ventilates patient at no less than 800 ml volume *(The examiner must witness for at least 30 seconds)*	1	
Connects reservoir and oxygen	1	
Adjusts liter flow to 15 liters/minute or greater	1	
The examiner indicates arrival of a second EMT. The second EMT is instructed to ventilate the patient while the candidate controls the mask and the airway		
Voices re-opening the airway	1	
Creates a proper mask-to-face seal	1	
Instructs assistant to resume ventilation at proper volume per breath *(The examiner must witness for at least 30 seconds)*	1	
Total:	**11**	

Critical Criteria

_____ Did not take, or verbalize, body substance isolation precautions

_____ Did not immediately ventilate the patient

_____ Interrupted ventilations for more than 20 seconds

_____ Did not provide high concentration of oxygen

_____ Did not provide, or direct assistant to provide, proper volume/breath
(more than two (2) ventilations per minute are below 800 ml)

_____ Did not allow adequate exhalation

(Reprinted with permission of the National Registry of Emergency Medical Technicians.)

SPINAL IMMOBILIZATION
SEATED PATIENT

Start Time: _____

Stop Time: _____   Date: _____

Candidate's Name: _____

Evaluator's Name: _____

	Points Possible	Points Awarded
Takes, or verbalizes, body substance isolation precautions	1	
Directs assistant to place/maintain head in the neutral in-line position	1	
Directs assistant to maintain manual immobilization of the head	1	
Reassesses motor, sensory and circulatory function in each extremity	1	
Applies appropriately sized extrication collar	1	
Positions the immobilization device behind the patient	1	
Secures the device to the patient's torso	1	
Evaluates torso fixation and adjusts as necessary	1	
Evaluates and pads behind the patient's head as necessary	1	
Secures the patient's head to the device	1	
Verbalizes moving the patient to a long board	1	
Reassesses motor, sensory and circulatory function in each extremity	1	
Total:	**12**	

Critical Criteria

_____ Did not immediately direct, or take, manual immobilization of the head

_____ Released, or ordered release of, manual immobilization before it was maintained mechanicall

_____ Patient manipulated, or moved excessively, causing potential spinal compromise

_____ Device moved excessively up, down, left or right on the patient's torso

_____ Head immobilization allows for excessive movement

_____ Torso fixation inhibits chest rise, resulting in respiratory compromise

_____ Upon completion of immobilization, head is not in the neutral position

_____ Did not assess motor, sensory and circulatory function in each extremity after voicing immobilization to the long board

_____ Immobilized head to the board before securing the torso

(Reprinted with permission of the National Registry of Emergency Medical Technicians.)

SPINAL IMMOBILIZATION
SUPINE PATIENT

Start Time: _____

Stop Time: _____   Date: _____

Candidate's Name: _____

Evaluator's Name: _____	Points Possible	Points Awarded
Takes, or verbalizes, body substance isolation precautions	1	
Directs assistant to place/maintain head in the neutral in-line position	1	
Directs assistant to maintain manual immobilization of the head	1	
Reassesses motor, sensory and circulatory function in each extremity	1	
Applies appropriately sized extrication collar	1	
Positions the immobilization device appropriately	1	
Directs movement of the patient onto the device without compromising the integrity of the spine	1	
Applies padding to voids between the torso and the board as necessary	1	
Immobilizes the patient's torso to the device	1	
Evaluates and pads behind the patient's head as necessary	1	
Immobilizes the patient's head to the device	1	
Secures the patient's legs to the device	1	
Secures the patient's arms to the device	1	
Reassesses motor, sensory and circulatory function in each extremity	1	
Total:	14	

Critical Criteria

_____ Did not immediately direct, or take, manual immobilization of the head

_____ Released, or ordered release of, manual immobilization before it was maintained mechanicall

_____ Patient manipulated, or moved excessively, causing potential spinal compromise

_____ Patient moves excessively up, down, left or right on the patient's torso

_____ Head immobilization allows for excessive movement

_____ Upon completion of immobilization, head is not in the neutral position

_____ Did not assess motor, sensory and circulatory function in each extremity after immobilization to the device

_____ Immobilized head to the board before securing the torso

(Reprinted with permission of the National Registry of Emergency Medical Technicians.)

IMMOBILIZATION SKILLS
TRACTION SPLINTING

Start Time: _____

Stop Time: _____ Date: _____

Candidate's Name: _____

Evaluator's Name: _____	Points Possible	Points Awarded
Takes, or verbalizes, body substance isolation precautions	1	
Directs application of manual stabilization of the injured leg	1	
Directs the application of manual traction	1	
Assesses motor, sensory and circulatory function in the injured extremity	1	
Note: The examiner acknowledges "motor, sensory and circulatory function are present and normal"		
Prepares/adjusts splint to the proper length	1	
Positions the splint next to the injured leg	1	
Applies the proximal securing device (e.g... ischial strap)	1	
Applies the distal securing device (e.g...ankle hitch)	1	
Applies mechanical traction	1	
Positions/secures the support straps	1	
Re-evaluates the proximal/distal securing devices	1	
Reassesses motor, sensory and circulatory function in the injured extremity	1	
Note: The examiner acknowledges "motor, sensory and circulatory function are present and normal"		
Note: The examiner must ask the candidate how he/she would prepare the patient for transportation		
Verbalizes securing the torso to the long board to immobilize the hip	1	
Verbalizes securing the splint to the long board to prevent movement of the splint	1	
Total:	**14**	

Critical Criteria
_____ Loss of traction at any point after it was applied

_____ Did not reassess motor, sensory and circulatory function in the injured extremity before and after splinting

_____ The foot was excessively rotated or extended after splint was applied

_____ Did not secure the ischial strap before taking traction

_____ Final Immobilization failed to support the femur or prevent rotation of the injured leg

_____ Secured the leg to the splint before applying mechanical traction

Note: If the Sagar splint or the Kendricks Traction Device is used without elevating the patient's leg, application of manual traction is not necessary. The candidate should be awarded one (1) point as if manual traction were applied.

Note: If the leg is elevated at all, manual traction must be applied before elevating the leg. The ankle hitch may be applied before elevating the leg and used to provide manual traction.

(Reprinted with permission of the National Registry of Emergency Medical Technicians.)

IMMOBILIZATION SKILLS
LONG BONE INJURY

Start Time: _____

Stop Time: _____   Date: _____

Candidate's Name: _____

Evaluator's Name: _____	Points Possible	Points Awarded
Takes, or verbalizes, body substance isolation precautions	1	
Directs application of manual stabilization of the injury	1	
Assesses motor, sensory and circulatory function in the injured extremity	1	
Note: The examiner acknowledges "motor, sensory and circulatory function are present and normal"		
Measures the splint	1	
Applies the splint	1	
Immobilizes the joint above the injury site	1	
Immobilizes the joint below the injury site	1	
Secures the entire injured extremity	1	
Immobilizes the hand/foot in the position of function	1	
Reassesses motor, sensory and circulatory function in the injured extremity	1	
Note: The examiner acknowledges "motor, sensory and circulatory function are present and normal"		
Total:	**10**	

Critical Criteria

_____ Grossly moves the injured extremity

_____ Did not immobilize the joint above and the joint below the injury site

_____ Did not reassess motor, sensory and circulatory function in the injured extremity before and after splinting

(Reprinted with permission of the National Registry of Emergency Medical Technicians.)

IMMOBILIZATION SKILLS
JOINT INJURY

Start Time: _____

Stop Time: _____   Date: _____

Candidate's Name: _____

Evaluator's Name: _____	Points Possible	Points Awarded
Takes, or verbalizes, body substance isolation precautions	1	
Directs application of manual stabilization of the shoulder injury	1	
Assesses motor, sensory and circulatory function in the injured extremity	1	
Note: The examiner acknowledges "motor, sensory and circulatory function are present and normal."		
Selects the proper splinting material	1	
Immobilizes the site of the injury	1	
Immobilizes the bone above the injured joint	1	
Immobilizes the bone below the injured joint	1	
Reassesses motor, sensory and circulatory function in the injured extremity	1	
Note: The examiner acknowledges "motor, sensory and circulatory function are present and normal."		
Total:	8	

Critical Criteria

_____ Did not support the joint so that the joint did not bear distal weight

_____ Did not immobilize the bone above and below the injured site

_____ Did not reassess motor, sensory and circulatory function in the injured extremity before and after splinting

(Reprinted with permission of the National Registry of Emergency Medical Technicians.)

BLEEDING CONTROL/SHOCK MANAGEMENT

Start Time: _____

Stop Time: _____   Date: _____

Candidate's Name: _____

Evaluator's Name: _____

	Points Possible	Points Awarded
Takes, or verbalizes, body substance isolation precautions	1	
Applies direct pressure to the wound	1	
Elevates the extremity	1	
Note: The examiner must now inform the candidate that the wound continues to bleed.		
Applies an additional dressing to the wound	1	
Note: The examiner must now inform the candidate that the wound still continues to bleed. The second dressing does not control the bleeding.		
Locates and applies pressure to appropriate arterial pressure point	1	
Note: The examiner must now inform the candidate that the bleeding is controlled		
Bandages the wound	1	
Note: The examiner must now inform the candidate the patient is now showing signs and symptoms indicative of hypoperfusion		
Properly positions the patient	1	
Applies high concentration oxygen	1	
Initiates steps to prevent heat loss from the patient	1	
Indicates the need for immediate transportation	1	
Total:	10	

Critical Criteria

_____ Did not take, or verbalize, body substance isolation precautions

_____ Did not apply high concentration of oxygen

_____ Applied a tourniquet before attempting other methods of bleeding control

_____ Did not control hemorrhage in a timely manner

_____ Did not indicate a need for immediate transportation

(Reprinted with permission of the National Registry of Emergency Medical Technicians.)

Evaluator's Name: _____

OROPHARYNGEAL AIRWAY	Points Possible	Points Awarded
Takes, or verbalizes, body substance isolation precautions	1	
Selects appropriately sized airway	1	
Measures airway	1	
Inserts airway without pushing the tongue posteriorly	1	
Note: The examiner must advise the candidate that the patient is gagging and becoming conscious		
Removes the oropharyngeal airway	1	

SUCTION

Note: The examiner must advise the candidate to suction the patient's airway		
Turns on/prepares suction device	1	
Assures presence of mechanical suction	1	
Inserts the suction tip without suction	1	
Applies suction to the oropharynx/nasopharynx	1	

NASOPHARYNGEAL AIRWAY

Note: The examiner must advise the candidate to insert a nasopharyngeal airway		
Selects appropriately sized airway	1	
Measures airway	1	
Verbalizes lubrication of the nasal airway	1	
Fully inserts the airway with the bevel facing toward the septum	1	
Total:	13	

Critical Criteria

_____ Did not take, or verbalize, body substance isolation precautions

_____ Did not obtain a patent airway with the oropharyngeal airway

_____ Did not obtain a patent airway with the nasopharyngeal airway

_____ Did not demonstrate an acceptable suction technique

_____ Inserted any adjunct in a manner dangerous to the patient

(Reprinted with permission of the National Registry of Emergency Medical Technicians.)

MOUTH TO MASK WITH SUPPLEMENTAL OXYGEN

Start Time: _____

Stop Time: _____   Date: _____

Candidate's Name: _____

Evaluator's Name: _____

	Points Possible	Points Awarded
Takes, or verbalizes, body substance isolation precautions	1	
Connects one-way valve to mask	1	
Opens patient's airway or confirms patient's airway is open (manually or with adjunct)	1	
Establishes and maintains a proper mask to face seal	1	
Ventilates the patient at the proper volume and rate *(800-1200 ml per breath/10-20 breaths per minute)*	1	
Connects the mask to high concentration of oxygen	1	
Adjusts flow rate to at least 15 liters per minute	1	
Continues ventilation of the patient at the proper volume and rate *(800-1200 ml per breath/10-20 breaths per minute)*	1	
Note: The examiner must witness ventilations for at least 30 seconds		
Total:	8	

Critical Criteria

_____ Did not take, or verbalize, body substance isolation precautions

_____ Did not adjust liter flow to at least 15 liters per minute

_____ Did not provide proper volume per breath
(***more than 2 ventilations per minute were below 800 ml***)

_____ Did not ventilate the patient at a rate a 10-20 breaths per minute

_____ Did not allow for complete exhalation

(Reprinted with permission of the National Registry of Emergency Medical Technicians.)

OXYGEN ADMINISTRATION

Start Time: _____

Stop Time: _____ Date: _____

Candidate's Name: _____

Evaluator's Name: _____	Points Possible	Points Awarded
Takes, or verbalizes, body substance isolation precautions	1	
Assembles the regulator to the tank	1	
Opens the tank	1	
Checks for leaks	1	
Checks tank pressure	1	
Attaches non-rebreather mask to oxygen	1	
Prefills reservoir	1	
Adjusts liter flow to 12 liters per minute or greater	1	
Applies and adjusts the mask to the patient's face	1	
Note: The examiner must advise the candidate that the patient is not tolerating the non-rebreather mask. The medical director has ordered you to apply a nasal cannula to the patient.		
Attaches nasal cannula to oxygen	1	
Adjusts liter flow to six (6) liters per minute or less	1	
Applies nasal cannula to the patient	1	
Note: The examiner must advise the candidate to discontinue oxygen therapy		
Removes the nasal cannula from the patient	1	
Shuts off the regulator	1	
Relieves the pressure within the regulator	1	
Total:	**15**	

Critical Criteria

_____ Did not take, or verbalize, body substance isolation precautions

_____ Did not assemble the tank and regulator without leaks

_____ Did not prefill the reservoir bag

_____ Did not adjust the device to the correct liter flow for the non-rebreather mask
(12 liters per minute or greater)

_____ Did not adjust the device to the correct liter flow for the nasal cannula
(6 liters per minute or less)

(Reprinted with permission of the National Registry of Emergency Medical Technicians.)

Start Time: _____

Stop Time: _____

Candidate's Name: _____   Date: _____

Evaluator's Name: _____

Note: If a candidate elects to initially ventilate the patient with a BVM attached to a reservoir and oxygen, full credit must be awarded for steps denoted by " ** " provided the first ventilation is delivered within the initial 30 seconds	Points Possible	Points Awarded
Takes of verbalizes body substance isolation precautions	1	
Opens the airway manually	1	
Elevates the patient's tongue and inserts a simple airway adjunct (oropharyngeal/nasopharyngeal airway)	1	
Note: The examiner must now inform the candidate "no gag reflex is present and the patient accepts the airway adjunct."		
** Ventilates the patient immediately using a BVM device unattached to oxygen	1	
** Hyperventilates the patient with room air	1	
Note: The examiner must now inform the candidate that ventilation is being properly performed without difficulty		
Attaches the oxygen reservoir to the BVM	1	
Attaches the BVM to high flow oxygen (15 liter per minute)	1	
Ventilates the patient at the proper volume and rate (800-1200 ml/breath and 10-20 breaths/minute)	1	
Note: After 30 seconds, the examiner must auscultate the patient's chest and inform the candidate that breath sounds are present and equal bilaterally and medical direction has ordered endotracheal intubation. The examiner must now take over ventilation of the patient.		
Directs assistant to hyper-oxygenate the patient	1	
Identifies/selects the proper equipment for endotracheal intubation	1	
Checks equipment · Checks for cuff leaks	1	
· Checks laryngoscope operation and bulb tightness	1	
Note: The examiner must remove the OPA and move out of the way when the candidate is prepared to intubate the patient.		
Positions the patient's head properly	1	
Inserts the laryngoscope blade into the patient's mouth while displacing the patient's tongue laterally	1	
Elevates the patient's mandible with the laryngoscope	1	
Introduces the endotracheal tube and advances the tube to the proper depth	1	
Inflates the cuff to the proper pressure	1	
Disconnects the syringe from the cuff inlet port	1	
Directs assistant to ventilate the patient	1	
Confirms proper placement of the endotracheal tube by auscultation bilaterally and over the epigastrium	1	
Note: The examiner must ask, "If you had proper placement, what would you expect to hear?"		
Secures the endotracheal tube (*may be verbalized*)	1	
Total:	21	

Critical Criteria

_____ Did not take or verbalize body substance isolation precautions when necessary

_____ Did not initiate ventilation within 30 seconds after applying gloves or interrupts ventilations for greater than 30 seconds at any time

_____ Did not voice or provide high oxygen concentrations (15 liter/minute or greater)

_____ Did not ventilate the patient at a rate of at least 10 breaths per minute

_____ Did not provide adequate volume per breath (maximum of 2 errors per minute permissible)

_____ Did not hyper-oxygenate the patient prior to intubation

_____ Did not successfully intubate the patient within 3 attempts

_____ Used the patient's teeth as a fulcrum

_____ Did not assure proper tube placement by auscultation bilaterally over each lung **and** over the epigastrium

_____ The stylette (if used) extended beyond the end of the endotracheal tube

_____ Inserted any adjunct in a manner that was dangerous to the patient

_____ Did not immediately disconnect the syringe from the inlet port after inflating the cuff

(Reprinted with permission of the National Registry of Emergency Medical Technicians.)

VENTILATORY MANAGEMENT
DUAL LUMEN DEVICE INSERTION FOLLOWING
AN UNSUCCESSFUL ENDOTRACHEAL INTUBATION ATTEMPT

Start Time: _____

Stop Time: _____

Candidate's Name: _____   Date: _____

Evaluator's Name: _____	Points Possible	Points Awarded
Continues body substance isolation precautions	1	
Confirms the patient is being properly ventilated with high percentage oxygen	1	
Directs the assistant to hyper-oxygenate the patient	1	
Checks/prepares the airway device	1	
Lubricates the distal tip of the device (*may be verbalized*)	1	
Note: The examiner should remove the OPA and move out of the way when the candidate is prepared to insert the device		
Positions the patient's head properly	1	
Performs a tongue-jaw lift	1	
☐ USES COMBITUBE ‖ ☐ USES THE PTL		
Inserts device in the mid-line and to the depth so that the printed ring is at the level of the teeth ‖ Inserts the device in the mid-line until the bite block flange is at the level of the teeth	1	
Inflates the pharyngeal cuff with the proper volume and removes the syringe ‖ Secures the strap	1	
Inflates the distal cuff with the proper volume and removes the syringe ‖ Blows into tube #1 to adequately inflate both cuffs	1	
Attaches/directs attachment of BVM to the first (esophageal placement)lumen and ventilates	1	
Confirms placement and ventilation through the correct lumen by observing chest rise, auscultation over the epigastrium and bilaterally over each lung	1	
Note: The examiner states, "You do not see rise and fall of the chest and hear sounds only over the epigastrium."		
Attaches/directs attachment of BVM to the second (endotracheal placement) lumen and ventilates	1	
Confirms placement and ventilation through the correct lumen by observing chest rise, auscultation over the epigastrium and bilaterally over each lung	1	
Note: The examiner states, "You see rise and fall of the chest, there are no sounds over the epigastrium and breath sounds are equal over each lung."		
Secures device or confirms that the device remains properly secured	1	
Total:	15	

Critical Criteria

_____ Did not take or verbalize body substance isolation precautions

_____ Did not initiate ventilations within 30 seconds

_____ Interrupted ventilations for more than 30 seconds at any time

_____ Did not hyper-oxygenate the patient prior to placement of the dual lumen airway device

_____ Did not provide adequate volume per breath (maximum 2 errors/minute permissible)

_____ Did not ventilate the patient at a rate of at least 10 breaths per minute

_____ Did not insert the dual lumen airway device at a proper depth or at the proper place within 3 attempts

_____ Did not inflate both cuffs properly

_____ **Combitube** - Did not remove the syringe immediately following the inflation of each cuff

_____ **PTL** - Did not secure the strap prior to cuff inflation

_____ Did not confirm, by observing chest rise and auscultation over the epigastrium and bilaterally over each lung, that the proper lumen of the device was being used to ventilate the patient

_____ Inserted any adjunct in a manner that was dangerous to the patient

(Reprinted with permission of the National Registry of Emergency Medical Technicians.)

VENTILATORY MANAGEMENT
ESOPHAGEAL OBTURATOR AIRWAY INSERTION FOLLOWING AN UNSUCCESSFUL ENDOTRACHEAL INTUBATION ATTEMPT

Start Time: _____

Stop Time: _____   Date: _____

Candidate's Name: _____

Evaluator's Name: _____

	Points Possible	Points Awarded
Continues body substance isolation precautions	1	
Confirms the patient is being ventilated high percentage oxygen	1	
Directs the assistant to hyper-oxygenate the patient	1	
Identifies/selects the proper equipment for insertion of EOA	1	
Assembles the EOA	1	
Tests the cuff for leaks	1	
Inflates the mask	1	
Lubricates the tube (*may be verbalized*)	1	
Note: The examiner should remove the OPA and move out of the way when the candidate is prepared to insert the device		
Positions the head properly with the neck in the neutral or slightly flexed position	1	
Grasps and elevates the patient's tongue and mandible	1	
Inserts the tube in the same direction as the curvature of the pharynx	1	
Advances the tube until the mask is sealed against the patient's face	1	
Ventilates the patient while maintaining a tight mask-to-face seal	1	
Directs confirmation of placement of EOA by observing for chest rise and auscultation over the epigastrium and bilaterally over each lung	1	
Note: The examiner must acknowledge adequate chest rise, bilateral breath sounds and absent sounds over the epigastrium		
Inflates the cuff to the proper pressure	1	
Disconnects the syringe from the inlet port	1	
Continues ventilation of the patient	1	
Total:	17	

Critical Criteria

_____ Did not take or verbalize body substance isolation precautions
_____ Did not initiate ventilations within 30 seconds
_____ Interrupted ventilations for more than 30 seconds at any time
_____ Did not direct hyper-oxygenation of the patient prior to placement of the EOA
_____ Did not successfully place the EOA within 3 attempts
_____ Did not ventilate at a rate of at least 10 breaths per minute
_____ Did not provide adequate volume per breath (maximum 2 errors/minute permissible)
_____ Did not assure proper tube placement by auscultation bilaterally and over the epigastrium
_____ Did not remove the syringe after inflating the cuff
_____ Did not successfully ventilate the patient
_____ Did not provide high flow oxygen (15 liters per minute or greater)
_____ Inserted any adjunct in a manner that was dangerous to the patient

(Reprinted with permission of the National Registry of Emergency Medical Technicians.)